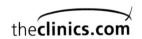

INFECTIOUS DISEASE CLINICS OF NORTH AMERICA

Infections and Rheumatic Diseases

GUEST EDITOR
Luis R. Espinoza, MD

CONSULTING EDITOR
Robert C. Moellering, Jr, MD

December 2006 • Volume 20 • Number 4

SAUNDERS

An Imprint of Elsevier, Inc.
PHILADELPHIA   LONDON   TORONTO   MONTREAL   SYDNEY   TOKYO

W.B. SAUNDERS COMPANY
A Division of Elsevier Inc.

Elsevier, Inc., 1600 John F. Kennedy Blvd., Suite 1800, Philadelphia, PA 19103-2899.

http://www.theclinics.com

INFECTIOUS DISEASE CLINICS   Volume 20, Number 4
OF NORTH AMERICA   ISSN 0891–5520
December 2006   ISBN-10: 1-4160-4225-3
Editor: Karen Sorensen   ISBN-13: 978-1-4160-4225-9

The ideas and opinions expressed in *Infectious Disease Clinics of North America* do not necessarily reflect those of the Publisher. The Publisher does not assume any responsibility for any injury and/or damage to persons or property arising out of or related to any use of the material contained in this periodical. The reader is advised to check the appropriate medical literature and the product information currently provided by the manufacturer of each drug to be administered to verify the dosage, the method and duration of administration, or contraindications. It is the responsibility of the treating physician or other health care professional, relying on independent experience and knowledge of the patient, to determine drug dosages and the best treatment for the patient. Mention of any product in this issue should not be construed as endorsement by the contributors, editors, or the Publisher of the product or manufacturers' claims.

Infectious Disease Clinics of North America (ISSN 0891–5520) is published in March, June, September, and December (For Post Office use only: volume 20 issue 4 of 4) by Elsevier Inc., 360 Park Avenue South, New York, NY 10010-1710. Business and Editorial Offices: 1600 John F. Kennedy Blvd., Suite 1800, Philadelphia, PA 19103-2899. Customer Service Office: 6277 Sea Harbor Drive, Orlando, FL 32887-4800. Periodicals postage paid at New York, NY and additional mailing offices. Subscription prices are $184.00 per year for US individuals, $308.00 per year for US institutions, $92.00 per year for US students, $216.00 per year for Canadian individuals, $373.00 per year for Canadian institutions, $243.00 per year for international individuals, $373.00 per year for international institutions, and $119.00 per year for Canadian and foreign students. To receive student rate, orders must be accompanied by name of affiliated institution, date of term, and the *signature* of program/residency coordinator on institution letterhead. Orders will be billed at individual rate until proof of status is received. Foreign air speed delivery is included in all *Clinics* subscription prices. All prices are subject to change without notice. **POSTMASTER:** Send address changes to *Infectious Disease Clinics of North America*, Elsevier Periodicals Customer Service, 6277 Sea Harbor Drive, Orlando, FL 32887-4800. **Customer Service: 1-800-654-2452 (US). From outside of the US, call 1-407-345-4000. E-mail: hhspcs@wbsaunders.com.**

Infectious Disease Clinics of North America is also published in Spanish by Editorial Inter-Médica, Junin 917, 1ᵉʳ A 1113, Buenos Aires, Argentina.

Reprints. For copies of 100 or more, of articles in this publication, please contact the Commercial Reprints Department, Elsevier Inc., 360 Park Avenue South, New York, New York 10010-1710. Tel. (212) 633-3813, Fax: (212) 462-1935, email: reprints@elsevier.com.

Infectious Disease Clinics of North America is covered in *Index Medicus, Current Contents/Clinical Medicine, Science Citation Alert, SCISEARCH,* and *Research Alert.*

Printed in the United States of America.

CONSULTING EDITOR

ROBERT C. MOELLERING, Jr, MD, Shields Warren-Mallinckrodt Professor of Medical Research, Harvard Medical School; Department of Medicine, Beth Israel Deaconess Medical Center, Boston, Massachusetts

GUEST EDITOR

LUIS R. ESPINOZA, MD, Professor and Chief, Section of Rheumatology, Department of Internal Medicine, Louisiana State University Health Sciences Center, New Orleans, Louisiana

CONTRIBUTORS

GRACIELA S. ALARCÓN, MD, MPH, Jane Knight Lowe Chair of Medicine in Rheumatology, Division of Clinical Immunology and Rheumatology, Department of Medicine, The University of Alabama at Birmingham, Birmingham, Alabama

RODOLFO E. BÉGUÉ, MD, Associate Professor of Pediatrics and Head, Division of Infectious Disease, Department of Pediatrics, Louisiana State University Health Sciences Center, New Orleans, Louisiana

JOHN D. CARTER, MD, Assistant Professor, Division of Rheumatology, Department of Medicine, University of South Florida, Tampa, Florida

INES COLMEGNA, MD, Section of Rheumatology, Department of Medicine, Louisiana State University Health Sciences Center, New Orleans, Louisiana

RAQUEL CUCHACOVICH, MD, Section of Rheumatology, Department of Medicine, Louisiana State University Health Sciences Center; Ochsner Clinic Foundation, New Orleans, Louisiana

LUIS R. ESPINOZA, MD, Professor and Chief, Section of Rheumatology, Department of Internal Medicine, Louisiana State University Health Sciences Center, New Orleans, Louisiana

ROBERT F. GARRY, PhD, Professor/Assistant Dean, Microbiology and Immunology, Director, Interdisciplinary Program in Molecular and Cellular Biology, Assistant Dean for Graduate Studies in Biomedical Sciences, Tulane University Health Sciences Center, New Orleans, Louisiana

IGNACIO GARCÍA-DE LA TORRE, MD, Head, Department of Immunology and Rheumatology, Hospital General de Occidente, Secretaría de Salud; Professor of

Immunology and Rheumatology, Centro Universitario de Ciencias de la Salud, Universidad de Guadalajara, Guadalajara, Jalisco, México

SERGE LARTCHENKO, MD, Section of Infectious Diseases, Department of Internal Medicine Louisiana State University Health Sciences Center, New Orleans, Louisiana

FRED A. LOPEZ, MD, Associate Professor and Vice Chair, Section of Infectious Diseases, Department of Internal Medicine, Louisiana State University Health Sciences Center, New Orleans, Louisiana

FRANCISCO MEDINA, MD, Rheumatology Department; and Research Unit on Autoimmune Diseases, Hospital de Especialidades, Centro Médico Nacional "Siglo XXI," Instituto Mexicano del Seguro Social, México City, Mexico

JOSÉ MORENO, MD, Chief, Research Unit on Autoimmune Diseases, Hospital de Especialidades, Centro Médico Nacional "Siglo XXI," Instituto Mexicano del Seguro Social, México City, Mexico

LETICIA PÉREZ-SALEME, MD, Infectology Department, Hospital de Especialidades, Centro Médico Nacional "Siglo XXI," Instituto Mexicano del Seguro Social, México City, Mexico

CARLOS PINEDA, MD, Research Subdirector, Instituto Nacional de Rehabilitación, Mexico City, Mexico

ALFONSO VARGAS RODRÍGUEZ, MD, Rheumatologist, Hospital Medica Sur, Centro Integral de Diagnóstico y Tratamiento, Mexico City, Mexico

LESLEY ANN SAKETKOO, MD, MPh, Clinical Fellow in Rheumatology, Section of Rheumatology, Department of Medicine, Louisiana State University Health Sciences Center; Department of Rheumatology, Ochsner Clinic Foundation, New Orleans, Louisiana

AJA M. SANZONE, MD, Fellow, Pediatric Infectious Diseases, Combined Fellowship Training Program of Tulane University and Louisiana State University Health Sciences Center, New Orleans, Louisiana

ANGÉLICA VARGAS, MD, Rheumatologist, Rheumatology Department, Instituto Nacional de Cardiología Ignacio Chávez, Mexico City, Mexico

CONTENTS

carbuncles), erysipelas, cellulitis, necrotizing fasciitis, pyomyositis, septic bursitis, and tenosynovitis.

Advances in the Management of Septic Arthritis

Ignacio García-De La Torre

Bacterial or septic arthritis is an important medical condition and is considered a rheumatologic emergency that can lead to rapid joint destruction and irreversible loss of function. Normal joints, diseased joints, and prosthetic joints are all vulnerable to bacterial infection. The mortality and morbidity of this condition are still considerable. Full recovery is possible, but poor outcome is common among those with pre-existing arthritis, especially rheumatoid arthritis. This article focuses on the risk factors and pathogenesis of nongonococcal bacterial arthritis; gonococcal arthritis and other forms of infectious arthritis, primarily in the context of a differential diagnosis and treatment, are also discussed.

Imaging of Osteomyelitis: Current Concepts

Carlos Pineda, Angélica Vargas, and Alfonso Vargas Rodríguez

Osteomyelitis frequently requires more than one imaging technique for an accurate diagnosis. Conventional radiography still remains the first imaging modality. MRI is the most sensitive and specific method for the detection of osteomyelitis, it provides more accurate information regarding the extent of the infectious process. Nuclear medicine is a highly sensitive but nonspecific technique, for the detection of osteomyelitis. Ultrasound represents a noninvasive method to evaluate the involved soft tissues and cortical bone and may provide guidance for diagnostic or therapeutic aspiration, drainage, or tissue biopsy. CT scan can be a useful method to detect early osseous erosion and to document the presence of sequestra. Positron emission tomography and single photon emission computed tomography are highly accurate techniques for the evaluation of chronic osteomyelitis, allowing differentiation from soft tissue infection.

Reactive Arthritis: Defined Etiologies, Emerging Pathophysiology, and Unresolved Treatment

John D. Carter

Reactive arthritis (ReA) is an inflammatory arthritis that arises after certain types of gastrointestinal or genitourinary infections. Approximately half of the patients with ReA experience spontaneous resolution of their symptoms within 6 months and half develop chronic ReA. The triggering microbes of ReA are gram-negative bacteria with a lipopolysaccharide component of their cell walls. All of these bacteria, or their bacterial products, have been demonstrated by polymerase chain reaction technology in the synovial tissue or fluid of patients with ReA; however, these findings have been questioned. Traditional therapies include nonsteroidal anti-inflammatory drugs, corticosteroids, and disease-modifying antirheumatic drugs; the role of antibiotics is not yet fully defined.

Systemic lupus erythematosus (SLE), scleroderma, and polymyositis/dermatomyositis (PM/DM) are autoimmune diseases with high morbidity and mortality. The important role infections play in these diseases has been documented in the literature over the years. This article reviews the role of infections in these three disorders, emphasizing in each (1) the predisposing factors for the development of infections, (2) the effect of infections on mortality, and (3) the most common microorganisms involved in these infectious processes.

Extrahepatic symptoms during chronic hepatitis C virus (HCV) infection are common and varied. Arthritis can be seen either as part of autoimmune processes (eg, associated with cryoglobulinemia) or independently. Whether the manifestation is specifically attributable to HCV infection or rather to the nonspecific result of a chronic inflammatory process is not clear. The literature available at this time is insufficient to guide the most appropriate course of treatment of HCV arthritis. Standard antirheumatic treatment can be considered, but with caution, because some of these medications occasionally may be hepatotoxic and response to therapy seems variable. Treatment decisions should be determined on a case-by-case basis.

Rheumatic complaints such as myalgias, arthralgias, arthritis and reactive arthritis are common in patients with HIV, and HIV positivity confers an increased susceptibility in populations with similar risk factors for HIV infection. With the advent of modern combined antiretroviral treatment, highly active antiretroviral therapy has had a profound beneficial effect on survival in HIV-infected patients, with lifelong control of HIV infection and normalization of life expectancy; but it has also contributed to an altered frequency and a different nature of rheumatic complications now being observed in this population, with new rheumatic complications, such as osteoporosis, osteonecrosis, gout, mycobacterial, mycotic osteoarticular infections, and neoplasia perhaps more prevalent. Rheumatologists, internists, and general physicians need to be aware of these changes to provide optimal diagnosis and how to disclose the results to their patients. They also need to be familiar with the management of HIV infection and to direct careful attention to the prevention of HIV transmission in health care facilities.

Role of Endogenous Retroviruses in Autoimmune Diseases

Ines Colmegna and Robert F. Garry

The human genome sequencing project and similar initiatives for other species have revealed that a large portion of vertebrate genomic DNA consists of genetic elements that are present in multiple copies. Human endogenous retroviruses (HERVs) represent a class of interspersed mobile repetitive elements known as retrotransposons. HERVs are closely related to certain members of the Retroviridae, an important family of human and animal viruses that includes HIV and human T-lymphotropic virus, causes of AIDS and adult T-cell leukemia, respectively. Recent studies have implicated HERVs in a wide variety of pathologic and physiologic processes. This article discusses studies that implicate HERVs in many human autoimmune diseases.

Impact of Biologic Agents on Infectious Diseases

Lesley Ann Saketkoo and Luis R. Espinoza

Until recently, inflammatory diseases, collagen vascular diseases, inflammatory bowel diseases, and multiple sclerosis were met with a limited offering for treatment. The introduction of biologic agents has revolutionized the approach to these diseases, offering many patients freedom from disease activity staving off resultant destruction to organs and joints with marked improvement in quality of life and disability. This article focuses on the development of serious infections associated with the use of biologic agents. Presented is a synthesis of case series, reports, and systematic reviews to elucidate implicated pathogens and clinical presentations in patients being treated with biologic agents and to form a cursory backbone for prevention and treatment strategies to which clinicians prescribing these agents or encountering patients already on these agents can readily refer. Maintenance of a high index of suspicion is imperative for the prevention and appropriate treatment of serious life-threatening infections in these patients.

FORTHCOMING ISSUES

RECENT ISSUES

ELSEVIER
SAUNDERS

Infect Dis Clin N Am
20 (2006) xi–xii

INFECTIOUS
DISEASE CLINICS
OF NORTH AMERICA

Preface

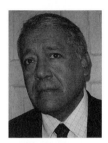

Luis R. Espinoza, MD
Guest Editor

The past few decades have seen many advancements in science that have helped define the role of infection in musculoskeletal diseases. Infection affects a considerable segment of the population, constitutes a significant cause of morbidity and mortality, and adds to the cost of caring for patients with musculoskeletal involvement. Unraveling the mystery of this important correlation aids clinical practitioners in the treatment and prevention of rheumatic diseases. This issue of the *Infectious Diseases Clinics of North America* is dedicated to a current overview of the interesting relationship between infections and the musculoskeletal system.

The opening article by Cuchacovich and colleagues reviews the role of the polymerase chain reaction in the identification of microbial components in a variety of tissues and its potential clinical applications and pitfalls in the diagnosis and management of several disorders. The next two articles, one by Lopez and Lartchenko and one by De La Torre, are devoted to the diagnosis and management of soft tissue infection and septic arthritis. Emphasis is placed on describing and discussing the predisposing risk factors and morbidity and mortality associated with these conditions in the era of newly introduced biologic agents.

An extensive and comprehensive review of imaging techniques in the diagnosis of osteomyelitis by Pineda and colleagues follows. An in-depth review of current imaging techniques with representative studies is presented.

Pathogenic aspects, including the potential role of HLA-B27 antigen, associated clinical syndromes, and diagnostic criteria and therapeutic modalities of reactive arthritis are discussed next by Carter. The potential benefits and adverse events of antibiotics and tumor necrosis factor-alpha are discussed in detail.

The next article by Alarcón presents an overview of the important role that infection plays in connective tissue disorders. Predisposing risk factors for the development of infection, the effect of infection on morbidity and mortality, and the most common microorganisms involved are thoroughly discussed. Sanzone and Begue next discuss the rheumatologic manifestations of hepatitis C. Hepatitis C can induce a variety of autoimmune and inflammatory musculoskeletal manifestations, and a comprehensive review follows.

The role of retroviruses in the development of arthritis and autoimmune disorders is discussed next. Medina and Moreno discuss the pandemic of HIV that began 25 years ago continues to be a significant health care problem in some parts of the world, especially in Central Africa. The changing clinical spectrum of the musculoskeletal involvement of HIV in developed countries, as well as the development of newer clinical syndromes, such as the immune reconstitution syndrome, is reviewed. Human endogenous retroviruses are extensively reviewed by Gary and Colmegna. Their classification is presented, and their potential implication in the causation of autoimmune disease is discussed.

The final article by Saketkoo and Espinoza discusses the infectious complications associated with the use of biologic agents, particularly tumor necrosis factor-alpha inhibitors. These agents have revolutionized the therapeutic management of rheumatoid arthritis and other connective tissue disorders. A systematic review of implicated pathogens, particularly tuberculosis, clinical presentation in patients being treated with these agents, as well as prevention and treatment strategies are presented.

This issue provides an overview of the major advances that have occurred in the field in the past four years and represents the concerted effort of experts on the topics discussed. I am most grateful to Karen Sorensen, Senior Clinics Editor at Elsevier for her confidence and support in the preparation of this issue.

Luis R. Espinoza, MD
Professor and Chief
Section of Rheumatology
Department of Internal Medicine
Louisiana State University Health Sciences Center
7th Floor, Box E-20
2020 Gravier Street
New Orleans, LA 70112-2822 USA

E-mail address: luisrolan@msn.com

INFECTIOUS
DISEASE CLINICS
OF NORTH AMERICA

Infect Dis Clin N Am
20 (2006) 735–758

Clinical Applications of the Polymerase Chain Reaction: An Update

Raquel Cuchacovich, MD[a,b]

[a]Section of Rheumatology, Department of Medicine, Louisiana State University Health
Sciences Center, 1542 Tulane Avenue, New Orleans, LA 70112, USA
[b]Ochsner Clinic Foundation, 1514 Jefferson Highway, New Orleans, LA 70121, USA

The development, in the past decade, of nucleic acid amplification (NAA) and detection methods has been found to be useful in the study of the etiopathogenesis, diagnosis, and management of a variety of clinical (including rheumatologic) disorders. A variety of molecular techniques have been developed that allow the amplification and detection of minute amounts of nucleic acid sequences from tissues or body fluids. These NAA methods can create millions of identical copies of DNA or RNA sequences present in clinical samples. The use of molecular technology has dramatically changed the approach to the laboratory diagnosis of many diseases. For example, these methods have been useful in the diagnosis of genetic disorders, such as sickle cell anemia, β-thalassemia, and cystic fibrosis. The recent development of NAA technology has also had significant impact on the diagnosis and management of many infectious diseases.

An association between infectious agents and rheumatic disorders has been established through such methods as polymerase chain reaction (PCR). Some rheumatic disorders are induced by viruses, such as parvovirus B19 (erosive rheumatoid arthritis [RA]); rubella (acute and chronic arthropathies); alpha viruses (acute infectious illness with fever, rash, arthritis, myalgia, encephalitis, epidemic polyarthritis, and chronic polyarthritis); adenoviruses (symmetric polyarthritis or a recurrent chronic polyarthritis); coxsackievirus (symmetric polyarthritis of small joints); hepatitis B (polyarteritis nodosa, cryoglobulinemia, transient arthritis); hepatitis C (type II

Portions of this article originally appeared in Cuchacovich R, Quinet S, Santos AM. Applications of polymerase chain reaction in rheumatology. Rheumatic Disease Clinics of North America 2003;29(1):1–20.

Section of Rheumatology, Department of Medicine, Louisiana State University Health Sciences Center, 1542 Tulane Avenue, New Orleans, LA 70112, USA.

E-mail address: rcucha@hotmail.com

doi:10.1016/j.idc.2006.09.003
id.theclinics.com

cryoglobulinemia, erosive RA, and polymyositis dermatomyositis); human T-cell lymphotropic virus type I–associated arthritis, polymyositis, Sjögren's syndrome, and RA); HIV-1 (reactive arthritis, psoriatic arthritis, spondyloarthropathy, and infiltrative lymphocytosis syndrome, and in some cases remission of systemic lupus erythematosus, RA, polymyositis). Gram-positive and gram-negative bacteria, such as *Streptococcus* sp, *Chlamydia trachomatis*, *Salmonella* sp, and *Shigella* sp have been found as triggering agents for rheumatic fever and reactive arthritis [1–13].

Several strategies for the amplification of nucleic acids have been described, including amplification of the nucleic acid target (eg, PCR, strand-displacement amplification, self-sustaining sequence replication); amplification of a nucleic acid probe (eg, ligase chain reaction, Q [b] replicase); and signal amplification (eg, branched-probe DNA assay). As these molecular methods are further refined and become more widely available in the next few years, physicians need to understand their clinical applications and be aware of their potential advantages, limitations, and clinical usefulness.

This article describes the principles behind PCR-based diagnosis and updates its clinical applications. It is beyond the scope of this article, however, to describe other NAA methods or to include a complete list of all PCR assays that have been developed; other recent reviews offer additional details.

Polymerase chain reaction

Molecular technologies have increased the speed of antigen detection methods. The most widely used of these methods is PCR, a technique that enables the amplification of specific sequences of nucleic acids. The technique was originally described by Saiki and coworkers and subsequently perfected by Mullis in 1987. PCR can amplify minute amounts of target DNA (10 to 100 copies in clinical samples) within a few hours. In the laboratory PCR is used for DNA sequencing, cloning, gene isolation, and analysis of gene expression, and for sequencing of mitochondrial and genomic DNA in the human genome organization project. PCR can be combined with other techniques to determine whether the amplification products contain a mutation, such as restriction enzyme digestion, allelic specific oligonucleotide hybridization, and single-strand conformation polymorphism analysis.

Applications in microbiology and infectious diseases have included the diagnosis of infection caused by slow-growing or fastidious microorganisms; detection of infectious agents that cannot be cultured; presence of novel microorganisms (*Tropheryma whippelii*) [14]; and recognition of newly emerging infectious diseases (nearly 100 kinds of organisms have been detected by PCR). The procedure also improves the accuracy of subtyping pathogens in epidemiologic studies, quantifies the viral load [15], and allows rapid identification of antimicrobial resistance. PCR can also be used to detect RNA viruses [16–18] (eg, hepatitis C virus); a specific messenger RNA (mRNA) transcribed by a microorganism; DNA virus in autoimmune conditions treated with immunosuppressive drugs [19–21]; and to identify cases of HIV patients with rheumatologic conditions (Box 1). It is important to understand how PCR-based techniques are used to detect the presence of infectious agents in which there are too few organisms present for detection by other means. This is illustrated by the use of PCR for the detection of *Mycobacterium* infection, especially tuberculosis in RA patients treated with tumor necrosis factor-α inhibitors. Tuberculosis among RA patients before the use of tumor necrosis factor-α inhibitors was approximately 6 cases

---

Box 1. Applications of PCR

Genetics
Detection of genetic defects associated with inherited diseases
Detection of mutations associated with genetic diseases
Determination of genetic susceptibility to a disease
Determination of disease risk to offspring in families with
    affected members
Detection of cancer and determination of the extent of residual
    disease
Ability to detect clonality with a high sensitivity (0.001%–0.1%)
Detection of gene polymorphism
Detection of nonself cells or occult neoplastic cells in tissues
Detection of genetic markers (receptor cell rearrangements,
    major histocompatibility complex system)
Forensic determination of identity

Infectious diseases
Ability to diagnose infections caused by slow-growing or
    fastidious microorganisms
Detection of infectious agents that cannot be cultured or
    organisms that have not yet been identified
Specie identification in the mycobacterium
Useful for screening, diagnosis, and management of viral
    infections (hepatitis viruses, human herpes virus 8, HIV)
Recognition of newly emerging infectious disease
Detection of RNA viruses (eg, hepatitis C virus) or specific mRNA
    transcribed by a microorganism
Recognition of viral load to monitor therapy
Detection of infections in autoimmune conditions treated with
    immunosuppressive drugs
Diagnosis of viral encephalitis
Identification of bacterial DNA for the diagnosis of septic arthritis
    and reactive arthritis
Allows rapid identification of antimicrobial resistance

per 100,000 patients; it has increased to 24 cases per 100,000 patients following the institution of tumor necrosis factor-α inhibitors. Tuberculosis has
been reported with the use of all tumor necrosis factor-α inhibitors including
etanercept, infliximab, and adalimumab. It is frequently caused by reactivation of latent tuberculosis, or new infection with *Mycobacterium avium* and
M avium-intracellulare. These nontuberculous mycobacteria have overlapping phenotypic properties that make their speciation difficult to determine
by conventional methods; also, their clinical picture can be atypical with isolated fever, and these presentations may lead to delays in the diagnosis with
subsequent dissemination. Smear can be negative 50% of the time, particularly in immunosuppressed individuals; cultures can take a long time, which
makes the diagnostic approach problematic. PCR can provide both rapid
results and an improved diagnostic accuracy of the involved mycobacteria
(*Mycobacterium tuberculosis* from nontuberculous mycobacteria) in the disease process, and lead to the right therapeutic approach in a short period of
time [8,11,22].

PCR is also used to detect mutations associated with genetic diseases, for
tissue typing, and to diagnose neoplastic diseases. It is also a valuable tool
for amplification of T-cell receptor genes to distinguish neoplastic proliferation from reactive T cells. Moreover, many diseases not traditionally
thought to be genetic are now being evaluated in terms of inherited suscep-
tibilities, or as genetically mediated maladaptive responses to external stimuli, such as autoimmune diseases.

PCR also facilitates antibody engineering, such as monoclonal drugs antibodies. The isolation of an individual antigen-binding B cell is sufficient to
isolate the relevant antibody-binding variable (V) region, by using oligonucleotide primers to amplify antibody V regions. In addition, the V region of
the monoclonal antibody can be fused to the constant region to produce the
desired isotype and subclass; by this method the entire antibody repertoire
in the form of recombinant antibody libraries can be obtained (see Box 1).

In the past few years a variant of this technique, called broad-range PCR,
has enabled researchers to identify a number of uncultivable microbial pathogens. This approach, which uses ribosomal RNA (rRNA) gene sequences
(which are found in all prokaryotes and eukaryotes and contain highly conserved regions interspersed with species-specific ones), makes it possible to
perform PCR on infected tissue containing extremely small numbers of
bacteria.

First, the highly conserved regions of the bacterial rRNA gene are used to
"prime" the synthesis of the remainder of the gene. The resulting PCR amplified product is then sequenced to identify bacteria-specific variable regions of the gene. Such an approach has enabled researchers to identify
a variety of microbes, including the etiologic agents of bacillary angiomatosis and Whipple's disease.

An enzymatic in vitro DNA method PCR can be coupled with a number
of other detection methods to identify any gene (by DNA) or its expression

(by mRNA) directly from clinical samples, regardless of the amount of target molecules present [23]. This application requires reverse transcription (RT) of the RNA isolated from the sample into DNA; the product of this reaction, termed "complementary DNA" (cDNA), then serves as the template for amplification by PCR. Caution must be exercised in these cases because RNA is a labile molecule and its degradation could lead to false-negative results. This process depends on a uniquely synthesized pair of oligonucleotide primers that flank and define the DNA segment of interest. In the initial step of the procedure, nucleic acid (eg, DNA) is extracted from the microorganism or clinical specimen of interest. A thermally stable DNA polymerase uses the target DNA strand to which the primer has bound as a template to synthesize a complementary strand of DNA in an automated instrument known as a "thermocycler." Heat (90°C–95°C) is used to separate the extracted double-stranded DNA into single strands (denaturation). Cooling to 55°C then allows primers specifically designed to flank the target nucleic acid sequence to adhere to the target DNA (annealing). The enzyme Taq polymerase and nucleotides are then added to create new DNA fragments complementary to the target DNA (extension). This completes one cycle of PCR. This process of denaturation, annealing, and extension is repeated numerous times in the thermocycler. At the end of a cycle, each newly synthesized DNA sequence acts as a new target for the next cycle, so that after 30 or more cycles, millions of copies of the original target DNA are created. The result is the accumulation of a specific PCR product with sequences located between the two flanking primers. Repeated cycles result in a 2n exponential increase of the template DNA, where n is the number of cycles. Detection of the amplified products can be done by visualization with agarose gel electrophoresis, an enzyme immunoassay format using probe-based calorimetric detection, or by fluorescence emission technology.

A major strength of PCR is that the DNA segment of interest does not need to be purified from the background DNA. Furthermore, PCR can be used to diagnose disease using almost any tissue or body fluid, including fresh and archival specimens. The exponential amplification of PCR provides for great sensitivity and the use of unique primers provides for the specificity. Unlike other assay systems in which sensitivity is often compromised for the sake of specificity, an increase in one of these parameters leads to increases in the other [24,25].

Variations on the standard polymerase chain reaction

Multiplex polymerase chain reaction

In multiplex PCR the assay is modified to include several primer pairs specific to different DNA targets to allow amplification and detection of a number of different sequences at the same time (eg, two pathogenic viruses from a single DNA sample). The procedure, however, requires optimum conditions to ensure that one PCR reaction is not dominant over the other. The products obtained in each reaction should vary in size to enable their visualization on the gel [26,27].

Reverse transcriptase polymerase chain reaction

RT-PCR is a semiquantitative, sensitive, and versatile method developed for the analysis of gene expression in cells and tissues. The procedure is a modification of PCR used when the initial template is RNA rather than DNA. In this case the enzyme reverse transcriptase, derived from retroviruses or the Moloney murine leukemia virus, converts the RNA target into a cDNA copy. Single-stranded cDNA molecules are converted into double-stranded DNA and cloned into appropriate vectors to generate cDNA libraries, used to isolate genes of interest. In addition to the controls used in a standard PCR, RT-PCR should also include a control in which the RT enzyme is omitted; this ensures that the RNA preparation does not contain residual contaminating genomic DNA. This cDNA can then be amplified by standard PCR methods as described previously.

RT-PCR can be used to amplify a much higher number of DNA copies present in bacteria, fungi, virus, or other proteins, and it may detect specific expression of certain genes during the course of infection or inflammation. The detection of cDNA using RT-PCR of mRNA encoded by a pathogen could be evidence of active infection, in contrast to the detection of DNA from nonviable organisms using standard PCR [28].

Quantitative reverse transcriptase polymerase chain reaction

It is possible to quantify the specific mRNA molecules using multiplex and mimic PCR. Multiplex PCR can also be used semiquantitatively to identify changes in concentrations of individual mRNA molecules relative to a housekeeping gene. Advantages of the technique are sensitivity, dynamic range of quantification, applicability to small clinical samples, elimination of radioisotopes and decay of labeled probes, speed, and multiplexing of assays for different mRNAs using the same RNA sample. Disadvantage of this approach, however, is that the level of transcription of some housekeeping genes may also be altered [29].

Nested polymerase chain reaction

The sensitivity of the PCR can be affected by the presence of low-quality templates; however, n PCR (or n RT-PCR) increase sensitivity and specificity. Two different amplifications are used. The first uses a set of primers that gives a large segment, which is the template for the next amplification, which uses another set of primers covering a smaller segment of the target nucleic acid that then anneals within the large segment. The specificity is increased because the formation of the final product depends on the binding of two separate pairs of primers, and the increased sensitivity results from the use of two cycles of amplification [30].

Inverse polymerase chain reaction

With the use of this procedure, it is possible to amplify sequences on either or both sides of the known region. The first step is the digestion of the sample DNA with a restriction enzyme. The target sequence should not contain restriction sites, so the enzyme is able to cut the DNA outside the known sequence; this is followed by the ligation of the restriction fragments. A second enzyme cuts within the known sequence, producing a linear DNA fragment. The known sequence is then amplified using standard PCR [28].

In situ polymerase chain reaction

Identification of individual cells expressing or carrying specific genes in a latent form in a tissue section under the microscope provides great advantages in recognition of a normal versus a dysregulated gene expression. Advantage of this technique is the finding of whether a specific gene is actively expressed within the cell by the expression of RNA copies of the gene within the cellular structure. Several types of tissues or cells can be evaluated (tissue cultured cells, peripheral blood leukocytes, any other single cell suspensions, paraffin fixed tissue); amplification of both DNA and RNA can be done; by the use of multiple labeled probes, various signals can be detected in a single cell; immunohistochemistry can be performed; the origin of the metastasis (RT-based in situ PCR), identity of the cell or structures affected by an infectious agent, and the association with mediators synthesized locally can potentially be determined. The validity of in situ amplification should be examined in every run [31].

Clinical applications of polymerase chain reaction

Diagnosis of infectious diseases

Newer DNA amplification methods have the potential significantly to influence the diagnosis and management of a variety of infectious diseases. Conventional laboratory diagnostic methods require a minimum of 24 hours and, in many cases, the time required is significantly longer. Moreover, cultures may yield no bacterial growth if there has been a delay in transporting the specimen to the laboratory, the number of viable infecting organisms is low, or the patient had been taking antibiotics at the time the culture specimen was obtained. In addition, certain pathogenic organisms, such as *Mycoplasma* sp, *Chlamydia* sp, rickettsia, and viruses, are not easily detected by routine culture methods and require specialized methods [32,33].

Rapid nonculture diagnostic tests relying on antigen detection by immuno-fluorescence or enzyme immunoassay, or using DNA probes, may have variable diagnostic sensitivities or specificities as compared with culture.

Molecular methods with amplification and detection of target nucleic acids generally have been found to have superior sensitivity and specificity and have the potential to provide results within hours of collecting the specimen [34–38]. Pilot studies have indicated the feasibility of designing broad-range multiplex PCR assays with the capability of detecting a panel of microorganisms from clinical specimens. Assays that are currently commercially available for use in diagnostic laboratories include tests for the detection of *C trachomatis*, *Chlamydia pneumoniae*, *M tuberculosis*, *Mycoplasma pneumoniae* (correlates with disease and establishes the diagnosis of atypical pneumonia), *Neisseria gonorrhoeae*, herpes simplex virus (HSV), cytomegalovirus, enterovirus, and other infectious agents. In addition, there are PCR assays available for monitoring the viral load of HIV, hepatitis C virus, and hepatitis B virus. Unfortunately, only a few of these commercially available assays have been extensively evaluated to determine the sensitivity, specificity, or clinical usefulness. There are reliable commercial probe systems for detection of *N gonorrhea*, *C trachomatis*, and papilloma virus. PCR assays have been found to be significantly more accurate, with sensitivities of 90% to 100% and specificities greater than 97% for the detection of *C trachomatis* from cervical or urethral specimens. The positive predictive values reported in these studies ranged from 89% to 100%. A major advantage of these tests is the ability to detect *Chlamydia* in urine specimens or urethral swabs. PCR testing of freshly voided urine was found to be the most sensitive (91%) and most specific (100%) method for detecting asymptomatic *C trachomatis* infection in men [39]. These assays also have been automated, allowing for the processing of large numbers of specimens. They may be used for diagnosis or screening for sexually transmitted diseases. A coamplification PCR assay for the direct detection of both *N gonorrhoeae* and *C trachomatis* from patients with sexually transmitted diseases has also been developed. The sensitivity and specificity of PCR detection of *N gonorrhoeae* from cervical and urethral specimens were found to be greater than 90% and 96%, respectively.

Direct amplification tests have also had a great impact on the rapid diagnosis of tuberculosis. Conventional culture methods for the isolation of mycobacteria generally take several weeks, whereas PCR takes only 24 hours. Commercial amplification assays have been found to have sensitivities of about 90% to 98%, as compared with culture of specimens that are smear positive for acid-fast bacilli (AFB). The performance of these amplifications, however, has been suboptimal for specimens without AFB seen on direct microscopic examination, with reported sensitivities as low as 46%. The specificity of PCR-based assays for *M tuberculosis* is excellent at >98%, and sensitivity is at least 80%. Although these assays cannot replace mycobacterial cultures, their ability rapidly to determine the presence of

M tuberculosis directly from respiratory tract specimens has enabled more rapid institution of effective therapy and implementation of important infection control and public health interventions [40–42]. *Mycobacterium* sp probes for the rapid identification of mycobacteria are now widely used to identify acid-fast organisms grown on solid media or in liquid media. Probes are available for *M tuberculosis*, *M avium complex*, *M kansasii*, and *M gordonae*. Mixed infections (*M tuberculosis* and *M avium-intracellulare*) can be identified. At present, two Food and Drug Administration (FDA)-approved NAA assays are widely available: the AMPLICOR M. Tuberculosis (Roche Diagnostic Systems, Branchburg, New Jersey) and the Amplified Mycobacterium Tuberculosis Direct Test (Gen-Probe, San Diego, California). The AMPLICOR assay uses PCR to amplify nucleic acid targets, is FDA approved in smear-positive respiratory samples, sensitivity ranges from 74% to 92% for smear-positive samples and 40% to 73% for smear-negative samples, specificity goes from 93% to 99%, and it has a negative predictive value of 100%. The Mycobacterium Tuberculosis Direct Test assay is an isothermal strategy for detection of *M tuberculosis* rRNA and is FDA approved for smear-positive and smear-negative respiratory specimens. It has sensitivity from 83% to 98% from smear-positive respiratory samples and from 70% to 81% from smear-negative respiratory samples; it is very helpful for confirming disease in intermediate- and high-risk patients and for excluding cases in low-risk patients.

The Centers for Disease Control and Prevention now recommends that AFB smear and NAA be performed on the first sputum smear collected. If smear and NAA are positive, pulmonary tuberculosis is diagnosed with near certainty. If the smear is positive and the NAA is negative, is recommended to test the sputum for inhibitors by spiking the sputum sample with an aliquot of lysed *M tuberculosis* and repeating the assay. If inhibitors are not detected, the process needs to be repeated on another sample and if it still remains negative, the patient most likely has nontuberculous mycobacterium. If smears are negative but clinical suspicion is high or intermediate, NAA should be done in a sputum sample, and if the sample test is positive a presumptive diagnosis of tuberculosis is made. If the smear is negative and the clinical suspicion is low NAA should not be done. Testing must be limited to those who have not been treated recently for active disease. The limitation of these NAA is that they give no drug susceptibility information; also, they detect nucleic acids from both living and dead organisms and may be false-positive for active disease. Assays that detect mRNA remain positive only while viable mycobacteria persist, so they are sensitive indicators of treatment response and drug susceptibility.

For extrapulmonary tuberculosis AFB smears and culture are less sensitive than in respiratory samples. Herein NAA play an important role in the diagnosis, although it is not completely defined. The sensitivity in nonrespiratory samples for Mycobacterium Tuberculosis Direct Test goes from 67% to 100%; in smear-negative samples, the sensitivity ranges from 52% to

100% in different studies. The AMPLICOR had a similar sensitivity, and the specificity of both assays remains high in nonrespiratory samples. The assays perform different based on the type of sample (spinal fluid, pleural fluid, ascitic fluid). Multidrug resistance in tuberculosis is a major public health problem. Coupling assays that detect gene mutations, such as line probe assays and molecular beacons, to PCR allows rapid detection of the drug-resistant mutations from smear-positive samples or from culture samples.

PCR also can be used to detect *Mycobacterium leprae* DNA present in small amounts or to identify the AFB when conventional techniques fail. In addition, PCR is able to detect *M leprae* after multidrug therapy has been started; because PCR allows early detection of the mycobacteria, treatment can be started even when histopathologic features of the disease are not present [22,43].

Although not FDA approved, PCR can identify different species of *Rickettsia*, such as *R rickettsii*, *Ehrlichia* sp, *Bartonella henselae* (bacillary angiomatosis), and spirochete in late secondary and tertiary cutaneous syphilitic lesions. Among viral pathogens that can be detected by PCR in addition to the ones already mentioned are HSV-1 and -2 from saliva and serum of patients with acute herpes labialis and from spinal fluid; PCR permits detection of either HSV serotype and provides a rapid and definitive diagnosis, has an extraordinary sensitivity greater than virus isolation, or direct detection of HSV antigens or nucleic acids. PCR assays also have established that HSV (mainly HSV-2) is the principal cause of benign recurrent lymphocytic meningitis and confirmed a strong association between HSV-1 infection and Bell's palsy. The clinical significance of small quantities of HSV DNA detected by PCR in the absence of infectious virus remains to be determined. Varicella zoster virus can be identified by multiplex RT-PCR from saliva, tear fluid, skin eruptions, and throat swabs. PCR detects the virus in very early clinical manifestations of the disease with skin biopsy specimens obtained from vesicular and nonvesicular erythematous regions.

In Kaposi's sarcoma the diagnosis can be difficult and PCR can be helpful, because it is highly sensitive and specific for the detection and quantification of human herpes virus 8. PCR is also useful in the detection of human papilloma viruses, such as human papilloma virus-5 (squamous cell carcinomas in renal transplant patients), human papilloma virus-16 (anogenital and cervical malignancies and verrucous carcinoma of the foot), and human papilloma virus-11 (anogenital verrucous carcinoma). PCR also detects other viruses, including parvovirus B19, and also confirms the presence of Epstein-Barr virus in T and B cells, and NK cell lymphomas (accurate classification of the lymphoma). In sudden acute respiratory syndrome, the virus genome was sequenced within weeks of discovery, providing sequence data for the development of RT-PCR based detection strategies.

In relationship to parasitic infections PCR can be used to aid in the diagnosis of *Leishmania infantum* (cutaneous leishmaniasis). For fungal infections probes also have simplified the identification of the dimorphic fungi, *Histoplasma capsulatum*, *Blastomyces dermatitis*, *Cryptococcus neoformans*, *Sporothrix schenckii*, *Trichophyton rubrum*, *Coccidioides immitis*, and *Candida albicans* [44].

Septic arthritis

The synovial fluid culture is positive in 90% of cases of nongonococcal bacterial arthritis, but Gram stains are positive in only 50% of cases, and clumps of stained or cellular debris may be mistaken for bacteria. Most infected joint effusions are purulent or very inflammatory with average leukocyte counts of 50 to 150,000 c/mL, predominately polymorphonuclear cells. Blood cultures are positive in 50% to 70% of patients with nongonococcal bacterial arthritis. In contrast, the synovial fluid Gram stain is positive in less than 25% of patients with gonococcal arthritis, and culture is positive in only 50%. The skin lesions and blood samples rarely yield positive cultures in disseminated gonococcus infection (DGI). A presumptive diagnosis of DGI is often made on the basis of characteristic signs, symptoms, and identification of *N gonorrhoeae* from a genitourinary source. Genitourinary cultures are positive in 70% to 90% of patients with DGI. The failure to recover *N gonorrhoeae* from a site of dissemination may be partly explained by the fastidious in vitro growth requirements of *N gonorrhoeae*. Immune mechanisms may also be responsible for the sterile synovitis and dermatitis. PCR has been used to detect *N gonorrhoeae* in patients with clinically typical but culture-negative gonococcal arthritis. The presence of gonococcal DNA, even in culture-negative synovial fluid, suggests that viable bacteria do indeed provoke the synovitis associated with DGI [45]. In a case of staphylococcal arthritis, PCR demonstrated persistent *Staphylococcus aureus* DNA in the synovial fluid for 10 weeks despite adequate antibiotic treatment and sterile synovial fluid [46,47]. Identification of bacterial DNA by PCR is most useful in patients with partly treated or culture-negative bacterial arthritis and in reactive arthritis [48]. PCR in synovial fluid also plays a role in potentially infected joint prostheses.

Reactive arthritis

A healthy but genetically predisposed individual may develop reactive arthritis after a suitable triggering infection. Most commonly the initial infection is localized in the digestive or urogenital tract, even by saprophyte flora; however, the list of microbes able to trigger reactive arthritis is not completely understood and the primary infection may also affect other organs. Despite intensive research, the pathogenic process is not completely understood; however, during the period of contracting the initial infection, incubation time, the primary illness, and the following interval period before the onset, critical immune reactions are thought to take place. A large variety of different microbes lead to a similar clinical entity; isolation of the causative microbe is only rarely possible, and the symptoms and signs of the primary or triggering infection actually may have been quite mild or even passed unnoticed [49,50]. Reactive arthritis is discussed in more detail elsewhere in this issue.

Arthritogenic microorganisms can be detected in synovial samples [51–56], not only of patients with reactive arthritis, but also can be found in other autoimmune conditions, such as RA (*C trachomatis, C pneumoniae, M pneumoniae,* and *M fermentans*) [57–59] and dermatomyositis (parvovirus B19) [60]. With the use of PCR, in the last few years several studies have shown that sometimes more than one microorganism can be present in the same joint [61–63]. This association has been observed for *C trachomatis* and *C pneumoniae, C trachomatis* and *Borrelia burgdorferi* [64], and for different species of pseudomonas in synovial samples from patients with spondyloarthropathy or unexplained arthritis.

Bacterial DNA of *C trachomatis* and *C pneumoniae* [65–68]; *Yersinia enterocolitica, Shigella flexneri,* and *Shigella sonnei; Salmonella typhimurium* and *Salmonella enteritidis; Pseudomonas* sp, *Bacillus serius, Campylobacter jejuni, U urealyticum, B burgdoferi,* and *T whippelii;* and RNA of *C trachomatis, C pneumoniae,* and *Yersinia pseudotuberculosis* has been found in patients with reactive arthritis and undifferentiated arthritis [69–71]. The search for *C trachomatis* in the urogenital tract in the first portion of the morning urine by PCR or ligand chain reaction is an acceptable and relatively easy diagnostic approach with a result comparable with urogenital swab analysis. RT-PCR can be used for highly unstable rRNA transcripts to identify viable bacteria in the synovial fluid and synovial tissue samples. Small amounts of sample are needed to perform these tests. PCR is not very sensitive for peripheral blood. There is no agreement on the best technique to detect *Chlamydia* by PCR, and standardization is still pending. None of the commercially available tests is sensitive enough to detect chlamydial DNA reliably in synovial fluid when compared with the amplification methods, such as nested PCR.

All known bacterial pathogens of humans belong to the eubacteria kingdom. This fact implies that the method to amplify 16S rDNA, such as PCR, could confirm the presence or absence of bacterial pathogens in a normally sterile body. Using this technique, bacterial DNA products seem to be derived from several bacterial species; however, all of them can be found in the human intestinal, urogenital, and respiratory tracts.

Uveitis

In acute anterior uveitis anti-*Klebsiella*, anti–*Y enterocolitica*, and anti-*Salmonella* antibodies have been found [1–5]. In posterior uveitis PCR is increasingly used in the detection of pathogenic organisms associated with many forms of ocular inflammatory and infectious diseases. PCR is able to diagnose viral uveitis, infectious endophthalmitis [72,73], and parasitic eye diseases [60]. The most common identifiable causes of posterior uveitis are infectious agents; in immunocompetent patients *Toxoplasma gondii* is the most common microorganism identified, whereas in immunosuppressed patients cytomegalovirus, varicella zoster virus, and HSV [74,75] are implicated in acute retinitis [76]. Although local antibody production and viral cultures are useful for the diagnosis, PCR can directly detect the RNA or DNA of the causative microorganism with higher specificity and sensitivity than the other methods [77,78].

Anterior segment and external eye disease

Although most of the bacterial causes of conjunctivitis and keratitis are readily cultured or detected by Gram staining, *C trachomatis*, adenoviruses [79], herpes simplex, and *T whippelii* cannot be detected by these methods [14]. PCR primer sets for these microorganisms, however, are able to diagnose these infections in a timely manner. In addition to the detection of infectious diseases of the eye, PCR can also be useful in the diagnosis of B-cell lymphoma that mimics a posterior uveitis and presents as an ocular inflammation in older patients. PCR has demonstrated usefulness for the diagnosis of viral retinitis, conjunctivitis, delayed-onset endophthalmitis, and posterior uveitis [80–82].

Viral disorders

NAA assays for the detection of viruses, such as HSV [83–85], cytomegalovirus, enterovirus, hepatitis C and B virus [16,86,87], and HIV [88,89], have proved to be useful for screening, diagnosis, and management. Most PCR assays for viral pathogens have sensitivity of 10 to 100 genomes, which corresponds to less than 1 plaque-forming unit in viral culture [90]. The Canadian Blood Services has adopted NAA methods to screen donated blood for hepatitis C and HIV because of the enhanced sensitivities of these assays. PCR detection of HSV in cerebrospinal fluid has become the gold standard for the diagnosis of herpes encephalitis or meningitis, with sensitivity and specificity of 95% and 94%, respectively, obviating the need for a brain biopsy. Enteroviruses are among the most common causes of aseptic meningitis. PCR for the diagnosis of enteroviral meningitis using cerebrospinal fluid samples has been found to be significantly more sensitive than conventional viral isolation (14% of specimens positive versus 10% positive, respectively) [91–93]. Moreover, the PCR assay can be completed within 1 day, whereas cultures for enteroviruses typically require up to 5 days for isolation of the virus. A PCR assay for cytomegalovirus is available for detection of the virus in plasma or cerebrospinal fluid specimens and has been useful in monitoring HIV and bone marrow transplant patients with cytomegalovirus infection.

The performance of this test has been comparable with that of antigen assays, with reported sensitivities and specificities of 95% to 98% and

98% to 100%, respectively. In contrast, the sensitivity of culture detection of cytomegalovirus is only 42%. Hepatitis G virus infection can be identified only through PCR testing, which indicates current infection; however, such testing is not readily available or standardized.

In addition to these diagnostic applications, NAA procedures have also been modified to allow for the quantitative measurement of viral load to monitor response to therapy for patients with HIV, cytomegalovirus, or hepatitis C virus infection [94]. For example, measuring HIV viral load in serum has had a major impact on the management of HIV-infected patients. Viral load measurement is of prognostic importance; it is used to predict progression of the disease and to assist in making treatment decisions.

PCR technology has also been used to identify infection by organisms that cannot be cultured. To accomplish this, investigators took advantage of the observation that portions of bacterial 16S rRNA sequences are highly conserved, whereas other regions are less well conserved and are species specific [95,96]. PCR amplification of 16S rRNA sequences of bacteria that cannot be cultured from tissues of patients with such diseases as Whipple's disease and bacillary angiomatosis enabled the discovery and identification of the etiologic agents [97]. Furthermore, using NAA methods, diseases previously thought to be noninfectious have been linked to infectious agents.

Cases

The following case scenarios may assist in understanding the clinical usefulness of PCR.

A 19-year-old student is admitted to a local hospital with a 2-week history of fever and monoarthritis involving the knee. Before her admission she had received two courses of oral antibiotic therapy for a presumed upper respiratory infection. Blood and synovial fluid cultures are negative. Should the patient continue with antibiotics? Should antibiotics be stopped because of lack of response?

A 60-year-old man with a 10-year history of RA, who has been receiving tumor necrosis factor antagonists for 2 years, is admitted to the hospital with low-grade fever, malaise, and cough. Three days ago he consulted his primary physician and a purified protein derivative was done that is 10 mm. A chest radiograph indicates the presence of disease in the upper left lobe airspace. Microscopic examination of a sputum specimen reveals a moderate number of AFB. Does this represent tuberculosis or the presence of nontuberculous bacteria?

Each of these clinical scenarios presents the physician with a problem that involves establishing a diagnosis of infection or reactive arthritis in a setting where routine laboratory investigations are likely to be nondiagnostic or do not provide results in a timely manner; however, the PCR will lead them in the right direction.

Detection of antimicrobial resistance

As many of the genetic mechanisms of antimicrobial resistance have become better understood, PCR-based methods have also been found accurately to identify antimicrobial resistance in clinical isolates and directly from patient specimens. Conventional culture and susceptibility test procedures for most pathogenic bacteria generally take 48 to 72 hours. Amplification of genetic determinants may be used to confirm antimicrobial resistance on the basis of the organism's genotype rather than relying on the variability of phenotypic expression of the resistance. Moreover, these tests can be done within hours, providing clinically relevant information days before conventional susceptibility test results become available [98].

PCR-based methods for the detection of antimicrobial resistance have been applied to bacteria including methicillin-resistant S aureus, vancomycin-resistant enterococci, and multidrug-resistant N tuberculosis. Detection of resistance to antiviral agents by molecular methods has also been described for acyclovir-resistant herpes viruses and HIV resistant to reverse transcriptase inhibitors and to protease inhibitors. Currently, none of these assays are available commercially but they have been used in a number of reference and research laboratories. The identification of methicillin resistance in S aureus represents an ideal application of NAA methods because the reliable detection of methicillin-resistant S aureus using culture and susceptibility tests may be problematic because expression of resistance (mec A gene) is usually heterogeneous and is influenced by culture conditions, especially in strains with low-level resistance [99,100]. Multiplex PCR and RT-PCR allow the identification of methicillin-resistant S aureus through the identification of the mec A and fem B genes.

Vancomycin-resistant enterococci have also emerged as important nosocomial pathogens in North American hospitals. PCR assays have been developed to recognize the vanA, vanB, and vanC genotypes and have demonstrated value in characterizing enterococci in the laboratory when conventional laboratory test results have been inconclusive [101,102].

Human genome amplification

The development of technically simple and reliable methods to detect sequence variations in specific genes is becoming more important as the number of genes associated with specific diseases grows. Applications of PCR to the human genome include (1) detection of genetic defects associated with inherited diseases (prenatal diagnosis); (2) determination of genetic susceptibility to disease; (3) gene polymorphism detection; (4) determination of the disease risk to offspring in families with affected members; (5) detection of cancer and the extent of residual disease; and (6) the forensic determination of identity [26,103–108]. One advantage of PCR in human genome testing is that only a few cells are required from biopsies, needle aspirations, or paraffin-embedded histologic sections [109]. PCR analysis of gene mutations is now widely used to identify the nature and location of the mutation. Several procedures can be used, such as allelic-specific oligonucleotide hybridization; density gradient electrophoresis; protein truncation test; single-strand conformation polymorphism analysis (sensitivity is 70%–90%); heteroduplex analysis (sensitivity 70%–90%); chemical mismatch cleavage; and RNase cleavage (sensitivity 40%–60%).

The genetic risk of several autoimmune diseases is linked to the major histocompatibility complex, with a particular association with certain susceptibility alleles. Identification of the HLA class I or II alleles has been done traditionally by serology in a complement-mediated microcytotoxicity assay. Several reports have compared the results of HLA typing by serology and by restriction fragment length polymorphism, and it has been suggested that 25% or more of alleles may be incorrectly assigned by serology. Moreover, the restriction fragment length polymorphism is more accurate and provides results more quickly (2 hours). The main disadvantages are cost and difficulty of implementation.

Genetic screening and counseling can be offered to couples at risk of bearing children with genetic diseases, or those with predisposing factors (spondyloarthropathy, HLA B27) [110]. Presymptomatic DNA screening is warranted when knowledge of the condition contributes to the health of the individual identified.

In the human genome there are around 10 million single nucleotide polymorphisms. These polymorphisms have been detected in genes responsible of nutrient transport, use, and function (folic acid, iron metabolism, and vitamin D receptor function). Nowadays errors that occur during the amplification process and limit the analysis of genetic alterations can be reduced by the introduction of hairpin-PCR, which separates genuine mutations from errors generated by misincorporation. The method is based on ligation of an artificial DNA hairpin to the DNA target of interest before the PCR.

The PCR (site directed mutagenesis–amplification-created restriction site) has been applied to the diagnosis of cancer and autoimmune diseases by identifying gene mutations in BRACA-1, ras oncogene, β-thalassemia, medium chain acyl coenzyme A dehydrogenase deficiency, hereditary hemochromatosis, and α_1-antitrypsin deficiency, and by increasing the sensitivity of residual disease detection. The detection of specific p53 mutations in microscopically normal tissue margins is correlated with recurrence; measuring these molecular margins may be useful in determining optimum therapy [111]. By amplifying either tumor-specific DNA abnormalities or tissue-specific mRNA, PCR (or RT-PCR) can detect micrometastases and circulating tumor cells. These and other PCR-based techniques have the potential to improve early detection and pretreatment staging, enhance diagnostic accuracy, identify patients at increased risk for recurrence or metastatic disease, and monitor the effectiveness of therapy. Combining DNA sequencing with PCR analyzes tumor samples rapidly and specifically for minute mutations in relation to clonal expression [112]. Multiplex PCR allows the identification of few neoplastic cells in a million normal cells, in this way providing information of effectiveness of treatment and risk of recurrent disease. RT-PCR has the ability to perform viral load determinations and viral genotyping for oncogenic viruses.

Limitations of polymerase chain reaction

Despite the obvious advantages of these newer procedures (Box 2), there may be potential limitations to DNA amplification technology in the diagnostic microbiology laboratory [113]. The accuracy and reproducibility of PCR assays depend on the technical expertise and experience of the operator. Specificity of the test may be affected by contamination of the specimen during laboratory processing, nonspecific primers being selected for the assay, and PCR conditions not being optimal and allowing nonspecific products to amplify. The most common sources of contamination are from other samples or from previous amplification procedures [114]. Contamination or amplification product carryover of even minute amounts of nucleic acid may result in generation of billions of DNA copies that may lead to false-positive test results [115,116]. For this reason laboratories should have separate

---

Box 2. Advantages and limitations of PCR

Advantages
Allows the amplification and detection of minute amounts
  of nucleic acid sequences in clinical samples
High sensitivity
High specificity
Good reproducibility
Versatility
Can provide results within a few hours
Widespread applicability to microbiology and study of infectious
  diseases
Able to analyze gene structure

Disadvantages
Potential false-negative results
Requires careful interpretation of results
A positive test is not validated for all infections
Expensive equipment
Cannot be used to study mutational analysis of large genes
Technically complex
Lack of standardization

rooms for different steps of the PCR procedure and must follow stringent quality control measures to prevent contamination or carryover. False-negative test results may occur because of the presence of substances in the specimen that inhibit nucleic acid extraction or amplification.

Certain specimen types (eg, blood) are more likely to contain such inhibitors. The assays may also lack sensitivity if there is a low inoculum of the microorganism present in the clinical specimen. This may be exacerbated if an inadequate sample or very small specimen volume (ie, <20 mL) is available for testing.

The PCR process relies on primer-mediated DNA replication and it has an absolute requirement for DNA sequence information. Another shortcoming is that the largest DNA fragments that can be reliably amplified are approximately 1000 base pairs in length, and considerably less if the source DNA was extracted from archival tissue blocks (because of partial degradation of the DNA).

PCR is not the tool of choice for performing exhaustive mutational analyses of large human genes that comprise many exons, such as the cystic fibrosis or breast cancer genes [24]. Interpretation of NAA test results is not always clear-cut. For example, assays may detect the residual DNA of a pathogenic microorganism even after successful treatment, and it is not clear whether this represents the presence of a small number of viable organisms or amplified DNA from nonviable organisms. PCR tests should not be used to monitor the effectiveness of a course of therapy and physicians must be aware of the laboratory testing procedures. In addition, the meaning of a positive PCR test result has not been validated for all infections. For example, it is uncertain whether a positive PCR test result for cytomegalovirus or *Chlamydia* from a patient's peripheral blood mononuclear cells or synovial fluid or tissue represents active disease, latent infection, or is reactive. Similarly, detection of pneumococcal DNA in blood samples has been reported in asymptomatic children colonized with *Streptococcus pneumococcus* and may not always indicate an invasive infection; however, the presence of viral RNA suggests that ongoing viral replication is occurring. Measuring viral RNA can facilitate the study of mechanisms of viral persistence and initially hidden viral replication. These observations suggest that there is a need for interpretative guidelines based on a correlation of NAA test results with clinical outcome. In such instances, detection of cDNA by RT-PCR of mRNA encoded by the pathogenic organism could be used as evidence of active infection.

The immediate availability of PCR testing in the clinical laboratory has been hindered by the following: (1) the complexity and time-consuming nature of the assays; (2) the need for personnel trained in molecular methods to perform the testing; and (3) the need to define an optimal protocol for each organism and to document the level of sensitivity and specificity of that protocol. Other important problems, such as contamination leading to false-positive reactions, the presence of inhibitors in clinical specimens, and assessing the clinical relevance of positive PCR assays, remain to be resolved [117].

Finally, it must be acknowledged that performance for a PCR assay is generally more expensive than conventional diagnostic laboratory methods. The requirement of separate rooms for pre- and post-PCR steps to reduce the risk of cross-contamination mean that molecular laboratories use an inordinate amount of laboratory space. The cost of these assays has been reported to be high.

Molecular technology involving NAA and detection is a promising tool for the rapid and accurate diagnosis of a variety of infectious diseases and for the confirmation or detection (or both) of antimicrobial resistance. A large number of PCR assays are still under development with the potential to provide accurate and rapid results when conventional methods are either not available, insensitive, or too slow. To date, evaluations of this technology have been generally limited by small samples and have not considered how these assays should fit into routine laboratory procedures, particularly in small, nonreference laboratories. As this technology continues to evolve, it is important to assess the cost effectiveness of these procedures and their real impact on patient management and outcomes.

References

[1] Phillips PE, Inman RD, Christian CL. Infectious agents in chronic rheumatic diseases. In: Koopman WJ, editor. Arthritis and allied conditions. 9th edition. Philadelphia: Lea & Febiger; 1979. p. 320.

[2] Phillips PE, Inman RD, Christian CL. Infectious agents in chronic rheumatic diseases. In: Koopman WJ, editor. Arthritis and allied conditions. 10th edition. Philadelphia: Lea & Febiger; 1985. p. 431–9.

[3] Phillips PE, Inman RD, Christian CL. Infectious agents in chronic rheumatic diseases. In: Koopman WJ, editor. Arthritis and allied conditions. 11th edition. Philadelphia: Lea & Febiger; 1989. p. 482–504.

[4] Phillips PE, Inman RD, Christian CL. Infectious agents in chronic rheumatic diseases. In: Koopman WJ, editor. Arthritis and allied conditions. 12th edition. Philadelphia: Lea & Febiger; 1993. p. 541–64.

[5] Phillips PE, Inman RD, Christian CL. Infectious agents in chronic rheumatic diseases. In: Koopman WJ, editor. Arthritis and allied conditions. 14th edition. Philadelphia: Lea & Febiger; 2001. p. 635–54.

[6] Espinoza L, Goldenberg DL, Arnett FC. Infections in the rheumatic diseases: a comprehensive review of microbial relations to rheumatic disorders. Orlando (FL): Grune & Stratton; 1988.

[7] Perl A. Mechanisms of viral pathogenesis in rheumatic disease. Ann Rheum Dis 1999;58: 454–61.

[8] Hochberg MC, Lebwohl MG, Plevy SE. The benefit/risk profile of TNF blocking agents: finding of a consensus panel. Semin Arthritis Rheum 2005;34:819–36.

[9] Belleza WG, Browne B. Pulmonary considerations in the immunocompromised patient. Emerg Med Clin North Am 2003;21:499–531.

[10] Marks DJ, Mitchison NA, Segal AW, et al. Can unresolved infection precipitate autoimmune disease? Curr Top Microbiol Immunol 2006;305:105–25.

[11] Bongartz T, Sutton AJ, Sweeting MJ. Anti-TNF antibody therapy in rheumatoid arthritis and the risk of serious infections and malignancies: systematic review and meta-analysis of rare harmful effects in randomized controlled trials. JAMA 2006;295:2275–85.

[12] Ebinger A, Rashid T. Rheumatoid arthritis is an autoimmune disease triggered by *Proteus* urinary tract infection. Clin Dev Immunol 2006;13:41–8.

[13] Pratesi F, Tommasi C, Anzilotti C. Deiminated Epstein-Barr virus nuclear antigen 1 is a target of anti-citrullinated protein antibodies in rheumatoid arthritis. Arthritis Rheum 2006; 54:733–41.

[14] O'Duffy JD, Griffing WL, Li CY, et al. Whipple's arthritis: direct detection of *Tropheryma whippelii* in synovial fluid and tissue. Arthritis Rheum 1999;42:812–7.

[15] Hawkins A, Davidson F, Simmonds P. Comparison of plasma viral loads among individuals infected with hepatitis C virus (HCV) genotypes 1, 2, and 3 by quantiplex HCV RNA assay versions 1 and 2, Roche, Monitor assay, and an in-house limiting dilution method. J Clin Microbiol 1997;35:187–92.

[16] Abe A, Inoue K, Tanaka T, et al. Quantitation of hepatitis B virus genomic DNA by real-time detection PCR. J Clin Microbiol 1999;37:2899–903.

[17] Cook L. Hepatitis C virus diagnosis and therapeutic monitoring: methods and interpretation. Clin Microbiol Newslett 1999;21:67–72.

[18] Hermida M, Ferreiro MC, Barral S, et al. Detection of HCV RNA in saliva of patients with hepatitis C virus infection by using a highly sensitive test. J Virol Methods 2002; 101:29–35.

[19] Bouza E, Garcia-Lechuz J, Munoz P. Infections in systemic lupus erythematosus and rheumatoid arthritis. Infect Dis Clin North Am 2001;15:335–61.

[20] Ley BE, Linton CJ, Bennett DM, et al. Detection of bacteraemia in patients with fever and neutropenia using 16S rRNA gene amplification by polymerase chain reaction. Eur J Clin Microbiol Infect Dis 1998;17:247–53.

[21] Wolf DG, Spector SA. Early diagnosis of human cytomegalovirus disease in transplant recipients by DNA amplification in plasma. Transplantation 1993;56:330–4.

[22] Franco Paredes C, Diaz Borjon A, Seuger MA. The ever-expanding association between rheumatologic diseases and tuberculosis. Am J Med 2006;119:470–7.

[23] Saiki RK, Gelfand DH, Stoffel S. Primer-directed enzymatic amplification of DNA with a thermostable DNA polymerase. Science 1988;239:487–91.

[24] Baumforth KRN, Nelson PN, Dugby JE, et al. The polymerase chain reaction. J Clin Pathol 1999;52:1–10.

[25] Eisenstein BI. The polymerase chain reaction: a new method of using molecular genetics for medical diagnosis. N Engl J Med 1990;322:178–83.

[26] Aubin JE, Liu F, Candeliere GA. Single-cell PCR methods for studying stem cells and progenitors. Methods Mol Biol 2002;185:403–15.

[27] Higuchi R, Dollinger G, Walsh PS, et al. Simultaneous amplification and detection of specific DNA sequences. Biotechnology 1992;10:413–7.

[28] Wolk D, Mitchell S, Patel R. Principles of molecular microbiology testing methods. Infect Dis Clin North Am 2001;15:1157–204.

[29] Orlando C, Pinzani P, Pazzagli M. Developments in quantitative PCR. Clin Chem Lab Med 1998;36:255–69.

[30] Porter-Jordan K, Rosenberg EI, Keiser JF. Nested polymerase chain reaction assay for the detection of cytomegalovirus overcomes false positives caused by contamination with fragmented DNA. J Med Virol 1990;30:85–91.

[31] Basgara O, Harris T. Latest development in in situ PCR. Methods Mol Biol 2006;334: 221–40.

[32] Relman DA. The identification of uncultured microbial pathogens. J Infect Dis 1993;168: 1–8.

[33] Relman DA. Detection and identification of previously unrecognized microbial pathogens. Emerg Infect Dis 1998;4:382–9.

[34] Cursons RTM, Jeyerajah E, Sleigh JW. The use of polymerase chain reaction to detect septicemia in critically ill patients. Crit Care Med 1999;27:927–40.
[35] Fredericks DN, Relman DA. Sequence-based identification of microbial pathogens: a reconsideration of Koch's postulates. Clin Microbiol Rev 1996;9:18–33.
[36] Fredericks DN, Relman DA. Application of polymerase chain reaction to the diagnosis of infectious disease. Infect Dis 1999;29:475–88.
[37] Tang YW, Procop GW, Persing DH. Molecular diagnostics of infectious diseases. Clin Chem 1997;43:2021–38.
[38] Tang YW, Persing DH. Molecular detection and identification of microorganisms. In: Murray EJ, Baron EJ, Pfaller MA, et al, editors. Manual of clinical microbiology. Washington: ASM Press; 1999. p. 215–44.
[39] Guaschino S, De Seta F. Update on *Chlamydia trachomatis*. Ann N Y Acad Sci 2000;900: 293–300.
[40] Beggs ML, Cave MD, Marlowe C, et al. Characterization of *Mycobacterium tuberculosis* complex direct repeat sequence for use in cycling probe reaction. J Clin Microbiol 1996; 34:2985–9.
[41] Salfinger M, Hale YM, Driscoll JR. Diagnostic tools in tuberculosis: present and future. Respiration (Herrlisheim) 1998;65:163–70.
[42] Woods GL. Molecular methods in the detection and identification of mycobacterial infections. Arch Pathol Lab Med 1999;123:1002–6.
[43] Lam A, Toma W, Schlesinger N. *Mycobacterium marinum* arthritis mimicking rheumatoidarthritis. J Rheumatol 2006;33:817–9.
[44] Sra K, Torres G, Rady P. Molecular diagnosis of infectious diseases in dermatology. J Am Acad Dermatol 2005;53:749–65.
[45] Liebling MR, Arkfeld DG, Michelini GA, et al. Identification of *Neisseria gonorrhoeae* in synovial fluid using the polymerase chain reaction. Arthritis Rheum 1994;37:702–9.
[46] Louie JS, Liebling MR. The polymerase chain reaction in infectious and post-infectious arthritis. Rheum Dis Clin North Am 1998;24:227–36.
[47] Van der Heyden IM, Wilbrink B, Vijl AE, et al. Detection of bacterial DNA in several synovial fluid samples obtained during antibiotic treatment from patients with septic arthritis. Arthritis Rheum 1999;42:198–203.
[48] Wilbrink B, Van der Heyden IM, Schouls LM, et al. Detection of bacterial DNA in joint samples from patients with undifferentiated arthritis and reactive arthritis, using polymerase chain reaction with universal 16S ribosomal RNA primers. Arthritis Rheum 1998;41: 535–43.
[49] Locht H, Krogfelt KA. Comparison of rheumatological and gastrointestinal symptoms after injection with *Campylobacter jejuni*/coli and enterotoxigenic *Escherichia coli*. Ann Rheum Dis 2002;61:448–52.
[50] Vittecoq O, Schaeverbeke T, Favre S. Molecular diagnosis of ureaplasma urealyticum in an immunocompetent patient with destructive reactive polyarthritis. Arthritis Rheum 1997; 40:2084–9.
[51] Ekman P, Kirveskari J, Granfors K. Modification of disease outcomes in *Salmonella*-infected patients by HLA-B27. Arthritis Rheum 2000;43:1527–34.
[52] Gaston JS, Cox C, Granfors K. Clinical and experimental evidence for persistent *Yersinia* infection in reactive arthritis. Arthritis Rheum 1999;42:2239–42.
[53] Inman RD, Johnston ME, Hodge M, et al. Postdysenteric reactive arthritis: a clinical and immunogenetic study following and outbreak of salmonellosis. Arthritis Rheum 1988;31: 1377–83.
[54] Kapasi K, Inman RD. ME epitope of HLA-B27 confers class I-mediated modulation of gram-negative bacterial invasion. J Immunol 1994;153:833–40.
[55] Kirveskari J, He Q, Holmstrom T. Modulation of peripheral blood mononuclear cell activation status during *Salmonella*-triggered reactive arthritis. Arthritis Rheum 1999;42: 2045–54.

[56] Schaeverbeke T, Lequen L, de Barbeyrae B, et al. Propionibacterium acnes isolated from synovial tissue and fluid in a patient with oligoarthritis associated with acne and pustulosis. Arthritis Rheum 1998;41:1889–93.

[57] Haier J, Nasralla M, Franco AR, et al. Detection of mycoplasmal infections in blood of patients with rheumatoid arthritis. Rheumatology (Oxford) 1999;38:504–9.

[58] Schaeverbeke T, Gilroy CB, Bebear C, et al. *Mycoplasma fermentans*, but not *M penetrans*, detected by PCR assays in synovium from patients with rheumatoid arthritis and other rheumatic disorders. J Clin Pathol 1996;49:824–8.

[59] Zhang L, Nikkari S, Skurnik M, et al. Detection of herpesvirus by polymerase chain reaction in lymphocytes from patients with rheumatoid arthritis. Arthritis Rheum 1993;36: 1080–6.

[60] Crowson AN, Magro CM, Dawood MR. A causal role for parvovirus B19 infection in adult dermatomyositis and other autoimmune syndromes. J Cutan Pathol 2000;27: 505–15.

[61] Braun J, Tuszervski M, Eggens U, et al. Nested polymerase chain reaction strategy simultaneously targeting DNA sequences of multiple bacterial species in inflammatory joint diseases. I. Screening of synovial fluid samples of patients with spondyloarthropathies and other arthritides. Rheumatol 1997;24:1092–100.

[62] Cuchacovich R, Japa S, Huang WQ, et al. Detection of bacterial DNA in Latin American patients with reactive arthritis by polymerase chain reaction (PCR) and sequencing analysis. J Rheumatol 2002;29:1426–9.

[63] Gerard HC, Wang Z, Wang GF, et al. Chromosomal DNA from a variety of bacterial species is present in synovial tissue from patients with various forms of arthritis. Arthritis Rheum 2001;44:1689–97.

[64] Schnarr S, Putschky N, Jendro MC, et al. *Chlamydia* and *Borrelia* DNA in synovial fluid of patients with early undifferentiated oligoarthritis: results of a prospective study. Arthritis Rheum 2001;44:2679–85.

[65] Bas S, Griffais R, Kvien TK, et al. Amplification of plasmid and chromosome chlamydia DNA in synovial fluid of patients with arthritis and undifferentiated seronegative oligoarthritis. Arthritis Rheum 1995;38:1005–13.

[66] Hannu T, Puolakkainen M, Leirisalo-Repo M. *Chlamydia* as a triggering infection in reactive arthritis. Rheumatology (Oxford) 1999;38:411–4.

[67] Schumacher HR Jr, Arayssi T, Crane M, et al. *Chlamydia trochomatis* nucleic acids can be found in the synovium of some asymptomatic subjects. Arthritis Rheum 1999;42:1281–4.

[68] Taylor-Robinson D, Gilvoy CB, Thomas BJ, et al. Detection of *Chlamydia trachomatis* DNA in joint of reactive arthritis patients by polymerase chain reaction. Lancet 1992; 340:81–2.

[69] Sigal LH. Synovial fluid-polymerase chain reaction detection of pathogens: what does it really mean? Arthritis Rheum 2001;44:2463–6.

[70] Wilkinson NZ, Kingsley GH, Jones HW, et al. The detection of DNA from a range of bacterial species in the joints of patients with a variety of arthritides using a nested, broad-range polymerase chain reaction. Rheumatology (Oxford) 1999;38:260–6.

[71] Wollenhaupt J, Schnarr S, Kuipers JG. Bacterial antigens in reactive arthritis and spondyloarthritis: rational use of laboratory testing in diagnosis and follow-up. Bailleres Clin Rheumatol 1998;12:627–47.

[72] Knox CM, Cervallos V, Margolis TP, et al. Identification of bacterial pathogens in patients with endophthalmitis by 16S ribosomal DNA typing. Am J Ophthalmol 1999;128:511–2.

[73] Knox CM, Chandler D, Short GA, et al. Polymerase chain reaction-based assay of vitreous samples for the diagnosis of viral retinitis: use in diagnostic dilemmas. Ophthalmology 1998;105:37–44.

[74] Cunningham ET Jr, Short GA, Irvine AR, et al. Acquired immunodeficiency syndrome-associated herpes simplex virus retinitis: clinical description and use of a polymerase chain reaction based array as a diagnostic tool. Arch Ophthalmol 1996;114:834–40.

[75] Yamamoto D, Pavan-Langston D, Kinoshita S, et al. Detecting herpes virus DNA in uveitis using the polymerase chain reaction. Br J Ophthalmol 1996;80:465–8.

[76] Abe T, Tsuchida K, Tamai M. A comparative study of the polymerase chain reaction and local antibody production in acute retinal necrosis syndrome and cytomegalovirus retinitis. Graefes Arch Clin Exp Ophthalmol 1996;234:419–24.

[77] Van Gelder RN. Frontiers of polymerase chain reaction diagnostics for uveitis. Ocul Immunol Inflamm 2001;9:67–73.

[78] Weinberg RS. Uveitis update on therapy. Ophthalmol Clin North Am 1999;12:71–81.

[79] Cooper RJ, Yeo AC, Bailey AC, et al. Adenovirus polymerase chain reaction assay for rapid diagnosis of conjunctivitis. Invest Ophthalmol Vis Sci 1999;40:90–5.

[80] Dabil H, Boley M, Schmitz TM, et al. Validation of a diagnostic multiplex polymerase chain reaction assay for infectious posterior uveitis. Arch Ophthalmol 2001;119:1315–22.

[81] Okhravi N, Adamson P, Carroll N, et al. PCR-based evidence of bacterial involvement in eyes with suspected intraocular infection. Invest Ophthalmol Vis Sci 2000;41:3474–9.

[82] Van Gelder RN. Application of the polymerase chain reaction to diagnosis of ophthalmic disease. Surv Ophthalmol 2001;46:248–58.

[83] Di Alberti L, Piatteli A, Artese L, et al. Human herpesvirus 8 variants in sarcoid tissues. Lancet 1997;350:1655–61.

[84] Mitchell PS, Espy MJ, Smith TF, et al. Laboratory diagnosis of central nervous system infections with herpes simplex virus by PCR performed with cerebrospinal fluid specimens. J Clin Microbiol 1997;35:2873–7.

[85] Tang YW, Mitchell PS, Espy MJ, et al. Molecular diagnosis of herpes simplex virus infections in the central nervous system. J Clin Microbiol 1999;37:2127–36.

[86] Choo QL, Kus G, Weiner AJ, et al. Isolation of a cDNA clone derived from a blood-borne non-A, non-B viral hepatitis genome. Science 1989;244:359–62.

[87] Detmer J, Lagier R, Flynn J, et al. Accurate quantification of hepatitis C virus (HCV) RNA from all HCV genotypes by using branched-DNA technology. J Clin Microbiol 1996;34: 901–7.

[88] Clarke JR, McClure MO. HIV-1 viral load testing. J Infect 1999;38:141–6.

[89] Moore PS, Gao SJ, Dominguez G, et al. Primary characterization of a herpesvirus agent associated with Kaposi's sarcomal. J Virol 1996;70:549–58.

[90] Read SJ, Burnett D, Fink C. Molecular techniques for clinical diagnostic virology. J Clin Pathol 2000;53:502–6.

[91] Backman A, Lantz P, Radstrom P, et al. Evaluation of an extended diagnostic PCR assay for detection and verification of the common causes of bacterial meningitis in CSF and other biological samples. Mol Cell Probes 1990;13:49–60.

[92] Lakeman FD, Whitley RJ, the National Institute of Allergy and Infectious Diseases Collaborative Antiviral Study Group. Diagnosis of herpes simplex encephalitis: application of polymerase chain reaction to cerebrospinal fluid from brain-biopsied patients and correlation with disease. J Infect Dis 1995;171:857–63.

[93] Thoren A, Widell A. PCR for the diagnosis of enteroviral meningitis. Scand J Infect Dis 1994;26:249–54.

[94] Saldanha J, Lelie N, Heath A. Establishment of the first international standard for nucleic acid amplification technology (NAT) assays for HCV RNA. WHO Collaborative Study Group. Vox Sang 1999;76:149–58.

[95] Relman DA. Universal bacteria 16S RNA amplification and sequencing in diagnostic molecular biology. In: Persing DH, Smith T, Tenover F, et al, editors. Diagnostic of molecular microbiology: principles and applications. Washington: American Society for Microbiology; 1993. p. 489–95.

[96] Relman DA, Falkow S. Identification of uncultured microorganisms: expanding the spectrum of characterized microbial pathogens. Infect Agents Dis 1992;1:245–53.

[97] Relman DA, Schmidt TM, MacDermott RP, et al. Identification of the uncultured bacillus of Whipple's disease. N Engl J Med 1992;327:293–301.

[98] Cockerill FR. Genetic methods for assessing antimicrobial resistance. Antimicrob Agents Chemother 1999;43:199–212.

[99] Bekkaoui F, McNevin JP, Leung CH, et al. Rapid detection of the mecA gene in methicillin-resistant staphylococci using a calorimetric cycling probe technology. Diagn Microbiol Infect Dis 1990;34:83–90.

[100] Cloney L, Marlowe C, Wong A, et al. Rapid detection of mecA in methicillin-resistant *Staphylococcus aureus* using cycling probe technology. Mol Cell Probes 1999;13:191–7.

[101] Modrusan Z, Marlowe C, Wheeler D, et al. Detection of vancomycin resistant genes vanA and vanB by cycling probe technology. Mol Cell Probes 1999;13:223–31.

[102] Patel R, Uhl JR, Kohner P, et al. Multiplex PCR detection of vanA, vanB, vanC-1, and vanC-2/3 genes in enterococci. J Clin Microbiol 1997;35:703–7.

[103] Barany F. Genetic disease detection and DNA amplification using cloned thermostable ligase. Proc Natl Acad Sci U S A 1991;88:189–93.

[104] Galeazzi M, Sebastiani GD, Morozzi G, et al. HLA class II DNA typing in a large series of European patients with systemic lupus erythematosus: correlations with clinical and autoantibody subsets. Medicine (Baltimore) 2002;81:169–78.

[105] Horton VA, Bunce M, Davies DR, et al. HLA typing for DR3 and DR4 using artificial restriction fragment length polymorphism PCR from archival DNA. J Clin Pathol 1995; 48:33.

[106] Lynas C, Hurlock NJ, Copplestone JA, et al. HLA-DR typing for kidney transplants: advantage of polymerase chain reaction with sequence-specific primers in a routine hospital laboratory. J Clin Pathol 1994;47:609–12.

[107] Ohtsuka T, Miyamoto Y, Yamakage A, et al. Quantitative analysis of microchimerism in systemic sclerosis skin tissue. Arch Dermatol Rev 2001;293:387–91.

[108] Shen DF, Zhuang Z, Le Hoang P, et al. Utility of microdissection and polymerase chain reaction for the detection of immunoglobulin gene rearrangement and translocation in primary intraocular lymphoma. Ophthalmology 1998;105:1664–9.

[109] Naber SP. Molecular pathology: detection of neoplasia. N Engl J Med 1994;331:1508–10.

[110] Weckmann AL, Granados J, Cardiel MH, et al. Immunogenetics of mixed connective tissue disease in a Mexican Mestizo population. Clin Exp Rheumatol 1999;17:91–4.

[111] Menke DM, Griesser H, Moder KG, et al. Lymphomas in patients with connective tissue disease: comparison of p53 protein expression and latent EBV infection in patients immunosuppressed and not immunosuppressed with methotrexate. Am J Clin Pathol 2000;113: 212–8.

[112] Wainscoat JS, Fey MF. Assessment of clonality in human tumors: a review. Cancer Res 1990;50:1355–60.

[113] Teba L. Polymerase chain reaction: a new chapter in critical care diagnosis. Crit Care Med 1999;27:860–9.

[114] Meier A, Persing DH, Finken M, et al. Elimination of contaminating DNA within polymerase chain reaction reagents: implications for a general approach to detection of uncultured pathogens. J Clin Microbiol 1993;31:646–52.

[115] Lo YM, Mehal WZ, Fleming KA. False-positive results and the polymerase chain reaction. Lancet 1998;2:679.

[116] Sankar G, Sommer SS. Removal of DNA contamination in polymerase chain reaction reagents by ultraviolet irradiation. Methods Enzymol 1993;218:381–8.

[117] Konet DS, Mezencio JM, Babcock G, et al. Inhibitors of RT-PCR in serum. J Virol Methods 2000;84:95–8.

ELSEVIER
SAUNDERS

Infect Dis Clin N Am
20 (2006) 759–772

INFECTIOUS
DISEASE CLINICS
OF NORTH AMERICA

Skin and Soft Tissue Infections

Fred A. Lopez, MD*, Serge Lartchenko, MD

*Section of Infectious Diseases, Department of Internal Medicine,
Louisiana State University Health Sciences Center, Box E7-17, 2020 Gravier Street,
New Orleans, LA 70112, USA*

Primary skin infections (ie, pyodermas) typically are initiated by some breach in the epidermis, resulting in infection by organisms, such as *Streptococcus pyogenes* and *Staphylococcus aureus*, that colonize the skin. Host-associated factors, such as immunosuppression, vasculopathy, neuropathy, or decreased lymphatic drainage, may predispose to skin infection. The clinical syndromes associated with skin infections are often characteristic and are defined most simplistically by anatomic distribution (Fig. 1). Although often mild and self-limited, skin infections can be more aggressive and involve deeper structures, including fascia and muscle. This article discusses skin and soft tissue infections, including impetigo, hair follicle-associated infections (ie, folliculitis, furuncles, and carbuncles), erysipelas, cellulitis, necrotizing fasciitis, pyomyositis, septic bursitis, and tenosynovitis.

Impetigo

Impetigo is a superficial skin infection that typically presents with multiple vesicular lesions on an erythematous base that eventually crust over. The microbiology of these infections consists primarily of *S aureus* and *S pyogenes*, either alone or in combination. Recent trends have shown an increasing incidence of *S aureus*–associated impetigo. Although usually seen in children aged 2 to 5 years, these infections can occur in individuals of any age. Impetigo is more common in humid and warm climates, but also can occur in cooler climates during the fall and summer months. It usually occurs on exposed parts of the body, including the face, extremities, and scalp. Predisposing factors include skin abrasions; minor trauma; burns; poor

This article is based in part on: Valeriano-Marcet J, Carter JD, Vasey FB. Soft tissue disease. Rheum Dis Clin North Am 2003;29:77–88; with permission.

* Corresponding author.
E-mail address: alopez1@lsuhsc.edu (F.A. Lopez).

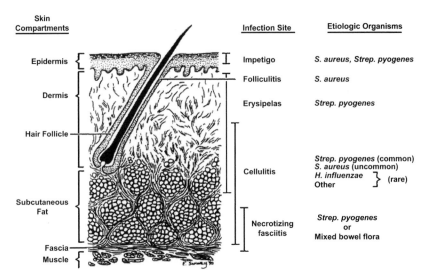

Fig. 1. Cutaneous anatomy, sites of infection, and infecting organisms. (*From* Feingold DS, Hirschmann JV. Approach to the patient with skin or soft tissue infection. Gorbach SL, Bartlett JG, Blacklow NR, editors. Infectious diseases. 3rd edition. Philadelphia: Lippincott Williams & Wilkins; with permission.)

hygiene; insect bites; diabetes mellitus; primary varicella infection; preexisting skin disease, such as eczema, atopic dermatitis, and cheilitis; hypogammaglobulinemia; and HIV infection [1]. Impetigo also can spread among people who are in close contact with each other (ie, children in day care centers and family members of the same household).

Two types of impetigo are described. The nonbullous form is most common and is more likely to be attributable to a mixed staphylococcal and streptococcal infection. Multiple ultimately vesiculopustular lesions cluster together before skin breakdown occurs with the development of a classic thick honey-colored crust. Regional lymphadenopathy without systemic signs often is present [2]. Pruritus and pain are not common. Bullous impetigo is less common than the nonbullous form and is seen primarily in newborns and infants. The microbiology typically consists of phage type II *S aureus* strains that secrete exfoliative toxin A. Initially vesicular, these lesions ultimately evolve into large yellow fluid-filled flaccid bullae. After rupture, thin light-brown crusts develop. Localized lymphadenopathy is less common than in the nonbullous form, and systemic signs usually are absent.

The differential diagnosis primarily includes herpes simplex virus infections and contact dermatitis. The diagnosis of impetigo usually is based on clinical findings. The identification of the organism from skin lesions or bullae-associated fluid by Gram staining and culture is pursued when the diagnosis is uncertain. Lesions should be de-crusted aseptically before the exudative material beneath is sampled for evaluation. Serologic antibody studies, such as anti-DNase B or antihyaluronidase B, are not considered routinely in this setting except when the diagnosis of acute poststreptococcal glomerulonephritis is entertained [3].

Topical therapy with mupirocin can be used to treat impetigo when there are a limited number of lesions [4]. When disease is more extensive and severe, oral penicillinase-resistant penicillins (ie, dicloxacillin) and first generation cephalosporins (cephalexin) for a total duration of 10 days are recommended because of their antistaphylococcal activity. As in many other skin-associated infections, the practitioner needs to be aware of the increased prevalence of methicillin-resistant *S aureus* (MRSA) causing infection in the community [5].

Folliculitis

Folliculitis refers to a circumscribed superficial pustular infection of the hair follicle. These pruritic lesions, which are up to 5 mm in diameter, often present as small red papules with a central area of purulence that may rupture and drain. Systemic signs and symptoms are rare. Lesions typically are located on the head, back, buttocks, and extremities. The most common organism isolated is *S aureus*. A condition known as hot tub folliculitis is attributable to hot tub or whirlpool water contaminated with *Pseudomonas aeruginosa*; the ear canal, the breast area, and other skin locations covered by a swim suit are commonly involved. A condition known as eosinophilic pustular folliculitis should be considered in the differential diagnosis of chronic excoriated-appearing follicular infections in HIV-infected patients who have a peripheral eosinophilia and CD4 count of less than $250/mm^3$ [6,7]. In normal hosts, folliculitis usually resolves spontaneously without systemic treatment, and the use of warm compresses for symptomatic relief and topical antibiotic therapy (ie, mupirocin, clindamycin, erythromycin) may be sufficient. Good hygiene is the best measure to prevent this type of infection.

Furuncles and carbuncles

Furuncles (ie, boils) are single hair follicle–associated inflammatory nodules extending into the dermis and the subcutaneous tissue, usually affecting moist, hairy, friction-prone areas of the body, such as the face, axillae, neck, and buttocks. Firm and tender, these nodular erythematous lesions may spontaneously drain purulent material. Fever and other constitutional symptoms rarely are present. The most common causative microorganism is *S aureus*, but the microbiology of furuncles depends on the location of the lesions. Risk factors for developing this condition include obesity, diabetes mellitus, atopic dermatitis, parenteral drug use, chronic kidney disease, impaired neutrophil function, use of corticosteroids, close exposure to others who have furuncles (ie, family members, contact sports), and malnutrition [8–11]. When the subcutaneous infection extends to involve multiple furuncles, the lesions are called carbuncles. Carbuncles are often located in the back of the neck, posterior trunk, or thigh. This multiseptate coalescence of multiple abscesses can be painful, and constitutional signs and symptoms, including fever and malaise, often are present. Purulent material may be expressed from multiple draining sinuses.

Severe complications of furuncular infections, such as bacterial endocarditis, have been reported [12]. If systemic involvement of any type is suspected, evaluation should include a complete blood count, blood cultures, and Gram stain and culture of purulent material. Small-sized furuncles usually can be managed by applying moist heat to encourage drainage. Incision and drainage is needed for carbuncles and larger furuncles [4]. Systemic antibiotics usually are reserved for individuals who have systemic signs of infection or associated cellulitis. Surgical consultation often is recommended for patients who have carbuncles.

Recently, a prospective study from 11 university-affiliated emergency departments reported an overall prevalence of MRSA in 59% of 422 patients who presented acutely with purulent skin and soft tissue infections [13]. This finding dictates a consideration of empiric coverage of MRSA in these infections in addition to incision and drainage when antibiotics are indicated [13]. Typically these *S aureus* isolates contain the *PVL* (Panton-Valentine Leukocidin) gene, exhibit a single pulsed-field electrophoretic pattern, and possess a type IV SCCmec element that confers methicillin resistance [14,15]. Patients who have recurrent furuncles may require eradication of *S aureus* from the nares with agents such as mupirocin ointment or oral clindamycin to decrease risk for infection [16].

Erysipelas

An infection of the upper dermis, erysipelas classically presents abruptly as a painful superficial cellulitis with associated fever, regional lymphadenopathy, and lymphangitis. A prodrome of a flu-like illness may precede the appearance of rash by several hours to 2 days. Distinct elevated borders surround brightly erythematous plaques that have no central clearing. Usually involving the lower extremities in more than 75% to 90% of cases, the face also is reported to be involved in 2.5% to 10% of cases [17,18]. Risk factors include tinea pedis, venous insufficiency, obesity, puncture sites, pressure ulcers, and lymphedema [19]. The microbiology associated with this infection is primarily *S pyogenes*. Other organisms reported to be associated with erysipelas include other beta-hemolytic streptococci (ie, Group B, C, or G), *S aureus*, enterococci, and, rarely, Gram-negative bacilli. The diagnosis remains clinically based; about 5% of patients are bacteremic and cultures from the skin are positive in less than 50% of cases [17]. Most patients can be treated as outpatients with oral antibiotics, such as penicillin, dicloxacillin, or cephalexin. Hospitalization can be considered for more severe cases, including patients who manifest systemic signs and symptoms, such as confusion and hypotension, or who are immunocompromised. Intravenous penicillin, cefazolin, nafcillin, or oxacillin can be considered for treatment of these patients. Rest, immobilization, moist heat, and elevation of the affected area are often recommended as supportive measures. Necrosis of the skin, abscess formation, bursitis, venous thrombophlebitis, osteitis, and septic arthritis are uncommon complications [20]. Recurrences occur in up to 29% of patients and appear more likely in the setting of leg ulcers, skin trauma, and tinea pedis [19,21].

Cellulitis

Cellulitis is a diffuse skin infection that involves the deep dermis and the subcutaneous fat tissues. Unlike erysipelas, which demonstrates superficial skin involvement with distinct margins, cellulitis is diffuse and spreading with no distinct demarcations. Although the inciting event typically is not discernable, predisposing factors include traumatic skin lesions, including puncture wounds, lacerations, surgical wounds, and burns; prior history of cellulitis; dermatophyte infections, such as tinea pedis; pressure ulcers; eczema; dermatitis; vascular insufficiency; lymphedema; presence of a foreign body; malnutrition; and immunosuppressive conditions, such as diabetes mellitus and cirrhosis [22,23]. Any cutaneous surface may be involved, but the most common site of infection is the lower extremity [24,25]. In immunocompetent hosts, the microorganisms most commonly implicated include Gram-positive cocci such as beta-hemolytic streptococci (particularly S pyogenes) and S aureus. In immunocompromised hosts, other microorganisms need to be included as potential pathogens. For example, Group B streptococcal-associated skin and soft tissue infections should be considered in adults who are pregnant, elderly, diabetic, cirrhotic, or have cancer [26,27]. A necrotic skin lesion with a hemorrhagic halo in a febrile neutropenic patient should include P aeruginosa in the microbiologic differential diagnosis. Likewise, Vibrio vulnificus infection should be considered in cirrhotic patients who present with hemorrhagic bullous lesions and septic physiology, particularly if there is a recent history of warm brackish water exposure or consumption of undercooked shellfish, such as oysters, that derive from warmer waters [28].

Patients who have cellulitis typically present with erythematous, edematous tender skin lesions that are warm to palpation. Regional lymphadenopathy and lymphangitis may be present. Systemic signs usually are more prominent in patients who have associated bacteremia. The differential diagnosis for cellulitis is broad and includes deep and superficial venous thromboses; gout; herpes zoster; angioedema; contact dermatitis; relapsing polychondritis; local reactions to chemicals, foreign bodies, and insect venom; and lymphedema, among others [29].

The diagnosis typically is determined clinically particularly when the cellulitis is considered uncomplicated (ie, lack of systemic signs, absence of immunocompromising conditions, and minimal skin surface area involved). A recent review of the available reported literature concluded that blood cultures do not assist diagnostics or therapeutics in immunocompetent adults who present with acute cellulitis [30]. Based on one analysis of 553 patients with community-acquired cellulitis, blood cultures are recommended when there is acute onset of infection in the geriatric patient associated with significant leukocytosis and high-grade fever or immunocompromised hosts [31]. Other possible diagnostic modalities for cellulitis include needle aspiration and skin biopsy, especially for patents who have strange exposures, refractory infections, or immunocompromising comorbidities. Unfortunately, cultures yield an organism in less than one third of samples obtained by needle aspiration or biopsy of infected tissue [32–37]. Swabbing ipsilateral tinea pedis–affected areas for bacterial culture may be helpful in identifying the microbiologic cause of cellulitis [38,39]. In general, imaging studies are not indicated in cellulitis unless a complicating factor (ie, foreign body, osteomyelitis, abscess, necrotizing fasciitis) or alternative diagnosis (ie, deep venous thrombosis) is being considered.

Treatment in most cases is directed against streptococci and *S aureus*. In the afebrile, immunocompetent patient who has a small area of involvement, oral antibiotic therapy consisting of dicloxacillin, cephalexin, clindamycin, or erythromycin can be considered if the community antibiotic-resistance profiles are favorable [4]. In immunocompetent patients who are more severely ill, initial parenteral antibiotics that can be used include nafcillin, oxacillin, or cefazolin [4]. The emergence of methicillin resistance in *S aureus* isolates from the community needs to be considered because these organisms are resistant to beta-lactam antibiotics, such as penicillins and cephalosporins. Agents such as trimethoprim-sulfamethoxazole, doxycycline or minocycline, clindamycin, linezolid, vancomycin, and daptomycin often are used to manage community-acquired MRSA skin infections. Immobilization and elevation of involved areas and treatment of underlying predisposing conditions is recommended. Surgical evaluation should be considered when the development of necrosis and gas is suspected or when there is no response to appropriate antibiotics.

Necrotizing fasciitis

Although uncommon, necrotizing fasciitis (NF) is an infectious diseases emergency. Predisposing conditions include diabetes mellitus, surgery, trauma, peripheral vascular disease, and injection drug use. Classification of this life-threatening infection has been proposed based on the microbiology of infection [40]. Type 1 necrotizing fasciitis refers to a mixed aerobic and anaerobic infection (ie, diabetic foot infection and Fournier's gangrene, for example). Facultative streptococci, staphylococci, enterococci, aerobic

Gram-negative bacilli, such as *Escherichia coli, Klebsiella, Pseudomonas, Enterobacter,* and *Proteus,* and anaerobes, such as *Peptostreptococcus, Bacteroides,* and *Clostridium* spp are the characteristic pathogens associated with these infections. Type II infections are monomicrobial, classically associated with the "flesh-eating" bacteria *S pyogenes.* Other bacteria capable of producing monomicrobial infection include *Streptococcus agalactiae, V vulnificus, Clostridium* spp, and *S aureus* [28,41]. Of note, *Aeromonas* spp– and *Streptococcus pneumoniae*–associated NF have been reported in patients who have underlying collagen vascular diseases [42–44].

Usually associated with antecedent skin infection or trauma, NF is rapid in onset with the sequential development of erythema, extensive edema, and severe, unremitting pain, often despite antibiotic therapy. Hemorrhagic bullous lesions, skin necrosis, and crepitus associated with gas in soft tissues also may develop. Systemic toxicity manifest by fever, hypotension, tachycardia, delirium, and multiple organ dysfunction is characteristic of severe cases. Anesthesia localizes at the infection site because of associated nerve necrosis. The legs and other extremities are the most common locations for NF, although any site can be involved, including the perineum, trunk, head and neck, and buttocks [45,46].

Early recognition of NF is essential. Plain films and CT scans can be helpful in demonstrating gas in the soft tissues when infection is attributable to anaerobic bacteria or the Enterobacteriaceae. Magnetic resonance imaging is reported to be more sensitive in identifying necrotizing skin and soft tissue infections and the extent of involvement [47–49]. No laboratory test is specific for the diagnosis of NF. A diagnostic scoring system for distinguishing these infections based on routine laboratory tests has been proposed. Titled the Laboratory Risk Indicator for Necrotizing Fasciitis (LRINEC) score, it uses factors that have been reported to be independently predictive of NF (total white cell count, hemoglobin, sodium, glucose, serum creatinine, and C-reactive protein) to create a score to assist physicians in the evaluation of NF [50]. The negative predictive value and positive predictive value of a cut-off score of 6 is reported to be 96% and 92%, respectively. The authors conclude that patients who have an LRINEC score greater than or equal to 6 should "be carefully evaluated for the presence of necrotizing fasciitis" [50]. Tissue oxygen saturation monitoring also has been reported to be helpful in identifying NF of the lower extremities in patients who do not have chronic venous stasis, peripheral vascular diseases, shock, or systemic hypoxia. A cut-off value of less than 70% for the involved tissue oxygen saturation demonstrated a sensitivity of 100% and a specificity of 97% [51].

When NF is suspected, surgical evaluation is needed. Definitive diagnosis of NF is made by visualization of affected fascia. The passage of a probe or finger without resistance across soft tissue that typically is adherent to deep fascial planes is characteristic [52]. Needle aspiration of involved soft tissue or blood cultures may yield the putative pathogen but is not specific for diagnosing necrotizing skin infections [53,54]. Frozen section full-thickness biopsy performed early in the course of infection may provide histopathologic confirmation of NF and prompt definitive surgical debridement [55]. Culture of intraoperatively-obtained tissue is most helpful in determining the microbial cause.

Surgery is not only diagnostic but also therapeutic. It is intended to preserve viable skin while removing necrotic tissue and ensuring hemostasis. Repeat intervention is recommended and multiple debridements may be required until evolving necrosis is no longer appreciated. Plastic surgical reconstruction with split-thickness skin grafting often is needed. In addition to surgery, polymicrobial-associated NF should be treated with a broad-spectrum antibiotic regimen consisting of ampicillin-sulbactam or piperacillin-tazobactam and ciprofloxacin and clindamycin [4]. Group A streptococcus-associated NF is best treated with penicillin plus clindamycin. The potential presence of S aureus may dictate the need for vancomycin because of the emergence of methicillin resistance in this organism. Overall mortality rates range from 17% to 40% and are increased when there is a delay in surgery or when toxic shock syndrome with NF secondary to S pyogenes is present [45,46,54,56].

Pyomyositis

Pyomyositis refers to purulent infection deep within a striated muscle group, often manifesting as an abscess. Infection does not result from a contiguous site but rather secondary to hematogenous seeding of injured muscle. Although usually involving one muscle group, multiple sites may be infected simultaneously in approximately 15% of cases [57]. Most commonly targeting the thigh, pyomyositis also can occur in the calf, upper extremity, gluteal, chest wall, and psoas muscles [57]. The incidence of this rare infection seems to be increasing in areas other than the tropics where it was originally described and it seems to be associated with immunocompromising conditions, such as HIV infection, malnutrition, concomitant parasitic or viral infection, diabetes mellitus, intravenous drug use, immunosuppressive drugs, rheumatologic diseases, cirrhosis, and malignancy [58,59]. Patients initially present with fever, swelling, and crampy pain at the involved muscle site before developing edema, tenderness, and "woody" induration. Diagnosis depends on a high index of clinical suspicion, and if not considered and addressed the infection can progress to sepsis and shock.

S aureus is the causative organism in most cases (ie, 75%–90%) [60]. Other organisms reported to cause pyomyositis include S pyogenes and other beta-hemolytic streptococci, S pneumoniae, Haemophilus influenzae, Gram-negative bacilli, anaerobes, mycobacteria, and fungi [61,62]. Blood cultures are positive in 5% to 30% of cases and are more likely to yield an organism in temperate climates [57,62,63]. Aspiration, Gram-stain, and culture of abscess material also may yield the causative organism.

Laboratory values are nonspecific, often revealing a neutrophilia, an elevated erythrocyte sedimentation rate, and normal aldolase and creatinine kinase levels. In the tropics, an eosinophilic leukocytosis is characteristic. Radiographic imaging is the most helpful noninvasive diagnostic test. Ultrasound, CT, and MRI (with gadolinium administration) are helpful, although the latter is most helpful in defining the extent of infection [64].

Once abscesses have formed, treatment consists of adequate drainage and antibiotics. Empiric antimicrobial therapy initially is broad in spectrum, particularly when the patient is immunocompromised, and should include anti–S aureus coverage. Pathogen-directed therapy is administered once culture and susceptibility testing results are available. Drainage can be performed percutaneously under ultrasound or CT guidance, but surgical drainage may be needed when infection is extensive or necrotic [59]. The usual duration of antibiotics is 3 to 6 weeks with the exact duration dictated by the patient's clinical course and serial radiographic imaging [59,62]. The reported mortality rate is 1% to 6% and patients usually recover with minimal sequelae [57,62].

Septic bursitis

Bursae are small sac-like cavities that contain fluid and are lined by a synovial membrane. They are located subcutaneously between bony prominences and tendons or in deeper fascial tissue between bone and muscle, essentially serving to reduce friction between these structures. Inflammation of bursae (ie, bursitis) can be caused by infection, particularly when the superficial subcutaneously located bursae are involved. These infections are typically secondary to local trauma and rarely attributable to hematogenous seeding. In addition to prior history of trauma to superficial bursae, other predisposing factors may include prior rheumatoid arthritis or gouty involvement of the bursae, alcoholism, diabetes mellitus, renal insufficiency, intravenous drug use, and other forms of immunosuppression [65,66]. Trauma often is occupationally associated, favoring situations that place pressure on the olecranon, prepatellar, and superficial infrapatellar bursae, the most common sites of septic bursitis [67,68].

Peribursal cellulitis, warmth, and erythema are common. Close inspection of the skin also may reveal lacerations, abrasions, and ecchymoses [67]. Fever and pain with movement of the associated joint also is characteristic of superficial bursitis. Interestingly, Smith and colleagues [69] have reported that in septic olecranon bursitis, a temperature of greater than or equal to 2.2°C between the affected and unaffected olecranon processes was 100% sensitive in distinguishing septic from nonseptic bursitis.

Like many other inflammatory conditions, a peripheral leukocytosis, an elevated C-reactive protein, and an elevated erythrocyte sedimentation rate are often present. Although radiographic evaluation may reveal abnormal accumulations of fluid, the presence of a foreign body, and the extent of infection, the diagnosis of septic bursitis requires sampling of the bursal fluid. The range of leukocytosis per mm^3 is broad and the absolute number usually is less than is present in septic arthritis. In one series of 32 patients with septic bursitis, the bursal fluid leukocyte count averaged 23,350/mm^3 with a standard deviation of 22,065/mm^3; more than 10% of patients had fewer than 2000 leukocytes/mm^3 [65]. Gram stain is positive in 50% or less of all cases [70]. Sensitivity of culture may be increased by directly inoculating bursa-associated fluid into liquid media versus direct culture methods [71]. Blood cultures also may be helpful in identifying the microbiologic cause of infection in deeper and more severe forms of septic bursitis [65]. More than 75% of septic bursitis cases are attributable to *S aureus*; other causes include streptococci, *Staphylococcus epidermidis*, enterococci, diphtheroids, and, rarely, Gram-negative bacilli [72]. Subacute and chronic infectious bursitis can be attributable to other organisms such as, *Brucella*, mycobacteria, *Prototheca*, and *Aspergillus*.

Treatment typically requires drainage and antibiotics. Initial antibiotics are dictated by Gram-stain evaluation of bursal fluid. If the Gram stain is negative, antistaphylococcal therapy is initiated with intravenous cefazolin, nafcillin or oxacillin, or vancomycin. Subsequent treatment then is dictated by culture and susceptibility results. Daily percutaneous drainage procedures are performed until sterility is attained and antibiotics usually are administered for at least 2 to 3 weeks. Indications for surgery include inadequate needle drainage of bursa, inability of needle to access bursa for drainage, necrosis, presence of foreign body, and refractory infection [67].

Infectious tenosynovitis

Infection of the synovial sheaths that surround a tendon is known as tenosynovitis. The flexor muscle–associated tendons and tendon sheaths of the hand are most commonly involved (flexor tenosynovitis). Penetrating trauma is the most common inciting event and infection then can travel rapidly from the digit to ulnar and radial bursae. Acute infection is most commonly attributable to *S aureus* and other skin-associated flora, such as streptococci, although the nature of the traumatic injury may impact the associated microbiology (ie, organisms associated with mammal bites, gardening, or fish handling) [59]. Nontraumatic causes of tenosynovitis are classically associated with disseminated gonococcal infection (DGI). In DGI, one or several tendons may be involved (extensor more often than flexor), usually targeting the ankles, toes, wrists, and fingers [73]. Chronic infectious flexor tenosynovitis is caused primarily by fungi and mycobacteria.

Patients who have acute flexor tenosynovitis present with erythematous fusiform swelling of an involved finger, which is held in a semiflexed position. Tenderness over the length of the tendon sheath and pain with extension of the finger also are typical [74]. Classically, patients who have DGI have fever, rash, tenosynovitis, and an asymmetric polyarthritis. The rash initially is macular, papular, or petechial before progressing to a pustular stage that can become hemorrhagic and necrotic. The lesions characteristically are few in number (ie, <20–30) and are distributed periarticularly over distal extremities.

Patients in whom there is clinical suspicion of flexor tenosynovitis should be evaluated by a hand surgeon and receive empiric antibiotics. The nature of the exposure and the underlying status of the host dictate the antimicrobial selection. Infection in an immunocompetent host resulting from a simple puncture would require at least Gram-positive skin flora coverage against staphylococci and streptococci. Pet bite–associated infectious tenosynovitis dictates expanded coverage to include Gram-negative organisms, such as *Pasteurella* and anaerobes. Imaging of the involved area, particularly with MRI, may be helpful in identifying the presence of gas, bone infection, foreign body, or fluid, and the extent of infection, but a definitive diagnosis requires evaluation of fluid from within the tendon sheath. Although some patients who present within 48 hours of developing trauma-associated flexor tenosynovitis can be treated with intravenous antibiotics and splinting alone, effective surgical drainage coupled with pathogen-directed therapy established by microbiologic evaluation of drainage material typically is required. DGI-associated tenosynovitis can be diagnosed with blood cultures. In addition, the organism may be detected in mucosal sites, such as the rectum, oropharynx, cervix, and urethra, and in the synovial fluid (when arthritis is present). Initial therapy with ceftriaxone intramuscularly or intravenously and hospitalization are recommended for patients who have DGI. Unless the diagnosis is excluded, treatment of concomitant chlamydial infection also should be administered. Intravenous therapy can be switched to oral antibiotics, such as cefixime, 24 to 48 hours after improvement begins to complete at least one week of treatment [75].

References

[1] Sadick NS. Current aspects of bacterial infections of the skin. Dermatol Clin 1997;15:341–9.
[2] Dillon HC. Impetigo contagiosa: suppurative and non-suppurative complications. I. Clinical, bacteriologic, and epidemiologic characteristics of impetigo. Am J Dis Child 1968;115: 530–41.
[3] Hirschmann JV. Impetigo: etiology and therapy. Curr Clin Top Infect Dis 2002;22:42–51.
[4] Stevens DL, Bisno AL, Chambers HF, et al. Practice guidelines for the diagnosis and management of skin and soft-tissue infections. Clin Infect Dis 2005;41:1373–406.
[5] Liassine N, Auckenthaler R, Descombes M-C, et al. Community-acquired methicillin-resistant *Staphylococcus aureus* isolated in Switzerland contains the Panton-Valentine Leukocidin or exfoliative toxin genes. J Clin Microbiol 2004;42:825–8.
[6] Parker SR, Parker DC, McCall CO. Eosinophilic folliculitis in HIV-infected women: case series and review. Am J Clin Dermatol 2006;7(3):193–200.
[7] Uthayakumar S, Nandwani R, Drinkwater T, et al. The prevalence of skin disease in HIV infection and its relationship to the degree of immunosuppression. Br J Dermatol 1997; 137:595–8.
[8] Rhody C. Bacterial infections of the skin. Prim Care 2000;27:459–73.

[9] Gilad J, Borer A, Smolyakov R, et al. Impaired neutrophil functions in the pathogenesis of an outbreak of recurrent furunculosis caused by methicillin-resistant *Staphylococcus aureus* among mentally retarded adults. Microbes Infect 2006;8:1801–5.

[10] Demircay Z, Eksioglu-Demiralp E, Ergun T, et al. Phagocytosis and oxidative burst by neutrophils in patients with recurrent furunculosis. Br J Dermatol 1998;138:1036–8.

[11] Kazakova SV, Hageman JC, Matava M, et al. A clone of methicillin-resistant *Staphylococcus aureus* among professional football players. N Engl J Med 2005;352:468–75.

[12] Bahrain M, Vasiliades M, Wolff M, et al. Five cases of bacterial endocarditis after furunculosis and the ongoing saga of community-acquired methicillin-resistant *Staphylococcus aureus* infections. Scand J Infect Dis 2006;38:702–7.

[13] Moran GJ, Krishnadasan A, Gorwitz RJ, et al. Methicillin-resistant *S. aureus* infections among patients in the emergency department. N Engl J Med 2006;355:666–74.

[14] Zetoka N, Francis JS, Nurenberger EL, et al. Community-acquired methicillin-resistant *Staphylococcus aureus*: an emerging threat. Lancet Infect Dis 2005;5:275–86.

[15] Fridkin SK, Hageman JC, Morrison M, et al. Methicillin-resistant *Staphylococcus aureus* disease in three communities. N Engl J Med 2005;352:1436–44 [erratum: N Engl J Med 2005;352:2362].

[16] Klempner MS, Styrt B. Prevention of recurrent staphylococcal skin infections with low-dose oral clindamycin therapy. JAMA 1988;260:2682–5.

[17] Eriksson B, Jorup-Ronstrom C, Karkkoonen K, et al. Erysipelas: clinical and bacteriologic spectrum and serological aspects. Clin Infect Dis 1996;23:1091–8.

[18] Bonnetblanc J-M, Bedane C. Erysipelas. recognition and management. Am J Clin Dermatol 2003;4:157–63.

[19] Dupuy A, Benchiki H, Roujeau JC, et al. Risk factors for erysipelas of the leg (cellulitis): case control study. BMJ 1999;318:1591–4.

[20] Coste N, Perceau G, Leone J, et al. Osteoarticular complications of erysipelas. J Am Acad Dermatol 2004;50:203–9.

[21] Jorup-Ronstrom C, Britton S. Recurrent erysipelas: Predisposing factors and costs of prophylaxis. Infection 1987;15:105–6.

[22] File TM Jr. Skin infections. In: Tan JS, editor. Expert guide to infectious diseases. Philadelphia: American College of Physicians–American Society of Internal Medicine; 2002. p. 605–17.

[23] Koutkia P, Mylonakis E, Boyce J. Cellulitis: evaluation of possible predisposing factors in hospitalized patients. Diagn Microbiol Infect Dis 1999;34:325–7.

[24] Ellis Simonsen SM, van Orman ER, Hatch BE, et al. Cellulitis incidence in a defined population. Epidemiol Infect 2006;134:293–9.

[25] Dong SL, Kelly KD, Oland RC, et al. ED management of cellulitis: a review of five urban centers. Am J Emerg Med 2001;19:535–40.

[26] Huang PY, Lee MH, Yang CC, et al. Group B streptococcal bacteremia in non-pregnant adults. J Microbiol Immunol Infect 2006;39:237–41.

[27] Edwards MS, Baker CJ. Group B streptococcal infections in elderly adults. Clin Infect Dis 2005;41:839–47.

[28] Lillis EA, Dugan V, Mills T, et al. A fish hook and liver disease: revisiting an old enemy. J La State Med Soc 2002;154:20–5.

[29] Falagas ME, Vergidis PI. Narrative review: diseases that masquerade as infectious cellulitis. Ann Intern Med 2005;142:47–55.

[30] Mills AM, Chen EH. Are blood cultures necessary in adults with cellulitis? Ann Emerg Med 2005;45:548–9.

[31] Perl B, Gottehrer NP, Raveh D, et al. Cost-effectiveness of blood cultures for adult patients with cellulitis. Clin Infect Dis 1999;29:1483–8.

[32] Epperly TD. The value of needle aspiration in the management of cellulitis. J Fam Pract 1986;23:337–40.

[33] Hook EW 3rd, Hooton TM, Horton CA, et al. Microbiologic evaluation of cutaneous cellulitis in adults. Arch Intern Med 1986;146:295–7.

[34] Newell PM, Norden CW. Value of needle aspiration in bacteriologic diagnosis of cellulitis in adults. J Clin Microbiol 1988;26:401–4.

[35] Sachs MK. The optimum use of needle aspiration in the bacteriologic diagnosis of cellulitis in adults. Arch Intern Med 1990;150:1907–12.

[36] Sigurdsson AF, Gudmunddsson S. The etiology of bacterial cellulitis as determined by fine-needle aspiration. Scand J Infect Dis 1989;21:537–42.

[37] Swartz MN. Cellulitis. N Engl J Med 2004;350:904–12.

[38] Semel JD, Goldin H. Association of athlete's foot with cellulitis of the lower extremities: diagnostic value of bacterial cultures of ipsilateral interdigital space samples. Clin Infect Dis 1996;23:1162–4.

[39] Bjornsdottir S, Gottfredsson M, Thorisdottir AS, et al. Risk factors for acute cellulitis of the lower limb: a prospective case-control study. Clin Infect Dis 2005;41:1416–22.

[40] Giuliano A, Lewis F, Hadley K, et al. Bacteriology of necrotizing fasciitis. Am J Surg 1977; 134:52–7.

[41] Miller LG, Perdreau-Remington F, Rieg G, et al. Necrotizing fasciitis caused by community-associated methicillin-resistant Staphylococcus aureus in Los Angeles. N Engl J Med 2005; 352:1445–53.

[42] Mok MY, Wong SY, Chan TM, et al. Necrotizing fasciitis in rheumatic diseases. Lupus 2006;15:380–3.

[43] Mendez EA, Espinoza LM, Harris M, et al. Systemic lupus erythematosus complicated by necrotizing fasciitis. Lupus 1999;8:157–9.

[44] Hill MD, Karsh J. Invasive soft tissue infections with Streptococcus pneumoniae in patients with systemic lupus erythematosus: case report and review of the literature. Arthr Rheum 1997;40:1716–9.

[45] Childers BJ, Potyondy LD, Nachreiner R, et al. Necrotizing fasciitis: a fourteen-year retrospective study of 163 consecutive patients. Am Surg 2002;68:109–16.

[46] Wong C-H, Chang H-C, Pasupathy S, et al. Necrotizing fasciitis: clinical presentation, microbiology, and determinants of mortality. J Bone Joint Surg 2003;85-A:1454–60.

[47] Brothers TE, Tagge DU, Stutley JE, et al. Magnetic resonance imaging differentiates between necrotizing and non-necrotizing fasciitis of the lower extremity. J Am Coll Surg 1998;187:416–21.

[48] Schmid MR, Kossmann T, Duewell S. Differentiation of necrotizing fasciitis and cellulitis using MR imaging. AJR Am J Roentgenol 1998;170:615–20.

[49] Saiag P, Le Breton C, Pavlovic M, et al. Magnetic resonance imaging in adults presenting with severe acute infectious cellulitis. Arch Dermatol 1994;130:1150–8.

[50] Wong CH, Khin L-W, Heng K-S, et al. The LRINEC (Laboratory Risk Indicator for Necrotizing Fasciitis) score: a tool for distinguishing necrotizing fasciitis from other soft tissue infections. Crit Care Med 2004;32:1535–41.

[51] Wang TL, Hung CR. Role of tissue oxygen saturation monitoring in diagnosing necrotizing fasciitis of the lower limbs. Ann Emerg Med 2004;44:222–8.

[52] Wilson B. Necrotizing fasciitis. Am J Surg 1970;18:416–31.

[53] Uman SJ, Kunin CM. Needle aspiration in the diagnosis of soft tissue infections. Arch Intern Med 1975;135:959–61.

[54] Kaul R, McGeer A, Low DE, et al. Population-based surveillance for group A streptococcal necrotizing fasciitis: clinical features, prognostic indicators, and microbiologic analysis of seventy-seven cases. Am J Med 1997;103:18–24.

[55] Stamenkovic I, Lew PD. Early recognition of potentially fatal necrotizing fasciitis: the use of frozen section biopsy. N Engl J Med 1984;310:1689–93.

[56] Ben-Abraham R, Keller N, Vered R, et al. Invasive group A streptococcal infections in a large tertiary center: epidemiology, characteristics, and outcome. Infection 2002;30:81–5.

[57] Crum NF. Bacterial pyomyositis in the United States. Am J Med 2004;117:420–8.

[58] Scriba J. Beitrag zur aetiologie der myositis acuta. Dtsch Z Chir 1885;22:497–502.
[59] Small LN, Ross JJ. Tropical and temperate pyomyositis. Infect Dis Clin N Am 2005;19: 981–9.
[60] Chauhan S, Jain S, Varma S, et al. Tropical myositis (myositis tropicans): current perspective. Postgrad Med J 2004;80:267–70.
[61] Gomez-Reino JJ, Aznar JJ, Pablos JL, et al. Nontropical pyomyositis in adults. Semin Arthritis Rheum 1994;23:396–405.
[62] Christin L, Sarosi GA. Pyomyositis in North America: case reports and review. Clin Infect Dis 1992;15:668–77.
[63] Chiedozi LC. Pyomyositis: review of 205 cases in 112 patients. Am J Surg 1979;137:255–9.
[64] Gordon BA, Martinez S, Collins AJ. Pyomyositis: characteristics at CT and MR imaging. Radiology 1995;197:279–86.
[65] Garcia-Porrua C, Gonzalez-Gay MA, Ibanez D, et al. The clinical spectrum of severe septic bursitis in northwestern Spain: a ten year study. J Rheumatol 1999;26:663–7.
[66] Ho G, Tice AD, Kaplan SR. Septic bursitis in the prepatellar and olecranon bursae, an analysis of 25 cases. Ann Intern Med 1978;89:21–7.
[67] Zimmermann B 3rd, Mikolich DJ, Ho G Jr. Septic bursitis. Semin Arthritis Rheum 1995;24: 391–410.
[68] Pien FD, Ching D, Kim E. Septic bursitis: experience in a community practice. Orthopedics 1991;14:981–4.
[69] Smith DL, McAfee JH, Lucas LM, et al. Septic and nonseptic olecranon bursitis. Utility of the surface temperature probe in the early differentiation of septic and nonseptic cases. Arch Intern Med 1989;149:1581–5.
[70] Valeriano-Marcet J, Carter JD, Vasey FB. Soft tissue disease. Rheum Dis Clin North Am 2003;29:77–88.
[71] Stell IM. Simple tests for septic bursitis: comparative study. BMJ 1998;316:1877–80.
[72] Cea-Pereiro JC, Garcia-Meijide J, Mera-Varela A, et al. A comparison between septic bursitis caused by *Staphylococcus aureus* and those caused by other organisms. Clin Rheumatol 2001;20:10–4.
[73] Rompalo AM, Hook EW, Roberts PL, et al. The acute arthritis dermatitis syndrome. Arch Intern Med 1987;147:281–3.
[74] Kanavel AB. Infections of the hand: a guide to the surgical treatment of acute and chronic suppurative processes in the fingers, hand and forearm. Philadelphia: Lea & Febiger; 1912.
[75] Centers for Disease Control. Sexually transmitted diseases treatment guidelines, 2006. MMWR 2006;55(RR11):1–94.

ELSEVIER
SAUNDERS

Infect Dis Clin N Am
20 (2006) 773–788

INFECTIOUS
DISEASE CLINICS
OF NORTH AMERICA

Advances in the Management of Septic Arthritis

Ignacio García-De La Torre, MD[a,b,*]

[a]*Department of Immunology and Rheumatology, Hospital General de Occidente,
Secretaría de Salud, Justo Sierra 2821, Guadalajara, Jalisco, C.P. 44690, México*
[b]*Department of Immunology and Rheumatology, Centro Universitario de Ciencias de la Salud,
Universidad de Guadalajara, Guadalajara, Jalisco 44690, México*

Bacterial or septic arthritis is an important medical condition and is considered a rheumatologic emergency that can lead to rapid joint destruction and irreversible loss of function. This term includes all joint infections caused by pyogenic bacteria and encompasses the terms pyogenic arthritis, suppurative arthritis, purulent arthritis, and pyarthrosis. Normal joints, diseased joints, and prosthetic joints are all vulnerable to bacterial infection. There are two peaks of incidence that seem to be age dependent: one under the age of 15 and the other over 55 years. The mortality and morbidity of this condition is still considerable. The mortality rates in adults range from 10% to greater than 50%. More than 30% of patients may be left with residual joint damage and with some joints, such as the hip, more than 50% may be irreversibly damaged. Delay in making the diagnosis has serious implications for prognosis. Full recovery is possible, but poor outcome is common among those with pre-existing arthritis, especially rheumatoid arthritis [1–5].

This article focuses on the risk factors and pathogenesis of nongonococcal bacterial arthritis; gonococcal arthritis and other forms of infectious arthritis, primarily in the context of a differential diagnosis and treatment, are also discussed.

Portions of this article originally appeared in García-De La Torre. Advances in the management of septic arthritis. Rheumatic Disease Clinics of North America 2003;29(1):61–75.

This work was supported in part by Grant G34022-M from Consejo Nacional de Ciencias y Tecnología and from Sistema Nacional de Investigadores, México.

* Department of Immunology and Rheumatology Hospital General de Occidente, Secretaría de Salud, Justo Sierra 2821, Guadalajara, Jalisco, C.P. 44690, Mexico.

E-mail address: igdlt@aol.com

Risk factors

Experimental evidence suggests that normal joints are very resistant to infections compared with diseased joints or prosthetic joints. Recognition of risk factors (systemic, local, and social) is important. Such factors act by increasing the risk of bacteremia, or reducing the body's capacity to eliminate organisms from the joint [6–8].

Systemic disorders that affect the host's response through an impaired immune system include diabetes mellitus, psoriasis, liver disease, chronic renal failure, malignancies, intravenous drug abuse, hemodialysis, alcoholism, patients with AIDS, hemophilia, organ transplantation, or hypogammaglobulinemia [9–13].

A high index of suspicion for septic arthritis should be considered in patients with other rheumatic diseases, such as rheumatoid arthritis, osteoarthritis, gout, pseudogout, and systemic lupus erythematosus. Of these, rheumatoid arthritis is the most common, probably because of the combination of joint damage and immunosuppressive medications. Polyarticular disease is common, functional outcomes are worse, and mortality is high in rheumatoid arthritis patients with septic joints. Diagnosis is often delayed because of the confusion of septic arthritis for a flare of rheumatoid arthritis [14,15].

Local factors, such as damage of a specific joint, may be the result of earlier trauma or recent joint surgery or arthroscopy; the presence of a prosthetic joint in the knee or the hip is an important predisposing factor for septic arthritis. Age is also important, with newborns and elderly people, especially those beyond the age of 80 years, being particularly vulnerable [1,16–19].

Social factors include occupational exposure to animals with respect to brucellosis [20], whereas the risk of tuberculosis is greatly increased in certain racial groups (eg, people from India) [21]. The past two decades, however, have seen a resurgence of tuberculosis in developed countries as a result of mass immigrations from endemic areas of the world; increasing numbers of immunocompromised individuals, including those with AIDS; increased infection rates in association with drug abuse, homelessness, and therapeutic noncompliance; and the emergence of drug-resistant mycobacteria [22].

In some cases, these risk factors are compounded (eg, patients with rheumatoid arthritis treated with immunosuppression or steroids are at higher risk for infection). It may also be difficult to distinguish infection from inflammatory synovitis, especially if the patient is receiving steroid therapy. Lethal infection and unusual organisms, such as *Listeria*, *Salmonella*, and *Actinobacillus ureae*, have been reported to cause septic arthritis in patients with rheumatoid arthritis receiving the novel anti–tumor necrosis factor-α therapy [23–26]. Box 1 lists the most common risk factors that predisposes to septic arthritis.

Box 1. Common risk factors in bacterial arthritis

Systemic disorders
Rheumatoid arthritis
Diabetes mellitus
Psoriasis
Liver diseases
Alcoholism
Chronic renal failure
Malignancies
Intravenous drug abusers
Hemodialysis patients
AIDS
Hemophilia
Organ transplantation
Hypogammaglobulinemia
Immunosuppressive drugs: glucocorticosteroids
Anti–tumor necrosis factor-α therapy

Local factors
Direct joint trauma
Recent joint surgery
Open reduction of fractures
Arthroscopy
Rheumatoid arthritis in a specific joint
Osteoarthritis
Prosthetic joint in knee or hip

Age
Newborns or elderly (>80 years old)

Social factors
Occupational exposure to animals (brucellosis)
Low social income: tuberculosis

Pathogenesis

In most cases bacterial arthritis is the consequence of occult bacteremia. In 1939 Shaffer and Bennett [27] showed that pneumococcal bacteremia in rabbits often caused pneumococcal arthritis, and other laboratory models of bacterial arthritis were subsequently described [28,29]. The synovium is highly vascular and contains no limiting basement membrane, promoting easy access of blood contents to the synovial space [30]. Certain bacteria, such as *Neisseria gonorrhoeae*, are particularly likely to infect a joint during a bacteremic episode. Pneumonia, pyelonephritis, or a skin infection is a common extra-articular site of infection causing bacteremic seeding in a joint.

Once the bacteria enter the closed joint space, they can trigger an acute inflammatory cell response within a few hours. The synovial membrane reacts with a proliferative lining-cell hyperplasia, and there is an influx of acute and chronic inflammatory cell, creating the characteristic acute, purulent joint inflammation. In a few days the inflammatory cells release cytokines and proteases, leading to cartilage degradation, inhibition of cartilage synthesis, and irreversible bone loss [31].

Less commonly, bacteria may also directly infect a joint from a deep penetrating wound; examples include plant thorn synovitis presenting as chronic synovitis caused by a foreign body reaction or acute pseudoseptic arthritis [32]; *Pantoea agglomerans*, a member of the family Enterobacteriaceae, was cultured from two cases of monoarthritis after plant thorn and wood sliver injuries [33]. Besides plant thorns and wood slivers, other material, such as nails and other sharp objects, can cause puncture wounds that penetrate a joint and result in the direct inoculation of bacteria into the joint [34]. Recently, a case of septic arthritis of the lumbar facet joint was reported in a patient with a long history of back pain who received acupuncture treatment; the diagnosis in this case was done with a bone and MRI scan [35].

Bacteria may be introduced during joint surgery. Orthopedic surgeons may encounter patients with joint infections as a result of trauma or surgical procedures. Some examples include penetrating injury or foreign body accidentally introduced into a joint; arthroscopic surgery; open reduction of fractures that involve the joint; and arthroplasty, including total joint replacement [36]. Late infections of prosthetic joints, defined as occurring a year or later after successful joint replacement, can result from contamination at the time of the implant surgery or as the result of bacterial seeding by transient bacteremia. This complication is also uncommon and the patients complain of pain in a previously painless total joint replacement [37,38].

Finally, infection resulting from the introduction of bacteria into the joint during intra-articular steroid injection is very uncommon and it has been found in one study to occur at a rate of 0.0002% [39]. The pathogenesis of these direct infections is identical to that of hematogenously acquired infections.

Microbiology

Virtually any microbial pathogen is capable of causing bacterial arthritis (Box 2). Among nongonococcal causes of acute bacterial arthritis, the gram-positive cocci are the major pathogens. *Staphylococcus aureus* is most common in both native and prosthetic joint infections, but *Staphylococcus epidermidis* is much more common in prosthetic infections than in native joint infections [30].

Box 2. Most common microorganisms causing septic arthritis

Gram-positive aerobes
   Staphylococcus aureus
   Streptococci: *Streptococcus pyogenes, Streptococcus*
     pneumoniae
Gram-negative bacilli
   Haemophilus influenzae
   Escherichia coli
Neisseria gonorrhoeae
Borrelia burgdorferi
Mycobacterial species
Fungal species
   Sporotrichosis
   Cryptococcus
   Blastomycosis
Anaerobes

In three recent large series, *S aureus* was the primary cause of bacterial arthritis in 40% of cases from England and Wales, 56% of cases from France, and 37% of cases from tropical Australia. *S aureus* causes 80% of joint infections in patients with concurrent rheumatoid arthritis and in those with diabetes. This microbe is also the primary pathogen in hip infections and in polyarticular septic arthritis [31]. In general, the causes of adult nongonococcal septic arthritis are 75% to 80% gram-positive cocci and 15% to 20% gram-negative bacilli.

After *S aureus*, the streptococci, including *Streptococcus pyogenes* (group B) and *Streptococcus pneumoniae*, are the most common gram-positive aerobes. Although pneumococcal arthritis has been uncommon in most series during the past 30 years, 10% of bacterial arthritis from a study from England and Wales over a 4-year period from 1990 to 1993 were caused by *S pneumoniae* [3]. In general, these microbes are important causes of bacterial arthritis in compromised hosts or in patients with serious genitourinary or gastrointestinal infections. Anaerobic infections are more common in prosthetic joint infections and in diabetics who develop septic arthritis. Also in most series, 10% to 20% of clinically diagnosed bacterial arthritis is never confirmed with positive synovial fluid or blood cultures [3,31].

Gram-negative bacilli are common causes of bacterial arthritis in intravenous drug users, in the elderly, and in patients with major immune deficiency. Gram-negative bacilli and *Haemophilus influenzae* are the most common pathogens in the newborn and in all children younger than 5 years of age. Before the widespread use of *H influenzae* vaccine, this microorganism was the most common cause of bacterial arthritis in young children between the ages of 1 month and 5 years. Bacterial arthritis caused by *H influenzae* is now extremely rare among children who have received the currently available vaccine. Overall, the age-specific incidence of infection caused by *H influenzae* among children younger than 5 years old has fallen by 70% to 80% since the introduction of *H influenzae* type b conjugate vaccines [40].

In the elderly, gram-negative microorganisms may be more common because of the comorbidities (eg, rheumatoid arthritis and diabetes mellitus) that predispose them to systemic gram-negative bacillary infections. Underlying joint diseases are also more prevalent among the elderly. HIV infection, however, has been associated with mycobacterial, fungal, and bacterial joint infections [41].

Patients with rheumatoid arthritis, especially those with severe disease, are at greater risk of septic arthritis as a complication of the rheumatoid disease. As a result of this, an emerging area of great importance and interest is infections and the use of biologic agents in the management of rheumatoid arthritis. Tumor necrosis factor blockade with infliximab (Remicade) or etanercept (Enbrel) has had a revolutionary impact in controlling the joint inflammation of some patients previously refractory to conventional disease-modifying antirheumatic drug therapy. Active bacterial infection, however, is a contraindication to the use of tumor necrosis factor suppression. Whether the more widespread use of these agents will affect the rate of septic arthritis in the rheumatoid population is unknown at this time [42–44].

Disseminated gonococcal infection is the most common form of bacterial arthritis in young, healthy sexually active adults in the United States. It occurs in approximately 1% to 3% of patients infected with *N gonorrhoeae*. It is an uncommon cause of bacterial arthritis in Europe, and in most countries the incidence varies with the patients' socioeconomic status. Most patients with this infection have arthritis or arthralgia as one of their principal manifestations. One study of 151 consecutive patients with acute nontraumatic arthritis or arthralgia seen at one hospital found that *N gonorrhoeae* was the most common cause of illness [45].

It is important to bear in mind that often the isolation of the organism responsible for the septic arthritis is difficult because of inadequate culture techniques or standards within the laboratory, or simply because of failure to collect blood or synovial fluid for laboratory examination.

Clinical features

The classical presentation of bacterial arthritis is as an acute, painful, hot and swollen single joint, occurring in approximately 80% to 90% of the cases. In some cases, however, a polyarticular pattern may occur (10%–20%), usually involving three or four joints and being asymmetric. The predilection is for a single large joint, typically the knee, which occurs in more than 50% of cases, but any joint may be involved. In the evaluation of a patient with an acute monoarthritis, septic arthritis is always a consideration, especially if the patient is febrile, appears toxic, or has an extra-articular site of bacterial infection [46].

Hip infections are more common in young children. The hip is often held in a flexed and externally rotated position and there is extreme pain on motion. It is often difficult to detect an effusion of the hip or the shoulder, although the joint is frequently warm and very tender [47]. The sacroiliac joint is involved in 10% of infections [48]; these are difficult to detect by physical examination and imaging studies have an important role in the diagnosis [49].

In some patients, the clinical and laboratory diagnosis of septic arthritis is often highly imprecise. The onset may be insidious, with few features of inflammation to alert the clinician to an underlying infection. In the spine, sacroiliac joints, and hips, pain may be the only presenting feature. In children and elderly people the clinical presentation is often nonspecific. Even when the typically indolent infection of joint tuberculosis is excluded, only half of the patients with bacterial arthritis may have fever or leukocytosis. A source of infection, often from the skin, lungs, or bladder is found in 50% of cases [1,30,31].

Polyarticular septic arthritis is most likely to occur in patients with rheumatoid arthritis or a systemic connective tissue disease or in patients with overwhelming sepsis. In patients with rheumatoid arthritis, an acute exacerbation of joint inflammation, whether monoarticular or polyarticular, must raise the suspicion of superimposed infection complicating rheumatoid disease [50].

In gonococcal infection the most common symptoms are migratory polyarthralgias, tenosynovitis, dermatitis, and fever [51,52]. Less than 50% of the patients with this type of infection present with a purulent joint effusion, most often of the knee or wrist. Multiple tendons of the wrist, ankles, and small joints may be inflamed and very tender. The skin lesions are typically multiple painless macules and papules, most often found on the arms, legs, or trunk.

The cornerstones for the diagnosis of septic arthritis are arthrocentesis and synovial fluid analysis. If the synovial fluid cell count is extremely high, in the range of 100,000 white blood cells/mm^3 or greater, treatment for presumed septic arthritis should be initiated pending culture result of the fluid. A negative gram-stained smear or a negative culture of the synovial fluid should be corroborated by negative blood cultures and, perhaps in the future, by a negative polymerase chain reaction test for bacterial DNA in the synovial fluid [53].

Predictors of mortality in a multivariate analysis include age over 65 years, confusion at presentation, and polyarticular disease. Predictors of joint damage include age over 65 years, diabetes mellitus, and infection with β-hemolytic streptococci [54].

Diagnosis

The key to the diagnosis of bacterial arthritis is the identification of bacteria in the synovial fluid by Gram stain or by culture. At the clinical suspicion of joint infection, synovial fluid aspiration should be performed. Gram stain, usually best seen on a concentrated sediment of centrifuged synovial fluid, culture, and leukocyte count and differential of the aspirated fluid often leads to the correct diagnosis. The synovial fluid of septic arthritis usually is purulent with an average leukocyte count of 50,000 to 150,000 cells/mm^3 (most of which are neutrophils). Gram stain smears are positive in only 60% to 80% of the time. The glucose levels in synovial fluid are often depressed and lactic acid and lactate dehydrogenase levels are raised in septic arthritis, but such values may also be seen in inflammatory joint disease (Table 1) [31,55,56].

Using blood culture bottles to culture synovial fluid specimens may increase the yield of the offending microorganism [57]. A recent study in 90 patients with acute joint effusions, however, found no significant differences in the yield of positive cultures with the use of conventional agar plate culture, culture with lysis and centrifugation tubes, or broth enrichment blood culture bottles. In patients with clinical signs of septic arthritis, the joint fluid cultures were positive by all three methods in eight patients and negative by all three methods in 19 patients [58].

Blood cultures are positive in about half of the patients with nongonococcal septic arthritis and should be obtained in any patient with suspected bacterial arthritis [59]. Negative cultures may occur in those who have received recent antimicrobial therapy or are infected with a fastidious organism, such as some streptococci or mycoplasma [30]. Other laboratory findings, such as an increased white blood cell count and an elevated erythrocyte sedimentation rate, are common but nonspecific. Measurements of erythrocyte

Table 1
Differential diagnosis of synovial fluid

Test	Normal	Non inflammatory	Inflammatory	Septic
Clarity	Transparent	Transparent	Translucent-opaque	Opaque
Color	Clear	Yellow	Yellow, opalescent	Yellow-green
Viscosity	High	High	Low	Variable
WBCs/mm^3	<200	200–2000	2000–10,000	>50,000
PMN%	<25	~25	>50	>75
Culture	Negative	Negative	Negative	Often positive
Glucose (mg/dL)	Nearly = to plasma	Nearly = to plasma	~25, lower than plasma	<25, even lower than plasma

Modified from McCarty DJ. Synovial fluid. In: Koopman WJ. Arthritis and allied conditions: a textbook of rheumatology. 14th edition. Philadelphia: Lippincott Williams and Wilkins; 2001. p. 83; with permission.

sedimentation rate or C-reactive protein may be more helpful in children with possible septic hips [17,48].

The coexistence of crystal-induced inflammation and bacterial infection must not be overlooked and a wet preparation for examination under polarizing microscopy is an essential test to be performed on the synovial fluid in addition to culturing for microorganisms. Fever can be caused by acute crystal-induced synovitis or acute flare of rheumatoid arthritis without infection [60]. When fever is present in a patient with an underlying inflammatory rheumatic disease, however, one must do an intensive search for complicating bacterial infection in the inflamed joint.

The usefulness of polymerase chain reaction in the diagnosis and management of many infectious diseases, including septic arthritis, is still being defined [61]. It seems to be useful in the detection of bacterial DNA in joint infections where the pathogens are fastidious, slow growing, or not able to be cultured. N gonorrhoeae and Mycoplasma are examples of such microorganisms. Polymerase chain reaction also may be useful in prosthetic joint infection, where the distinction between septic and aseptic loosening must be made before surgical revision can be undertaken [62]. Determination by polymerase chain reaction of bacterial DNA in serial samples of synovial fluid can confirm the eradication of infection or the persistence of infection. In the first case polymerase chain reaction becomes negative, and in the later polymerase chain reaction remains positive with high-intensity signal.

If synovial fluid cannot be obtained with closed-needle aspiration, the joint should be aspirated under CT or fluoroscopic or ultrasound guidance. Certain joints, such as the hip or sacroiliac joints, may require surgical arthrotomy for diagnostic aspiration. In acute septic arthritis, radiographs are usually normal at presentation but should be obtained in all patients because associated osteomyelitis or concurrent joint disease may rarely be present. In addition, a baseline radiograph is often useful for comparison purposes should the response to therapy be delayed or poor [63].

Scintigraphy, CT scanning, or MRI is far more sensitive than plain films in early septic arthritis. CT is more useful to detect effusions and inflammation in joints that are difficult to examine, especially in the hip, sternoclavicular, and sacroiliac joints. MRI demonstrates adjacent soft tissue edema and abscesses and may be especially helpful in detecting septic sacroiliitis [49,63].

Differential diagnosis

The differential diagnosis of bacterial arthritis includes various inflammatory joint diseases (Box 3). The crystal-induced arthritis gout and pseudogout (calcium pyrophosphate dihydrate deposition disease) are the two most important forms of acute arthritis that may be difficult to differentiate from bacterial arthritis on clinical examination [46]. Patients with gout may have a monoarthritis with shaking chills, high fever, and leukocytosis. A history of recurrent monoarthritis, typical podagra, and the presence of tophi or

---

Box 3. Differential diagnosis of septic arthritis

Crystal-induced arthritis
    Gout
    Pseudogout
Rheumatoid arthritis
    Pseudoseptic arthritis
Chronic seronegative arthritis
    Reiter's syndrome
    Psoriatic syndrome
    Ankylosing spondylitis
    Arthritis associated with inflammatory bowel disease
Lyme disease
Mycobacterial and fungal arthritis

---

radiologic evidence of chondrocalcinosis, however, are most predictive of crystal-induced arthritis. The only definitive diagnostic test is the demonstration of the characteristic urate crystals of gout or the calcium pyrophosphate dihydrate crystals of pseudogout. In rare cases, patients have concurrent crystal-induced and bacterial arthritis. For this reason, one must routinely culture and look for crystal in the synovial fluid from any joint with an acute effusion of unknown etiology [64].

Any form of chronic inflammatory joint disease, such as Reiter's syndrome, psoriatic arthritis, ankylosing spondylitis, and arthritis associated with inflammatory bowel disease, can present with a new swollen joint that can simulate bacterial arthritis. In these rheumatic diseases the familial clustering is related to the presence of the histocompatibility antigen HLA-B27 in 50% to 95% of cases. Most patients with these conditions may have some of the following clinical features: recent genitourinary or gastrointestinal signs or symptoms, conjunctivitis or uveitis, enthesopathy or skin or mucous membrane lesions, and predilection for the sacroiliac joints [31].

Another rheumatoid disease that in some cases is important to differentiate from bacterial arthritis is rheumatoid arthritis. This disease is typically a symmetrical, chronic polyarthritis, but in some patients an acute or subacute exacerbation of one or few joints is common. The correct diagnosis may be difficult to establish because the clinical findings may be somewhat atypical. Some patients with rheumatoid arthritis and bacterial arthritis may present little fever or peripheral blood leukocytes. Rheumatoid arthritis alone, however, may present with a pseudoseptic arthritis picture, including an explosive acute synovitis with a marked synovial fluid leukocytosis. For this reason, Gram stain and culture of synovial fluid are essential when evaluating the new onset of synovitis in these patients [65].

Lyme disease may present with an acute or chronic monoarthritis, especially of the knee. Early symptoms include the typical erythema migrans skin lesions and transient polyarthralgias with viral-like features, including fever, headaches, and a variety of neurologic signs. Patients are generally from or have visited an endemic area, and seasonal exposure contributes. Joint effusions may be massive but often resolve without treatment and then recur. Chronic persistent synovitis develops in 20% of patients with untreated Lyme disease. At the time of arthritis, almost all patients should have IgG antibodies to *Borrelia burgdorferi*, which should be confirmed by a more specific method, such as Western blot [66,67].

Several other infectious diseases that cause arthritis also should be included in the differential diagnosis of bacterial arthritis. Mycobacterial and fungal arthritis are much less common than bacterial arthritis, but during the past decade have reemerged in the context of the worldwide epidemic of HIV infection. Eighty percent of joint infections in England and Wales from 1990 to 1992 were caused by mycobacteria [3]. An indolent chronic monoarthritis is often the only symptom of mycobacterial and fungal arthritis. In both, there is a predilection for weight-bearing joints and the spine. There are usually no systemic symptoms and joint swelling is marked but signs of acute joint inflammation are absent or mild. Synovial fluid cultures are positive in 80% to 90% of tuberculosis and fungal arthritis. In cases of tuberculosis, caseating or noncaseating granulomas are present in 90% of synovial biopsies [68].

Treatment

Once septic arthritis is suspected and the proper samples for microbiologic studies are collected, appropriate antibiotic treatment and adequate joint drainage should begin immediately. Because septic arthritis is so rapidly destructive, however, broad-spectrum antibiotics are usually recommended until culture data are available. The choice of which antibiotic agent to use should be based on the Gram stain and the age and risk factors of the patient. If the initial Gram stain of the synovial fluid shows gram-positive cocci, the drugs of choice are cefazolin, 1 to 2 g intravenously every 8 hours, for community-acquired infections and vancomycin, 30 mg/kg intravenously daily in two divided doses, for hospital or nursing home-acquired infection. The total vancomycin dose should not exceed 2 g/d unless serum levels are monitored [69].

If the initial Gram stain of the synovial fluid shows gram-negative bacilli, therapy should be initiated with a third-generation cephalosporin, such as ceftazidime (1 to 2 g intravenously every 8 hours); ceftriaxone (2 g intravenously every 24 hours); or cefotaxime (2 g intravenously every 8 hours). Ceftazidime should be given with an aminoglycoside, such as gentamicin, when *Pseudomonas aeruginosa* is considered to be a likely pathogen.

Modifications of these initials regimens can be made when the culture and susceptibility results of the synovial fluid or blood culture isolate are available [31].

The duration of antimicrobial therapy cannot be generalized for all patients. It is generally suggested to give parenteral antibiotics for at least 14 days followed by oral therapy for an additional 14 days. Selected patients with infections caused by organisms that are susceptible in vitro to oral agents with high bioavailability, however, such as a fluoroquinolone, can be successfully treated with a short course of 4 to 7 days of parenteral therapy followed by 14 to 21 days of oral therapy. Longer courses of parenteral antimicrobial therapy for up to 3 to 4 weeks may be necessary to cure selected patients with difficult-to-treat pathogens, such as *P aeruginosa* or *Enterobacter* sp [31,69].

In patients with gonococcal infection it is suggested to initiate treatment with an agent known to have activity against strains of *N gonorrhoeae* that are prevalent in the community. Oral therapy can be used in patients who refuse hospitalization or with mild illness, but even in these cases it is advisable that the first dose of therapy should be administered parenterally. Because penicillin-resistant strains of *N gonorrhoeae* are now widespread in both the western and eastern hemispheres, the initial therapy of choice is ceftriaxone (1 g either intravenously or intramuscularly) or another third-generation cephalosporin, such as cefotaxime (1 g intravenously every 8 hours). Quinolones, such as ciprofloxacin (500 mg by mouth twice a day) and ofloxacin (400 mg orally once daily), have shown efficacy and safety in the treatment of both uncomplicated and complicated gonococcal infections. The duration of treatment should be for a minimum of 3 days. Patients with the triad of tenosynovitis, dermatitis, and arthralgia or synovitis who have small or absent joint effusions typically respond dramatically and quickly to treatment. In contrast, patients with purulent arthritis may require therapy for 7 to 14 days. All patients treated for gonococcal infection should also receive a 7-day course of doxycycline (100 mg orally twice a day) to cover the possibility of concurrent infection with *Chlamydia trachomatis* [70].

Most joints can be drained with closed-needle aspiration, although daily aspiration may be necessary. If adequate drainage cannot be obtained by needle aspiration, either arthroscopy or open drainage is necessary. Initial open surgical drainage is usually necessary in hip infections, especially in children. Arthroscopy is often preferred in knee or shoulder infections because of easier irrigation and better visualization of the joint [47,48,71].

After initial treatment, serial synovial fluid analysis should demonstrate that the fluid has become sterile and that the total leukocyte count is decreasing. If not, more definitive joint drainage or an alteration in the antimicrobial regimen should be considered. Infected knees often continue to accumulate synovial fluid and require daily aspiration for 7 to 10 days. Attention should also be paid to joint position and immediate joint mobilization by means of continuous passive motion devices that are necessary to prevent contractures and promote optimal nutrition to the articular cartilage.

Prognosis

The prognosis of bacterial arthritis has not changed much in the past few decades despite more effective antibiotics and improved methods of joint drainage. The outcome is directly related to host factors, such as previous joint damage, the virulence of the infecting organism, and the speed with which adequate treatment is begun. In addition, inflammation and destruction of joints may continue even in those with sterile joints despite effective antimicrobial therapy. This may be caused by the persistence of bacterial DNA within the joint, which has been shown to induce arthritis in an animal model of septic arthritis [31,72].

It is extremely difficult to predict the functional outcome of individual patients during and at the conclusion of treatment. A recent study evaluated 121 adults and 31 children with bacterial arthritis. A poor joint outcome, as defined by the need for amputation, arthrodesis, prosthetic surgery, or severe functional deterioration, occurred in one third of the patients. Adverse prognostic factors included older age, pre-existing joint disease, and an infected joint containing synthetic material. Mortality resulting from bacterial arthritis is dependent on the presence of comorbid conditions, such as advanced age, coexistent renal or cardiac disease, and immunosuppression. The mortality rates in most series have ranged from 10% to 15% [73]. Physicians must always first consider septic arthritis in the evaluation of any patient with acute arthritis.

Summary

Septic arthritis still continues to be a common and serious problem at major urban medical centers and is one of the most rapidly destructive forms of acute arthritis. The yearly incidence of bacterial arthritis varies from 2 to 10 per 100,000 in the general population to 30 to 70 per 100,000 in patients with rheumatoid arthritis and in patients with joint prostheses. Irreversible loss of joint function may develop in up to 50% of the patients. Despite better antimicrobial agents and improved hospital care, the fatality rate for this medical problem has not changed substantially during the past 30 years.

An understanding of the risk factors and the pathogenesis of nongonococcal bacterial arthritis and other forms of infectious arthritis, primarily in the context of a differential diagnosis and treatment, are important to avoid the delay in making a correct diagnosis and to improve the prognosis.

Acknowledgment

I thank Ignacio Garcia-Valladares for his technical assistance in the preparation of this article.

References

[1] Cooper C, Cawley MID. Bacterial arthritis in an English health district: a 10 year review. Ann Rheum Dis 1986;45:458–63.

[2] Bacterial arthritis [editorial]. Lancet 1986;2:721–2.

[3] Ryan MJ, Kavanagh R, Wall PG, et al. Bacterial joint infections in England and Wales: analysis of bacterial isolates over a four year period. Br J Rheum 1997;36:370–3.

[4] Gupta MN, Sturrock RD, Field M. A prospective 2-year study of 75 patients with adult-onset septic arthritis. Rheumatology 2001;40:24–30.

[5] Nade S. Septic arthritis. Best Pract Res Clin Rheumatol 2003;17:183–200.

[6] Goldenberg DL, Chisholm PL, Rice PA. Experimental models of arthritis: morphological and histopathological characterization of the arthritis after intraarticular injections of *Neisseria gonorrhoeae*, *Staphylococcus aureus*, group A Streptococcus, and *Escherichia coli*. J Rheumatol 1983;10:5–11.

[7] Schurman DJ, Mirra J, Ding A, et al. Experimental *E. coli* arthritis in the rabbit: a model of infection and post-infectious inflammatory synovitis. J Rheumatol 1977;4:118–28.

[8] Keefer CS, Parker F Jr, Myers WK. Histological changes in the knee joint in various infections. Arch Pathol 1934;18:199–215.

[9] Goldenberg DL, Cohen AS. Acute infectious arthritis: a review of patients with a non-gonococcal joint infection. Am J Med 1976;60:369–77.

[10] Roca RP, Yoshikawa TT. Primary skeletal infections in heroin users: a chemical characterization, diagnosis and therapy. Clin Orthop 1979;144:238–48.

[11] Mitchell WS, Brooks PM, Stevenson RD, et al. Septic arthritis in patients with rheumatoid disease: a still under-diagnosed complication. J Rheumatol 1976;3:124–33.

[12] Douglas GW, Levin RU, Sokolof L. Infectious arthritis complicating neoplastic disease. N Engl J Med 1964;270:299–302.

[13] Franz A, Webster AD, Furr PM, et al. Mycoplasmal arthritis in patients with primary immunoglobulin deficiency: clinical features and outcome in 18 patients. Br J Rheumatol 1997;36:661–8.

[14] Gardner GC, Weisman MH. Pyarthrosis in patients with rheumatoid arthritis: a report of 13 cases and a review of the literature from the past 40 years. Am J Med 1990;88:503–11.

[15] Blackburn WD, Dunn TL, Alarcon GS. Infection versus disease activity in rheumatoid arthritis: eight years' experience. South Med J 1986;79:1238–41.

[16] Armstrong RW, Bolding F, Joseph R. Septic arthritis following arthroscopy: clinical syndromes and analysis of risk factors. Arthroscopy 1992;8:213–23.

[17] Klein DM, Barbera C, Gray ST, et al. Sensitivity of objective parameters in the diagnosis of pediatric septic hips. Clin Orthop 1997;338:153–9.

[18] Kallio MJ, Unkila-Kallio L, Aalto K, et al. Serum C-reactive protein, erythrocyte sedimentation rate and white blood cell count in septic arthritis of children. Pediatr Infect Dis J 1997;16:411–3.

[19] Wilkins RF, Healy RA, Decker JL. Acute infectious arthritis in the aged and chronically ill. Arch Intern Med 1996;106:354–67.

[20] Brucellosis in Britain [editorial]. BMJ 1984;289:817.

[21] Hasley JP, Reebak JS, Barnes CG. A decade of skeletal tuberculosis. Ann Rheum Dis 1982;41:7–10.

[22] Niall DM, Murphy PG, Fogarty EE, et al. Puncture wound related pseudomonas infections of the foot in children. Ir J Med Sci 1997;166:98–101.

[23] Baghai M, Osmon DR, Wolk DM, et al. Fatal sepsis in a patient with rheumatoid arthritis treated with etanercept. Mayo Clin Proc 2001;76:653–6.

[24] Kaur PP, Derk CT, Chatterji M, et al. Septic arthritis caused by *Actinobacillus ureae* in a patient with rheumatoid arthritis receiving anti-tumor necrosis factor-alpha therapy. J Rheumatol 2004;31:1663–5.

[25] Rachapalli S, O'Daunt S. Septic arthritis due to *Listeria monocytogenes* in a patient receiving etanercept. Arthritis Rheum 2005;52:987.

[26] Katsarolis I, Tsiodras S, Panagopoulos P, et al. Septic arthritis due to *Salmonella enteritidis* associated with infliximab use. Scand J Infect Dis 2005;37:304–6.

[27] Shaffer MF, Bennett GA. The passage of type III rabbit virulent pneumococci from the vascular system into joints and certain other body cavities. J Exp Med 1939;70:293–302.

[28] Rigdon RH. Pathogenesis of arthritis following intravenous injection of staphylococci in the adult rabbit. Am J Surg 1942;55:553–61.

[29] Lewis GW, Cluff LE. Synovitis in rabbits during bacteremia and vaccination. Bull Johns Hopkins Hosp 1965;116:175–90.

[30] Goldenberg DL, Reed JI. Bacterial arthritis. N Engl J Med 1985;312:764–71.

[31] Goldbenberg DL. Septic arthritis. Lancet 1998;351:197–202.

[32] Stevens KJ, Theologis T, McNally EG. Imaging of plant-thorn synovitis. Skeletal Radiol 2000;29:605–8.

[33] De Champs C, Le Seaux S, Dubost JJ, et al. Isolation of *Pantoea agglomerans* in two cases of septic monoarthritis after plant thorn and wood silver injuries. J Clin Microbiol 2000;38:460–1.

[34] Gredlein CM, Silverman ML, Downey MS. Polymicrobial septic arthritis due to *Clostridium* species: case report and review. Clin Infect Dis 2000;30:590–4.

[35] Daivajna S, Jones A, O'Malley M, et al. Unilateral septic arthritis of a lumbar facet joint secondary to acupuncture treatment: a case report. Acupunct Med 2004;22:152–5.

[36] Tong DC, Rothwell BR. Antibiotic prophylaxis in dentistry: a review and practice recommendations. JAMA 2000;131:366–74.

[37] Stinchfield FE, Bigliani LU, Neu HC, et al. Late hematogenous infection of total joint replacement. J Bone Joint Surg 1980;62:1345–50.

[38] Poss R, Thornhill TS, Ewald FC, et al. Factors influencing the incidence and outcome of infection following total joint arthroplasty. Clin Orthop 1984;182:117–26.

[39] Gray RG, Tenenbaum J, Gottlieb NL. Local corticosteroid injection treatment in rheumatic disorders. Semin Arthritis Rheum 1981;10:231–54.

[40] Adams WG, Deaver KA, Cochi SL, et al. Decline of childhood *Haemophilus influenza* type b (Hib) disease in the Hib vaccine era. JAMA 1993;269:221–6.

[41] Kaandorp CJ, van Schaardenburg D, Krijnen P, et al. Risk factors for septic arthritis in patients with joint disease: a prospective study. Arthritis Rheum 1995;38:1819–25.

[42] O'Dell JR. Anticytokine therapy: a new era in the treatment of rheumatoid arthritis? N Engl J Med 1999;340:310–2.

[43] Lipsky PE, van der Heijde DM, St. Clair EW, et al. Infliximab and methotrexate in the treatment of rheumatoid arthritis: anti-tumor necrosis factor trial in rheumatoid arthritis with concomitant therapy study group. N Engl J Med 2000;343:1594–602.

[44] Keane J, Gershon S, Wise RP, et al. Tuberculosis associated with infliximab, a tumor necrosis factor alpha-neutralizing agent. N Engl J Med 2001;345:1098–104.

[45] Rompalo AM, Hook EW III, Roberts PL. The acute arthritis-dermatitis syndrome: the changing importance of *Neisseria gonorrhoeae* and *Neisseria meningitides*. Arch Intern Med 1987;147:281–3.

[46] Baker DG, Schumacher HR Jr. Acute monoarthritis. N Engl J Med 1993;329:1013–20.

[47] Morgan DS, Fisher D, Merianos A, et al. An 18 year clinical review of septic arthritis from tropical Australia. Epidemiol Infect 1996;117:243–328.

[48] Le Dantec L, Maury F, Flipo RM, et al. Peripheral pyogenic arthritis: a study of one hundred seventy-nine cases. Revue Rheum 1996;63:103–10.

[49] Zimmerman B III, Mikolich DJ, Lally EV. Septic sacroiliities. Semin Arthritis Rheum 1996; 26:592–604.

[50] Dubost JJ, Fis I, Denis P, et al. Polyarticular septic arthritis. Medicine (Baltimore) 1993;72: 296–310.

[51] O'Brien JP, Goldenberg DL, Rice PA. Disseminated gonococcal infection: a prospective analysis of 49 patients and a review of pathophysiology and immune mechanisms. Medicine (Baltimore) 1983;62:395–406.

[52] Wise CM, Morris CR, Wasilauskas BL, et al. Gonococcal arthritis in an era of increasing penicillin resistance: presentation and outcomes in 41 recent cases (1985–1991). Arch Intern Med 1994;154:2690–5.

[53] Louie JS, Liebling MR. The polymerase chain reaction in infectious and post-infectious arthritis: a review. Rheum Dis Clin North Am 1998;24:227–36.

[54] Weston VC, Jones AC, Bradbury N, et al. Clinical features and outcome of septic arthritis in a single UK Health District 1982–1991. Ann Rheum Dis 1999;58:214–9.

[55] Shmerling RH, Delbanco TL, Tosteson ANA, et al. Synovial fluid tests: what should be ordered? JAMA 1990;264:1009–14.

[56] McCarty DJ. Synovial fluid. In: Koopman WJ, editor. Arthritis and allied conditions a textbook of rheumatology, vol. 1. 14th edition. Philadelphia: Lippincott Williams and Wilkins; 2001. p. 83.

[57] Von Essen R. Culture of joint specimens in bacterial arthritis: impact of blood culture bottle utilization. Scand J Rheumatol 1997;26:293–300.

[58] Kortekangas P, Aro HT, Lehtonen OP. Synovial fluid culture and blood culture in acute arthritis: a multi-case report in 90 patients. Scand J Rheumatol 1995;24:44–7.

[59] Esterhai JL Jr, Gelb I. Adult septic arthritis. Orthop Clin North Am 1991;22:503–14.

[60] Pinals RS. Polyarthritis and fever. N Engl J Med 1994;330:769–74.

[61] Post JC, Ehrlich GD. The impact of the polymerase chain reaction in clinical medicine. JAMA 2000;283:1544–6.

[62] Mariani BD, Martín DS, Levine MJ, et al. The Coventry Award: polymerase chain reaction detection of bacterial infection in total knee arthroplasty. Clin Orthop 1996;331:11–22.

[63] Forrester DM, Feske WI. Imaging of infectious arthritis. Semin Roentgenol 1996;31:239–49.

[64] Ilahi OA, Swarna U, Hamill RJ, et al. Concomitant crystal and septic arthritis. Orthopaedics 1996;19:613–7.

[65] Singleton JD, West SG, Nordstrom DM. Pseudoseptic arthritis complicating rheumatoid arthritis: a report of six cases. J Rheumatol 1991;18:1319–22.

[66] Steere AC, Malawista SE, Snydman DR, et al. Lyme arthritis: an epidemic of oligoarticular arthritis in children and adults in three Connecticut communities. Arthritis Rheum 1977;20: 7–17.

[67] Steere AC. Lyme disease. N Engl J Med 2001;345:115–25.

[68] Bocanegra TS. Mycobacterial, Brucella, fungal and parasitic arthritis. In: Klippel JH, Dieppe PA, editors. Rheumatology, vol. 2. 2nd edition. London: Mosby International; 1998. p. 6.

[69] Hamed KA, Tam JY, Prober CG. Pharmacokinetic optimization of the treatment of septic arthritis. Clin Pharmacokinet 1996;21:156–63.

[70] Mahowald ML. Gonococcal arthritis. In: Klippel JH, Dieppe PA, editors. Rheumatology, vol. 2. 2nd edition. London: Mosby International; 1998. p. 6.

[71] Ho G Jr. How best to drain an infected joint: will we ever know for certain? J Rheumatol 1993;20:2001–3.

[72] Deng GM, Nilsson IM, Verdrengh M, et al. Intra-articularly localized bacterial DNA containing CpG motifs induces arthritis. Nat Med 1999;5:702–5.

[73] Kaandorp CJ, Krijnen P, Moens HJ, et al. The outcome of bacterial arthritis: a prospective community-based study. Arthritis Rheum 1997;40:884–92.

ELSEVIER
SAUNDERS

Infect Dis Clin N Am
20 (2006) 789–825

INFECTIOUS
DISEASE CLINICS
OF NORTH AMERICA

Imaging of Osteomyelitis:
Current Concepts

Carlos Pineda, MD[a],*, Angélica Vargas, MD[b],
Alfonso Vargas Rodríguez, MD[c]

[a]Instituto Nacional de Rehabilitación, Avenida México-Xochimilco No. 289,
Arenal de Guadalupe, Tlalpan, Mexico City, 14389, Mexico
[b]Rheumatology Department, Instituto Nacional de Cardiología Ignacio Chávez,
Juan Badiano No. 1, Sección XVI, Tlalpan, Mexico City, 14080, Mexico
[c]Centro Integral de Diagnóstico y Tratamiento, Hospital Medica Sur,
Puente de Piedra No. 150, Toriello Guerra, Tlalpan, Mexico City, Mexico

Osteomyelitis is defined as infection in bone. The root word osteon
(bone) and myelo (marrow) are combined with -itis (inflammation) to define
the clinical state in which bone is infected with microorganisms. It is a
heterogeneous disease in its pathophysiology, clinical presentation, and
management. Progressive destruction of bone and the formation of sequestra are characteristics of this disease. The clinical diagnosis in the late stages
is achieved easily; an accurate early diagnosis is more challenging. Prompt
and precise diagnosis can determine morbidity and extent of the infection.
Imaging techniques play a key role in diagnosis and follow-up.

Adult osteomyelitis most commonly arises from open fractures, diabetic
foot infections (Fig. 1), or the surgical treatment of closed injuries [1]. In
children, osteomyelitis is one of the more common invasive bacterial infections leading to hospitalization and prolonged antibiotic administration.
Single or multiple bones can be infected; involvement of multiple osseous
sites seems to be particularly common in infants (Fig. 2). Most cases of osteomyelitis in children arise hematogenously, occurring characteristically in
the metaphysis of long bones, such as the femur, tibia, and humerus [2]. Preceding blunt trauma to the site of bone infection is common, but the role of
trauma in the pathogenesis of osteomyelitis in children remains unclear [3].

Currently, there are different classification systems to describe osteomyelitis. Lew and Waldvogel [4] classify cases as either hematogenous or

* Corresponding author.
E-mail address: carpineda@yahoo.com (C. Pineda).

0891-5520/06/$ - see front matter © 2006 Elsevier Inc. All rights reserved.
doi:10.1016/j.idc.2006.09.009   *id.theclinics.com*

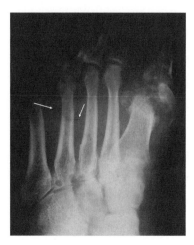

Fig. 1. Foot infection in a patient who has diabetes mellitus and gout. The radiograph reveals soft tissue swelling, osteolysis, osteosclerosis, and fragmentation. Radiolucent areas within the soft tissues are related to the presence of gas (*arrows*).

secondary to a contiguous focus of infection. The latter may be further subdivided as with or without vascular insufficiency. Either hematogenous or contiguous focus osteomyelitis may be further classified as acute or chronic. An alternative classification system proposed by Cierny and colleagues [5] considers the quality of the host, the bone's anatomic nature, and treatment and prognostic factors, resulting in four anatomic disease types (stages 1–4) and three physiologic host categories (A, B, and C) (Box 1).

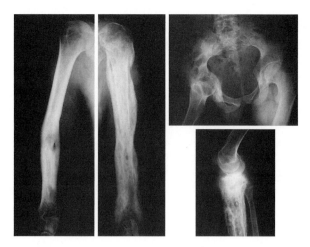

Fig. 2. Chronic multifocal osteomyelitis in a 23-year-old man who developed fever, upper and lower extremity pain, and progressive limp since he was 16 years old. Radiographs reveal multiple sites of osteomyelitis characterized by diffuse periostitis, sequestra, and involucrum formation. Contamination from a contiguous source of infection resulted in right hip septic arthritis.

Box 1. Cierny-Mader staging system for osteomyelitis

Anatomic type
   Stage 1: Medullary osteomyelitis
   Stage 2: Superficial osteomyelitis
   Stage 3: Localized osteomyelitis
   Stage 4: Diffuse osteomyelitis

Physiologic class
A Host
   Normal host

B Host
   Systemic compromise (Bs)
   Local compromise (Bl)
   Systemic and local compromise (Bls)

C Host
   Treatment worse than the disease

Systemic or local factors that affect immune surveillance, metabolism, and local vascularity
Systemic (Bs)
   Malnutrition
   Renal, hepatic failure
   Diabetes mellitus
   Chronic hypoxia
   Immune disease
   Malignancy
   Extremes of age
   Immunosuppression or neuropathy
   Immune deficiency

Local (Bl)
   Chronic lymphedema
   Venous stasis
   Major vessel compromise
   Arteritis
   Extensive scarring
   Radiation fibrosis
   Small vessel disease
   Complete loss of sensation
   Tobacco abuse

The traditional Waldvogel's system has the advantage of greater simplicity and familiarity, whereas the Cierny-Mader system is both specific and dynamic, suggesting treatment and altering therapy depending on patient response or change in status.

The clinical stages of osteomyelitis frequently are designated as acute, subacute, and chronic [6]. This designation does not imply that definitive divisions exist between one stage and another, nor does it signify that all cases of osteomyelitis progress through each of these phases. The relatively abrupt onset of clinical symptoms and signs during the initial stage of infection indicates clearly the acute osteomyelitic phase; if this acute phase passes without complete elimination of infection, subacute or chronic osteomyelitis can become apparent. The transition from acute to subacute and chronic osteomyelitis can indicate that therapeutic measures have been inadequate or inappropriate or that the organisms are especially resistant to accepted modes of therapy.

The organisms and special situations

The distribution of osteomyelitis is influenced dramatically by the age of the patient, the specific causative organism, and the presence or absence of any underlying disorder or situation. In infants and children, acute osteomyelitis most commonly is caused by hematogenous spread. *Staphylococcus aureus* is the most common causative agent, followed by β-hemolytic streptococcus, *Streptococcus pneumoniae*, *Escherichia coli*, and *Pseudomonas aeruginosa* [7,8]. The incidence of infection by *Haemophilus influenzae* has declined dramatically because of widespread HIB vaccination [8–10]. Although any bone can be affected, the most commonly involved are the metaphyses of long bones, especially the distal femur and proximal tibia, followed by the distal humerus, distal radius, proximal femur, and proximal humerus [11]. *S aureus* is also the most prevalent infecting organism later in life in osteomyelitis of the mature skeleton, and Gram-negative rods are found in the elderly. Fungal osteomyelitis is a complication of catheter-related fungemia, the use of illicit drugs contaminated by *Candida* sp, and prolonged neutropenia. *P aeruginosa* can be isolated from injectable drug users and from patients who have urinary catheters in place for long periods of time.

The most common form of musculoskeletal tuberculosis is tuberculous spondylitis. Isolated extraspinal bone infection by *Mycobacterium tuberculosis* is less common. The most frequent form of musculoskeletal involvement, excluding the spine, is within muscles and soft tissues [12].

Osteomyelitis is a relatively uncommon complication of HIV-positive patients. Hematogenous dissemination of *S aureus*, however, is the most common source of infection in these individuals, especially in intravenous drug abusers, but *Salmonella* in these patients also has been reported. In a series of 560 HIV-positive patients, 12 cases of osteomyelitis were caused by either *S aureus* or *Salmonella* infection [13]. Other bacteria, such as *Neisseria gonorrhoeae* [14], *Cryptococcus neoformans*, and *Nocardia asteroids* [15] also have been reported. All bones can be affected, in addition to the spine and vertebral bodies [15–17]. In these patients, some uncommon forms of bone infections, such as bacillary angiomatosis from an unusual bacillus (*Bartonella henselae*) [18] and *M tuberculosis* have been documented [19–21].

Terminology

Infective osteitis indicates contamination of the bone cortex. Infective periostitis implies contamination of the periosteal cloak that surrounds the bone. Descriptive terms have been applied to certain radiographic and pathologic characteristics that are encountered during the course of osteomyelitis. A sequestrum (Fig. 3) represents a segment of necrotic bone that is separated from living bone by granulation tissue. Sequestra may reside in the marrow for protracted periods of time, harboring living organisms that have the capability of evoking an acute flare-up of the infection. An involucrum denotes a layer of living bone that has formed about dead bone; it can become perforated by tracts. An opening in the involucrum is termed cloaca (Fig. 4). Tracts leading to the skin surface from the bone are termed sinuses, although they sometimes are described as fistulae. A bone abscess (Brodiés abscess) is a sharply delineated focus of infection. It is lined by granulation tissue and frequently is surrounded by eburnated bone [22].

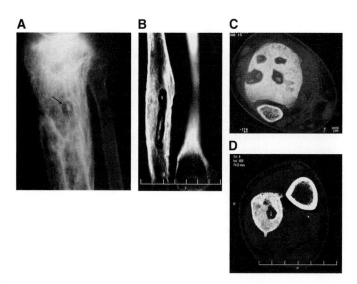

Fig. 3. Chronic osteomyelitis: sequestration. Routine radiography and CT in different patients. (*A*) In this tibia, chronic osteomyelitis is associated with a radiodense sharply marginated focus within a lucent cavity (*arrow*). (*B*) Coronal reformatted image. (*C, D*) Transaxial images. CT scanning can be used to identify sequestered bone as in these tibiae. (*Courtesy of* Sergio Fernández Tapia, MD, Tampico, Mexico.)

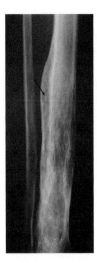

Fig. 4. Hematogenous osteomyelitis of a tubular bone in the adult. An involucrum is defined as a layer of living bone that has formed about the dead bone. It can surround and eventually merge with the parent bone. In this case, radiograph shows extensive periostitis of the tibia surrounding sclerotic bone (*arrow*). (*Courtesy of* Sergio Fernández Tapia, MD, Tampico, Mexico.)

Pathogenesis

Acute osteomyelitis presents as a suppurative infection accompanied by edema, vascular congestion, and small-vessel thrombosis. As the infection spreads within the intramedullary cavity, increased pressure causes extension to the cortex by Havers and Volkmann's canals with subsequent spread to the subperiosteal space and through the periosteum into the adjacent soft tissues. In osteomyelitis, elevation of the periosteum is prominent in infants and children (immature skeleton), whereas in adults, the periosteum is more firmly attached to the bone, resulting in less elevation [23]. When both the medullary and the periosteal blood supplies are compromised, large areas of sequestra may be formed [24]. The coexistence of infected, nonviable tissues and an ineffective host response leads to the chronicity of this disease. Pathologic features of chronic osteomyelitis are the presence of necrotic bone, the formation of new bone, and the exudation of polymorphonuclear leukocytes joined by large numbers of lymphocytes, histiocytes, and occasionally plasma cells [25]. The involucrum often is perforated by openings through which pus may track into the surrounding soft tissues and eventually drain to the skin surfaces, forming a chronic sinus.

The clinical picture of osteomyelitis may be confusing, and laboratory findings, including an elevated erythrocyte sedimentation rate and leukocytosis, are nonspecific for bone infection in its early stage or can even be normal. Serial blood cultures are positive in 32% to 60% of cases [26–28]. Cultures of blood and material aspirated by needle of the involved bone yield positive findings in up to 87% of cases [29,30], and the yield from subperiosteal aspiration approaches 90% [8,31]. Clinical presentation of pediatric osteomyelitis may be even more elusive. Infection in the neonate and infant is usually clinically silent. Toddlers may present with limping, pseudoparalysis, or pain on passive movement. The earliest soft tissue changes include swelling, heat, and redness [32].

Because delay in the treatment of osteomyelitis significantly diminishes the cure rate and increases the rate of complications and morbidity, several imaging modalities have been used for early detection of osteomyelitis, including conventional radiography, several nuclear medicine or scintigraphic techniques, CT, MRI, and ultrasonography (US). Although these infections often are suspected clinically, imaging is used to confirm the presumed clinical diagnosis and to provide information regarding the exact site and extent of the infectious process. In musculoskeletal infections, the diagnostic imaging evaluation and the resulting information can be extremely helpful to the clinician planning medical or surgical treatment.

Imaging findings

Conventional radiography

Plain radiographs are the first step in the imaging assessment of osteomyelitis because they may suggest the correct diagnosis, exclude other pathology, or provide clues for other pathologic conditions. It takes from 10 to 21 days for an osseous lesion to become visible on conventional radiographs, because a 30% to 50% reduction of bone density must occur before radiographic change is apparent. It is the insensitivity of this technique in the early diagnosis of bone infection that has prompted the use of alternative methods, such as scintigraphy and MR imaging, for the prompt recognition of osteomyelitis [22].

Radiographic evidence of significant osseous destruction in hematogenous pyogenic osteomyelitis is delayed for a period of days to weeks. Initial and subtle radiographic changes in the soft tissues may appear within 3 days of bacterial contamination of bone; however, focal deep soft tissue swelling in the metaphyseal region of infants and children may be the first important radiographic sign. Such swelling, which is temporally related to the vascular changes and edema of the early osteomyelitic process, results in displacement of the lucent tissue planes from the underlying bone. In the neonate, this displacement is difficult to detect because of the lack of subcutaneous fat and the presence of poorly defined fascial planes. A few days after the appearance of the initial soft tissue changes, muscle swelling and obliteration of the soft tissue planes can be observed. The deep muscles and soft tissues are affected first, followed later by involvement of the more superficial muscles and subcutaneous tissue [22].

In pyogenic infection, radiographically evident bone destruction and periostitis can be delayed for 1 to 2 weeks after intraosseous lodgment of the organisms. At all early stages, the degree of bony involvement that is visible on the radiograph is considerably less than is evident on pathologic examination. Eventually, large destructive lesions become evident on the radiograph (Fig. 5). In the child, these lesions appear as enlarging, poorly defined lucent shadows of the metaphysis surrounded by varying amounts of eburnation; the lucent lesions can extend to the growth plate and, on rare occasions, may violate it (Fig. 6). In addition, destruction progresses horizontally, reaching the cortex, and periostitis follows.

In the infant, the epiphyses are unossified or only partially ossified, so that radiographic recognition of epiphyseal destruction can be extremely difficult. Metaphyseal lucent lesions, periostitis, and a joint effusion are helpful radiographic clues. In the adult, soft tissue alterations are more difficult to detect on radiographic examination. Epiphyseal, metaphyseal, and diaphyseal osseous destruction create radiolucent areas of varying size, which are associated with mild periostitis. Cortical resorption can be identified as endosteal scalloping, intracortical lucent regions or tunneling, and poorly defined subperiosteal bony defects or gaps.

Single or multiple radiolucent abscesses can be evident during subacute or chronic stages of osteomyelitis. These abscesses now are defined as circumscribed lesions showing predilection for (but not confinement to) the ends of tubular bones; they are found characteristically in subacute pyogenic osteomyelitis, usually of Staphylococcal origin. Brodie's abscesses (Fig. 7) are especially common in children, more typically boys. In this age group, they appear in the metaphysis, particularly that of the distal or proximal portions of the tibia. Abscesses vary from less than 1 cm to more than

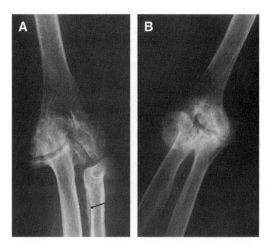

Fig. 5. Variola (Smallpox) osteomyelitis and septic arthritis. AP (*A*) and oblique (*B*) views of the elbow. The presence of symmetric changes, epiphyseal extension and destruction, predilection for the elbow, and extensive diaphyseal osteoperiostitis of tubular bones (*arrow*) suggest the diagnosis of osteomyelitis variolosa.

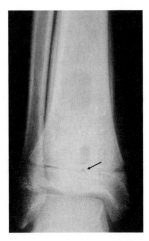

Fig. 6. In this child who had pain and swelling of the ankle, initial radiographs at the time of clinical presentation do not reveal osseous destruction. Four weeks later, a lytic metaphyseal focus in the distal tibia readily is apparent. It extends to the growth cartilage. The presence of multilayered type of periostitis is also seen. (*Courtesy of* Sergio Fernández Tapia, MD, Tampico, Mexico.)

4 cm in diameter. The wall of the abscess is lined by inflammatory granulation tissue that is surrounded by spongy bone eburnation. The fluid in the abscess may be purulent or mucoid; bacteriologic examination of the fluid may or may not reveal the infecting organisms. Closed needle biopsy or aspiration guided by imaging techniques can be useful in establishing

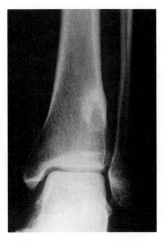

Fig. 7. Brodie's abscess. Anteroposterior radiograph of the tibia. Observe the elongated radiolucent lesion with surrounding sclerosis not extending to the closing growth plate. (*Courtesy of* Sergio Fernández Tapia, MD, Tampico, Mexico.)

a bacteriologic diagnosis of osteomyelitis. Material should be obtained for both histologic diagnosis and appropriate tissue culture (Fig. 8). Radiographs outline radiolucency with adjacent sclerosis. This lucent region commonly is located in the metaphysis, where it may connect with the growth plate by a tortuous channel. A circular or elliptic radiolucent lesion without calcification that is smaller or larger than 2 cm is characteristic of a cortical abscess, a circular lucent area with or without calcification smaller than 2 cm is typical of an osteoid osteoma, and a linear lucent shadow without calcification is characteristic of a stress fracture [22]. In any skeletal location, CT or MR imaging can be used to better assess the extent of the abscess and any signs of its reactivation. Radiographic detection of this channel is important; identification of a metaphyseal defect connected to the growth plate by such a tract ensures the diagnosis of osteomyelitis. When an abscess is located in the cortex, its radiographic appearance, consisting of a lucent lesion with surrounding sclerosis and periostitis, simulates that of an osteoid osteoma or a stress fracture.

The periosteal reaction (PR) of bone deserves a special mentioning. It is observed in a wide variety of benign, malignant, and systemic conditions, and in periods of normal growth and in response to injury. PR can be classified broadly as lamellated (linear-single or multiple), solid, spiculated, Codman's triangle, and expanded shell, based on radiographic appearances. The differential diagnosis of multiple layered PR (onion-skin image) includes osteomyelitis, Ewing's sarcoma, osteosarcoma, hypertrophic osteoarthropathy, and Langerhans cell histiocytosis [33]. When an underlying process persists, the matrix between multiple lamellations or between a single layer and the cortex eventually ossifies, giving rise to a continuous, solid

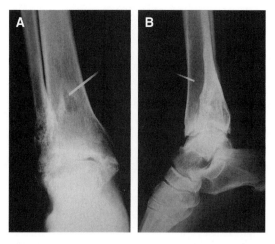

Fig. 8. Distal tibial bone biopsy and aspiration. AP (*A*) and lateral (*B*) views. Closed needle biopsy and aspiration accomplished with fluoroscopic guidance confirm the presence of *S aureus* osteomyelitis.

layer of periosteal new bone. Solid PR is associated with osteomyelitis, LCH, chondroblastoma, and healing fractures. Codman's triangle typically is associated with osteosarcoma and osteomyelitis. This cuff of reactive bone at the extreme ends of a lesion represents periosteal elevation by pus, hemorrhage, or the leading edge of a neoplastic lesion [33].

In the axial skeleton, hematogenous spread of infection frequently leads to a focus in the anterior subchondral regions of the vertebral body adjacent to the intervertebral disc. Extension to the ventral surface of the vertebra can be associated with infection of the adjacent longitudinal ligaments, but more typically discal perforation soon ensues. At this stage, radiographs may be entirely normal. Soon (1 to 3 weeks), however, a decrease in height of the intervertebral disc is accompanied by loss of normal definition of the subchondral bone plate and enlarging destructive foci within the neighboring vertebral body. The combination of rapid loss of intervertebral disc height and adjacent lysis of bone is most suggestive of an infectious process. With further spread of infection, progressive destruction of the vertebral body and the intervertebral disc becomes evident, and the process soon contaminates the adjacent vertebra. Such involvement of two contiguous vertebral bodies almost uniformly is associated with transdiscal infection and rarely is the result of multicentric involvement.

After a variable period (10 to 12 weeks), regenerative changes appear in the bone with sclerosis or eburnation. The osteosclerotic response is variable in severity and has been used in the past as a helpful sign in differentiating pyogenic from tuberculous infection. Although such sclerosis is indeed common in pyogenic (nontuberculous) spondylitis, it also may be evident in tuberculosis, particularly in black patients. Furthermore, some people who have pyogenic spinal infection do not reveal significant eburnation, particularly when symptoms and signs have not been of long duration, so that using the presence or absence of bony sclerosis as a foolproof way of differentiating tuberculous and nontuberculous spondylitis can lead to an erroneous diagnosis. More helpful in this differentiation is a combination of findings that strongly indicates tuberculous spondylitis (Fig. 9), including the presence of a slowly progressive vertebral process with preservation of intervertebral discs, subligamentous spread of infection with erosion of anterior vertebral margins, large and calcified soft tissue abscesses, and the absence of severe bony eburnation.

A radiographic–pathologic correlation of osteomyelitis is summarized in Table 1.

The sensitivity for plain film radiography has been reported to range from 43% to 75%, and the specificity from 75% to 83% [24,34–37]. Radiographs, when positive, are helpful, but negative radiographic findings are unreliable to exclude the diagnosis of osteomyelitis in patients who have violated bone. In these situations, radiographic findings are nonspecific, being diagnostic in as few as 3% to 5% of culture-positive cases [25,38].

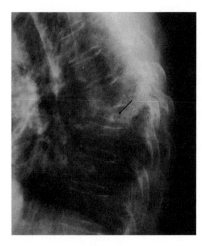

Fig. 9. Tuberculous spondylitis: Vertebra plana and kyphosis. In this patient, a wafer-like remnant of the infected vertebral body can be seen (*arrow*). Abnormal kyphosis is present. The adjacent vertebrae appear normal.

Sinography

Opacification of a sinus tract can produce important information that influences the choice of therapy. In this technique, a small flexible catheter is placed within a cutaneous opening. Retrograde injection of contrast material defines the course and extent of the sinus tract and its possible communications with neighboring structures (Fig. 10). Sinography may be combined with CT for better delineation of the sinus tracts.

Conventional tomography

The major role of this technique in osteomyelitis is the detection of sequestra in cases of chronic osteomyelitis, as these pieces of necrotic bone can be obscured by the surrounding osseous abnormalities on conventional radiography. Because the presence of pieces of sequestered bone suggests activity of the infectious process, their detection is important to the infectious diseases and orthopedic specialists to guide the therapeutic options (Fig. 11).

Radionuclide techniques

Bone scintigraphy has been used widely for examination of patients suspected of having osteomyelitis. All nuclear medicine modalities use one or more of the stages of the functional cataract of inflammation or infection, which are activated as a part of the defense mechanisms of the host.

Bone scan

The bone scan typically becomes positive within 24 to 48 hours after the onset of symptoms [39,40]. The first examination of choice is a three-phase

Table 1
Radiographic–pathologic correlation in osteomyelitis

Radiographic abnormality	Pathologic abnormality
Soft tissue swelling with obliteration of tissue planes and mass formation	Vascular changes, edema of soft tissues, and infectious penetration of periosteum
Periostitis and involucrum	Subperiosteal abscess formation with lifting of the periosteum and bone formation
Increasing lysis, cortical lucency	Infection in haversian and Volkmann's canals of cortex
Osteoporosis, bone lysis, and cortical lucency	Infection in medullary space, haversian and Volkmann's canals with abscess formation and trabecular destruction
Single or multiple radiolucent cortical or medullary lesions with surrounding sclerosis	Localized cortical and medullary abscess
Sequestration	Thrombosis of metaphyseal vessels and interruption of periosteal vessels with cortical necrosis
Sinus tracts	External migration of dead pieces of cortex with breakdown of skin and subcutaneous tissue

Data from Resnick D, Niwayama G. Osteomyelitis, septic arthritis and soft tissue infection: mechanisms and situations. In: Resnick D, editor. Diagnosis of bone and joint disorders. 3rd edition. Philadelphia: WB Saunders; 1995. p. 2335.

bone scan. This examination is readily performed after injection of 25 mCi of methylene diphosphonate. The patient is imaged with a nuclear medicine gamma camera. The initial or flow phase is acquired at a rate of 2 seconds per frame, followed by blood pool phase images approximately 5 to 10 minutes after injection. Delayed static images of the area of interest are performed 3 hours after injection. Abnormal findings for osteomyelitis typically include increased flow activity, blood pool activity, and positive uptake on 3-hour images. The intensity of uptake becomes more focal and intense at the area of interest, and when positive on all three phases is highly sensitive for osteomyelitis (73% to 100% sensitivity) [40–43]. In a recent metaanalysis the pooled sensitivity reached 61% but the specificity was the lowest (25%) compared with leukocyte scintigraphy and MRI [44].

This technique has high sensitivity for osteomyelitis and can differentiate cellulitis from osteomyelitis reliably when no complicating conditions are present. Cellulitis is only positive on the first two phases and has a normal (not increased) uptake on the 3-hour images. The specificity for osteomyelitis decreases, however, when other conditions are present simultaneously. These include recent trauma, surgery, placement of orthopedic devices, or diabetes [45–47]. In these conditions the specificity of a three-phase bone scan decreases; most reports are between 73% and 79% but have been reported as low as 38%. These complicating conditions may cause a positive bone

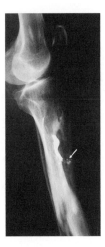

Fig. 10. Sinography. Chronic osteomyelitis. A small flexible catheter was placed within a cuta-neous opening (*arrow*). Retrograde opacification of a sinus tract confirmed the communication with an abscess in the midportion of the tibia.

scan but the findings are of lower specificity. Further imaging generally is re-quired to assess more accurately possible osteomyelitis in these conditions.

Gallium scan

Infection also has been identified by injection of 5 mCi of gallium [48]. The mechanisms that favor the increased uptake of radiogallium are not

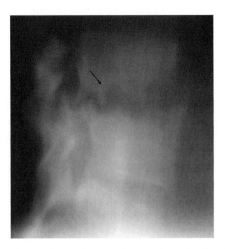

Fig. 11. Conventional tomography of the spine in a patient who has *S aureus* endocarditis. A lateral tomogram of L4–L5 region shows a large osteolytic area involving the disc space and contiguous vertebral bodies, with surrounding sclerosis (*arrow*).

fully understood, but are probably related to gallium attachment to serum proteins, particularly transferrin produced by leucocytes and siderophores produced by infected microorganisms. This product has improved specificity compared with the three-phase bone scan alone [46,49]. Imaging typically is performed 48 hours after injection but occasionally can be performed at 24 hours. Gallium has occasional false positives from fractures and tumor uptake, and has marked excretion through the gastrointestinal tract. Although more specific than a three-phase bone scan, image quality suffers slightly compared with a three-phase bone scan and takes longer. Alternatively, the bone scan has the relative advantage of being very sensitive and, if negative, effectively excludes the diagnosis of osteomyelitis. The reported sensitivity for gallium scan has ranged from 25% to 80%, with a specificity of 67% [50–52].

A gallium scan can be obtained in conjunction with technetium (Tc) scan in the same patient, and the information that is obtained may be more useful than that of either examination alone [53]. After administration of Tc agents, scans can be obtained within a few hours, documenting the presence of an inflammatory process; optimal scanning with gallium, however, may necessitate a delay of 10 to 24 hours. Gallium scans may reveal abnormal accumulation in patients who have active osteomyelitis when Tc scans reveal decreased activity ("cold" lesions) or perhaps normal activity. Furthermore, gallium accumulation seems to correlate more closely with activity in cases of osteomyelitis than does Tc uptake [53].

White blood cell scan

The white blood cell scan (WBCS) was done originally with Indium[111]-labeled white blood cells and more recently with ^{99m}Tc hexamethylpropyleneamine oxime (HMPAO)–labeled white cells [54]. The indium product has a higher radiation dose to the patient, takes 24 hours to perform, and the images have extensive noise. This product was available in clinical trials earlier than the HMPAO WBCS with a reported sensitivity of more than 90% and a specificity of 78% [50]. This technique was shown to be useful in complicated and uncomplicated patients. Similar sensitivity and specificity were found with the HMPAO technique. In an effort to improve the specificity of bone imaging, complementary scintigraphy may be performed using autologous polymorphonuclear neutrophils (PMN) labeled with ^{99m}Tc HMPAO. The diagnosis relies in the congruent spatial distribution of the images in both methods. In some instances, however, there is an uncommon scintigraphic pattern represented by absence of uptake of ^{99m}Tc HMPAO PMN. In a retrospective study by Galpérine and coworkers [55], 17 cases of cold ^{99m}Tc HMPAO PMN scintigraphy but with positive ^{99}Tc HMDP and proven bacterial orthopedic infected hardware were analyzed. All the patients had a cold image over the hip and the causative agent was *Staphylococcus*. There is no reasonable explanation for the phenomenon; the authors suggest that in the case of cold HMPAO in conjunction with positive HMDP, the former should be considered as a false negative and require further study. The advantages of the Tc WBCS that make it preferable for clinical use include same day study and result, lower radiation dose, and better image quality and resolution.

All these studies require withdrawal of 50 mL of blood and separation of the white cell component from the rest of the blood with radiolabeling of the white blood cells. After reconstitution of the radiolabeled cells in saline, the cells are reinjected into the patient. Labeled leukocyte studies by in vitro method using ^{111}In-oxine, ^{99m}Tc HMPAO, and ^{99m}Tc-stannous colloid have the inherent limitation of personnel safety: risks of infection and cross-contamination. To overcome these problems, attempts have been made to target leukocytes directly by in vivo labeling techniques. There are several receptors present on the leukocytes and the granulocytes that can be targeted with suitable ligands, such as monoclonal antibodies, antibody fragments, or peptides. Currently there is ongoing investigation under these categories with anti-NCA90-Fab (Leukoscan), murine MoAb IgG$_1$ (Granuloscient; CISBio International), anti-CD15 antigen (Neutrospect, ^{99m}Tc-fanolesomab; LeuTech), and the receptor-binding agent DPC-11870 that targets the leukotriene B4 receptor, which is abundantly expressed in the granulocyte cell surface [56].

The main advantage of the WBCS, however, is the marked improvement in specificity compared with bone scans, particularly when complicating conditions are superimposed. The specificity increases to 80% to 90% when compared with the bone scan. Several authors have reported a loss of sensitivity of leukocyte scintigraphy when imaging chronic osteomyelitis in the axial skeleton. The nonspecific uptake of labeled leukocytes has been suggested to be attributable to the presence of hematopoietic bone marrow in the axial skeleton. The decreased uptake of labeled cells in infections of the axial skeleton is poorly understood, but microthrombotic occlusion and inflammatory compression of the blood vessels may prevent labeled cells from reaching the site of infection. The sensitivity of leukocyte scintigraphy decreased from 84% to 21% for chronic osteomyelitis in the axial skeleton [44].

A drawback of nuclear medicine is its limited spatial resolution with less ability to clearly delineate areas of complex anatomy, such as the foot and ankle. The circulatory compromise that predisposes individuals to distal extremity infection also may limit the delivery of isotopes distally. Although three-phase bone scintigraphy has an accuracy of 90% or greater for the diagnosis of osteomyelitis in otherwise normal bone, the specificity of the test decreases in the setting of preexisting conditions, such as fracture, presence of orthopedic hardware, and neuropathic joint disease [42]. Nuclear medicine can image patients who have prostheses without interference from artifact. Another advantage of nuclear medicine over other imaging modalities is that pediatric patients rarely require sedation, children can be scanned more than once after the injection of the radiopharmaceutical, and multiple foci of disease can be demonstrated [57].

Radiolabeled antibiotics

The use of radiolabeled antibiotics is fast emerging as a promising diagnostic test for the detection of infective lesions because of their specific binding to the bacterial component [58]. The main advantage of these agents may be the differentiation between infection and sterile inflammatory lesions [59,60]. The normal Infecton (ciprofloxacin labeled with Tc-99m) image shows high uptake by the kidneys with excretion to the urinary bladder, moderate uptake by the liver and spleen, and no uptake by bone or bone marrow [61]. In a population of 102 patients who had various infections undergoing an Infecton scan, the authors reported an overall sensitivity and specificity of the method of 83% and 91%, respectively [61]. More recently, Malamitsi and coworkers [62] evaluated 45 patients who had known or suspected bone infection with Infecton scans. Almost all were also subjected to a three-phase ^{99m}Tc-methylene diphosphonate bone scan and most of them to a ^{99m}Tc-human polyclonal immunoglobulin scan, in addition to a gallium-67-citrate scan, plus CT or MRI or both. The sensitivity and specificity of Infecton scintigraphy were found to be 97.2% and 80%, respectively, with positive and negative predictive values of 94.6% and 88.9% [62]. Siaens and coworkers [63] investigated the differences and advantages of ^{99m}Tc-enrofloxacin versus Infecton in a murine model of musculoskeletal infections, their results showing less uptake of Infecton by normal tissue.

Labeled immunoglobulins

A Tc-99m–labeled murine immunoglobulin M monoclonal antigranulocyte antibody that binds to human polymorphonuclear leukocyte CD15 antigens has been evaluated. The initial report is promising, with possibly better diagnostic results than other techniques, initial sensitivity of 91%, and specificity of 70% [42]. Rubello and coworkers [64] performed 253 Leukoscan examinations in a group of 220 consecutive patients who had suspected bone infections. The examination was performed by acquiring early (Protocol A = 4 h) and delayed (Protocol B = 18–24 h) planar images. The radiotracer uptake intensity in the infected site was graded using a four-point visual scale compared with the contralateral body region in the case of the peripheral skeleton or the nearest vertebrae in the case of spondylodiscitis. Sensitivity was equal in both protocols (84.2%) but specificity was higher in delayed images (85.7% versus 76.2%). In patients who had an early high uptake Leukoscan intensity, further delayed images appear unnecessary for the purpose of diagnosing infection. In contrast, in patients who have an early mild Leukoscan uptake intensity only, delayed imaging seems to be recommended for improving specificity.

Streptavidin/^{111}In-biotin

Streptavidin, a 65-kDa protein, accumulates at sites of inflammation and infection as a result of increased capillary permeability. In addition to being used by bacteria for their growth, biotin forms a stable, high-affinity noncovalent complex with avidin. Lazzeri and coworkers [65] explored the usefulness of this technique for the detection of early vertebral osteomyelitis in a series of 55 patients. Thirty-two of the patients underwent MRI and 24 underwent CT scan. DTPA-conjugated biotin was radiolabeled by incubating 500 µg of DTPA-biotin with 111 MBq of ^{111}In-chloride. Two-step scintigraphy was performed by first infusing 3 mg streptavidin intravenously, followed 4 hours later by ^{111}In-biotin. Imaging was begun 60 minutes later. Streptavidin/^{111}In-biotin scintigraphy was positive in 32 of 34 patients who had spinal infection (94.12% sensitivity) and negative in 19 of 21 patients who did not have infection (95.24% specificity). The sensitivity for MRI and CT were 54.17% and 35.29% with a specificity of 75% and 57.14%, respectively. The only false positive result observed with streptavidin/^{111}In-biotin scintigraphy corresponded to the site of a spinal malignancy. These results suggest that streptavidin/^{111}In-biotin scintigraphy is an efficacious method for the detection of vertebral osteomyelitis in the first 2 weeks after the onset of symptoms.

More than 400,000 hip and knee arthroplasties are performed annually in the United States. Differentiating infection from aseptic loosening, the most common cause of joint arthroplasty failure, is extremely important because the management of these two conditions differs markedly. Bone marrow imaging with a combination of ^{111}In-labeled leukocytes and ^{99m}Tc sulfur colloid has an accuracy of more than 90% and is the preferred radionuclide procedure for diagnosing prosthetic joint replacement infection [66,67].

Cross-sectional imaging

Computed tomography

CT provides images with high spatial and contrast resolution of bone and surrounding soft tissue, and exceptional cortical bony detail. It can provide a good definition of cortical bone destruction, periosteal reaction (Fig. 12), and soft tissue changes. Postcontrast images are more useful for soft tissue abnormalities than for bony changes. Increased density of the medullary cavity can be seen replacing the normal low-density fatty marrow, but this finding is nonspecific and may be seen not only in infections but also in neoplasms, hemorrhage, fractures, or irradiation [68]. It is the best method of detection of small foci of gas within the medullary canal, an infrequent but reliable diagnostic sign of osteomyelitis [69]; areas of cortical erosion or destruction; tiny foreign bodies serving as a nidus for infection; and involucrum and sequestration formation [69–72].

The primary applications of CT to the evaluation of infections of the musculoskeletal system are the delineation of the osseous and soft tissue extent of the disease process, especially in areas of complex anatomy, such as the vertebral column, and the guidance of interventional procedures (biopsies and aspirations), particularly of the spine (Fig. 13) and sacroiliac joints.

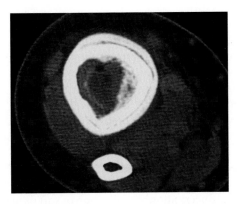

Fig. 12. Infective periostitis. Transaxial CT scan of the tibia and fibula shows a well-defined shell of lifted periosteum surrounding an area of abnormal medullary bone. (*Courtesy of* Sergio Fernández Tapia, MD, Tampico, Mexico.)

In chronic osteomyelitis, CT demonstrates abnormal thickening of the affected cortical bone, with sclerotic changes, encroachment of the medullary cavity, and the abnormal chronic draining sinus. CT provides excellent multiplanar reconstructions of the axial images allowing delineation of even the subtlest osseous changes. The CT is superior to MRI in the detection of sequestra (see Fig. 3) and identifies even small devitalized bony fragments. Because resection of necrotic bone with thorough debridement of infected bone and excision of soft tissue fistulae are two major aims of surgical treatment, CT has considerable importance in determining operative therapy [73]. One limitation of CT is in the assessment of body parts with metallic implants because of beam-hardening artifact [35]. The sensitivity and specificity of CT for diagnosis of osteomyelitis has not been established clearly, but it is known to be lower than the sensitivity of MRI [69]. Its use in clinical practice should be limited to specific circumstances and it should not be used as part of the regular osteomyelitis imaging. CT is not routinely useful for diagnosis in prosthetic joints, because artifacts diminish image resolution [11].

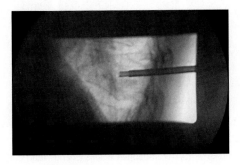

Fig. 13. Craig needle vertebral body biopsy. With the use of fluoroscopic guidance a T10–T11 bone biopsy was obtained. A diagnosis of *S aureus* osteomyelitis was established.

Ultrasound

US is a useful tool in musculoskeletal infections; it can be helpful to differentiate acute or chronic infection from tumors or noninfective inflammatory conditions with similar clinical presentation, to localize the site and extent of infection, and to identify precipitating factors as foreign bodies or fistulae. Moreover, sonography can provide guidance for diagnostic or therapeutic aspiration, drainage, or biopsy (Fig. 14) [74]. US may detect features of osteomyelitis several days earlier than conventional radiographs [75], predominately in children [48,76,77].

In osteomyelitis, typically US usefulness was limited because of its restricted visualization of outer cortical and juxtacortical tissues [23]. Nevertheless, new high-resolution transducers allow visualization of soft tissues close to the bone and bone surface itself, particularly in the extremities [75]. Until now, however, evaluation of osseous involvement has required additional imaging (MRI, CT, nuclear medicine), and a normal US does not exclude bone infection [78].

The earliest sign of acute osteomyelitis on US is juxtacortical soft-tissue swelling associated with early periosteal elevation or thickening. This abnormality is followed by increase in periosteal reaction, and in up to two thirds of cases it is accompanied by a layer of subperiosteal exudates and, rarely, abscess formation. Periosteal abscess should be suspected if a hypo- to hyperechogenic change contiguous to bone surface with adjacent structure displacement is demonstrated (Fig. 15) [75]; in the appropriate clinical settings, these collections confirm the clinical diagnosis of osteomyelitis [79]. Finally, cortical erosions can become apparent on US [80].

US assessment is likely to be more sensitive in children who have suspected acute osteomyelitis. In the immature skeleton, periosteal reaction is greatest, mainly in tubular bones, because of its relatively weak attachment to the subjacent bone [81].

In chronic osteomyelitis, US is not only valuable in making the diagnosis but also can be used to assess involvement of the adjacent soft tissues and

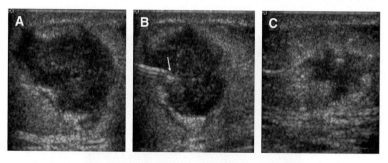

Fig. 14. US-guided needle aspiration of an abscess. Longitudinal scans of a soft tissue mass located on the upper left arm. (*A*) Well-defined heterogeneous fluid collection within the soft tissues. (*B*) Needle aspiration (*arrow*) yielded 30 mL of purulent material. (*C*) Postprocedure scan demonstrated marked reduction in the abscess size.

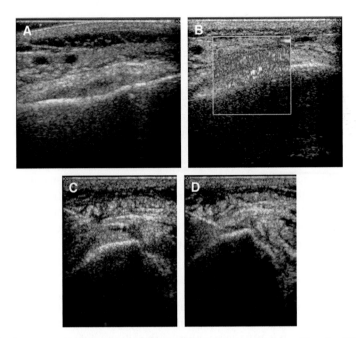

Fig. 15. *S aureus* periosteal abscess. (*A*) Longitudinal US scan. (*B*) Power Doppler US. (*C, D*) Transverse scans during needle aspiration. US demonstrated a hyperechogenic area contiguous to the tibial shaft with soft tissues displacement. Power Doppler shows a hyperemic area consistent with an active periosteal abscess.

guide placement of a percutaneous drainage catheter. Soft tissue abscess related to chronic osteomyelitis is identified as a hypo- or anechoic fluid collection. After US localization of the abscess, a needle can be placed into the collection under sonographic guidance. The collection is then aspirated (Fig 14).

There are several limitations in the radiologic diagnosis of osteomyelitis reactivation because of the concurrent presence of bone changes induced by infection and by bone remodeling. In this regard, US can help in the evaluation of a chronic osteomyelitis reactivation, which may be associated with soft tissue abscess, fistula, or sinus tract formation [80]. Fluid collection adjacent to the cortex with its extension into the marrow cavity through a cortical break is almost pathognomonic of reactivated chronic osteomyelitis [82]. Collections in contact with the cortex in absence of soft tissue or muscle intervening are suggestive of active disease [83].

Special conditions

US may be useful in differentiating septic arthritis from osteomyelitis, especially in the case of septic hip and its differences with proximal femur or pelvis osteomyelitis [84]. US is a reliable noninvasive technique that can be helpful for the diagnosis of reactivation of posttraumatic chronic osteomyelitis in adults [82].

This technique also is helpful for evaluating musculoskeletal soft tissues next to orthopedic hardware and in cases of osteomyelitis complicating metal fixation in an extremity, without significant degradation by metallic artifact [82]. It can demonstrate loosening of metallic hardware and fluid collection or sinus tracts in the soft tissues of the involved extremity [78]. Ultrasonography is a relatively inexpensive imaging method for osteomyelitis evaluation; in the future, higher resolution equipment and color Doppler and power Doppler sonography may increase the usefulness and accuracy of this method.

In patients who have sickle cell disease with osteomyelitis suspicion, US should be the initial imaging investigation. In children who have sickle cell disease, subperiosteal fluid concentrations of 4 mm or more in depth seem to be diagnostic [85]; however, less pronounced concentrations (<4 mm) should be distinguished from acute osteomyelitis and can occur in association with medullary infarction [75]. US also may be used to distinguish infection from infarction in these patients [2].

Magnetic resonance imaging

MRI has been used widely for evaluation of musculoskeletal infections; spatial resolution makes it useful in differentiating between bone and soft tissue infection, which is often a problem with radionuclide scans [86]. MRI is highly sensitive for detecting osteomyelitis as early as 3 to 5 days [2,84,87] with satisfactory specificity [88], because of the excellent contrast provided between the abnormal areas and the normal bone marrow. It has been demonstrated in several studies that MRI sensitivity is greater than that of plain films and CT, and similar to that of radionuclide studies [86,89–92]. MRI sensitivity for the diagnosis of osteomyelitis generally has been reported between 82% and 100%, and specificity between 75% and 96%.

MRI is the modality of choice in cases of well-established osteomyelitis and in determining the extent of infection, especially of eventual epidural abscess or phlegmon, the intramedullary involvement, and consecutive neural compression [88]. In addition it is a useful tool in the evaluation of the presence of intraosseous abscess [78], except when multiple lesions are suspected [11]. Furthermore, MRI helps the orthopedic surgeon to plan the optimal surgical management [93,94], allowing better planning for open or percutaneous drainage of fluid collections and surgical debridement [95,96]. MRI also contributes to the assessment of the extent of devitalized tissue and to the definition of the critical adjacent structures (spine, physes, joint spaces, and so forth) that require modified management to avoid morbidity and complications [97–99].

Initial MRI screening usually includes T1-weighted and T2-weighted spin-echo pulse sequences. Different pulse sequences and imaging protocols can be used in the evaluation of the musculoskeletal system; depending on the pulse sequences used, major differences can be noted on the signal intensity and appearance of normal and abnormal tissues.

Acute osteomyelitis

In the acute phase of osteomyelitis, the edema and exudates within the medullary space produce an ill-defined low-signal intensity on the T1-weighted images and a high signal on T2-weighted and STIR or fat-suppressed sequences. Usually the surrounding soft tissues are also abnormal, with ill-defined planes. The cortical bone can be disrupted and can have abnormally increased signal intensity. The absence of cortex thickening in acute osteomyelitis helps to differentiate it from a chronic infection of bone. Bone marrow findings are nonspecific; other conditions, such as trauma with bone bruise, fracture, infarct, ischemia, and neoplastic processes, may have the same signal intensity alterations as seen in osteomyelitis.

Suppression of fat signal in MRI has proven to extend the dynamic range of tissue contrast, eliminating the strong interfering signal of fat on T1- and T2-weighted images, and post-intravenous contrast injection images (gadolinium). These advantages of fat suppression have been extensively used in clinical practice [100–112]. Because of the superior visualization of inflammatory edema, the most suitable sequences for screening acute osteomyelitis are the short tau inversion recovery (STIR) or the T2-weighted fat-suppressed fast spin-echo (SE) sequence [34]. On STIR or fat-suppressed sequences osteomyelitis looks hyperintense [84,113]. STIR images generally have a lower spatial resolution than conventional T1- and T2-weighted images and cannot be used to differentiate fluid collections, such as abscesses, from circumscribed soft tissue edema [34,114] (Fig. 16). Fat suppressed sequences can help in the visualization of lesions with relatively high water content, such as osteomyelitis, edema, and tumors [115–117]; these sequences must be supplemented by T1-weighted SE images, which provide excellent anatomic detail.

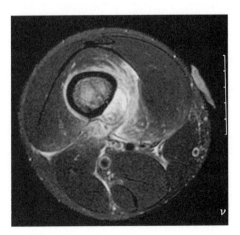

Fig. 16. This 43-year-old man developed pain in the thigh and a limp. Transaxial T2-weighted (TR/TE, 2000/80) SE image demonstrates high signal intensity within the soft tissues. Bone marrow abnormalities are manifested as focal areas of high signal intensity consistent with early stages of osteomyelitis. (*Courtesy of* Sergio Fernández Tapia, MD, Tampico, Mexico.)

STIR and T2-weighted TSE images with fat suppression consistently show perosseous edema. Strong peripheral contrast enhancement confirms the presence of an abscess. Necrotic sequestra depict low-intensity regions without contrast enhancement on STIR and T2-weighted images, in contrast to the high signal intensity of an abscess [73].

Gadolinium may define areas of necrosis [73,84] and also is useful to demonstrate abscess on T1-weighted images (Fig. 17) [2]. Sinus tracts can extend from the marrow and bone, through the soft tissues, and out the skin as high signal intensity areas on T2-weighted images [1].

In acute osteomyelitis intra- and extramedullary fat globules can be seen in MRI; this nonpathognomonic sign has been suggested to be secondary to an increased intramedullary pressure, which leads to septic necrosis, lipocyte death, and free fatty globule release [118].

In patients who have septic arthritis who fail to respond to appropriate antibiotic therapy within 48 hours, osteomyelitis must be suspected and MRI should be considered [84]. Subperiosteal fluid collections may be seen, with low signal intensity on the T1-weighted sequences and intermediate to high signal intensity on the T2 and fat-suppressed images.

Subacute osteomyelitis

Brodie's abscess, single or multiple radiolucent abscesses, can be evident during subacute or chronic stages of osteomyelitis. It is best diagnosed by the combination of conventional radiography and MRI [73]. The central abscess cavity is of low signal intensity on T1-weighted images and high signal

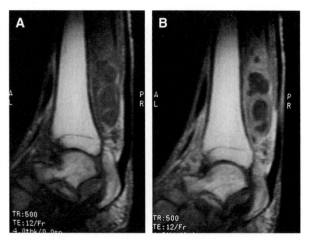

Fig. 17. (*A*) Sagittal T1-weighted MRI (TR/TE, 500/12) shows a soft tissue abscess in the posterior aspect of the distal tibia. (*B*) Gadolinium enhanced T1-imaging demonstrates the extent of the infectious process without associated bony abnormalities. (*Courtesy of* Sergio Fernández Tapia, MD, Tampico, Mexico.)

intensity on STIR and T2-weighted images. The bone marrow surrounding the Brodie's abscess often demonstrates reactive hyperemia. High signal intensity on T2-weighted images around the area of an abscess reflects the hyperemic bone marrow. The granulation tissue lining the inner wall of the abscess has low signal intensity on T1. The high signal intensity of the granulation tissue surrounded by the low signal intensity band of bone sclerosis creates a "double-line effect," with peripheral ring enhancement with gadolinium administration and high T2 signal intensity [114,119,120]. This central abscess with the surrounding granulation tissue, outer ring of fibrotic reaction [121], and a peripheral rim of endosteal reaction produces a target appearance with four distinct layers that are more evident after gadolinium injection [122]. The rim sign (peripheral low signal intensity) in subacute and chronic osteomyelitis has been reported in 93% of patients who have chronic osteomyelitis and in less than 1% of patients who have acute infection [116].

It has been demonstrated that MRI is as sensitive as ^{99}Tc methylene diphosphonate bone scintigraphy in demonstrating osteomyelitis and because of its spatial resolution it is more specific and more sensitive than other techniques in demonstrating soft tissue infections [123]. One study compared the results achieved with plain radiography, CT, and indium-111 labeled leukocyte scanning with MRI in patients who had suspected osteomyelitis or soft tissue infections; results suggested that MRI is more accurate for detection of this kind of infection than plain radiography and CT. Patients who had nonmagnetic devices were better evaluated with MRI than CT [121]. In 50% of cases, subacute osteomyelitis is confused with a tumor; bone erosions and periosteal reaction with reactive bone formation also can be confused with osteosarcoma or Ewing sarcoma [32].

Chronic osteomyelitis

In chronic osteomyelitis, low signal intensity (on T1- and T2-weighted images) areas of devascularized fibrotic scarring in the marrow may be seen, instead of the usual high intensity T2 signal in the bone marrow (Fig 18) [124]. Bone sclerosis with cortical thickening from periosteal apposition and focally reduced bone marrow cavity predominate. Sinus tracts may be present. Also, a relatively sharp, well-defined interface between the normal and abnormal marrow (poorly defined, wide transition zone in acute osteomyelitis) may be seen [125].

Gadolinium-enhanced T1-weighted imaging is crucial for identification of sequestra, which do not enhance. The pattern of contrast enhancement may allow the discrimination of fibrovascular scar from infectious foci, helping in the discrimination between acute and chronic osteomyelitis [119,126] (Fig. 19). MRI can be useful to differentiate osteomyelitis from a neoplasm, such as chondroblastoma, osteoid osteoma, enchondroma, or eosinophilic granuloma.

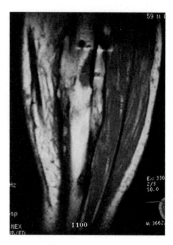

Fig. 18. Chronic active osteomyelitis MRI. Coronal T1-weighted image of the upper leg shows thickening of the cortical bone associated with low signal intensity areas in the bone marrow. An artifact related to a previously removed metal fixation device is seen. (*Courtesy of* Sergio Fernández Tapia, MD, Tampico, Mexico.)

Special situations

In patients who have a history of chronic posttraumatic osteomyelitis and suspected reactivation of bone infection, MRI has a sensitivity of 100%, a specificity of 60%, an accuracy of 79%, a positive predictive value of 69%, and a negative predictive value of 100% [127].

Vertebral osteomyelitis can be detected early by MRI (before evident changes appear in radiographic studies) as soft tissue swelling and bone destruction [88]. Involvement of two adjacent vertebrae may be demonstrated 1 to 3 weeks before radiographic or tomographic evidence of bone destruction. The endplates are ill defined; the vertebral disc and adjacent vertebral bodies are hypointense on T1-weighted SE noncontrast images and hyperintense on STIR and T2-weighted SE images (Fig. 20) [128]. Early extension of inflammatory edema outside the limits of the vertebral bodies and the annulus fibrosus into the paravertebral fat causes low signal intensity on T1-weighted SE noncontrast images and hyperintense postcontrast and on STIR images [88].

In tuberculosis arthritis bone erosions are revealed more frequently than in pyogenic arthritis. The pannus of granulation tissue erodes and destroys cartilage and eventually bone [129]; this process is not uniformly distributed, so that areas of cartilaginous destruction may be intermixed with relatively normal areas. In general, the progression of joint space loss is more prominent with pyogenic arthritis than with tuberculosis arthritis because bacterial proteolytic enzymes accelerate articular cartilage destruction [130]. On MRI mycobacterial arthritis displays intermediate to low signal intensity

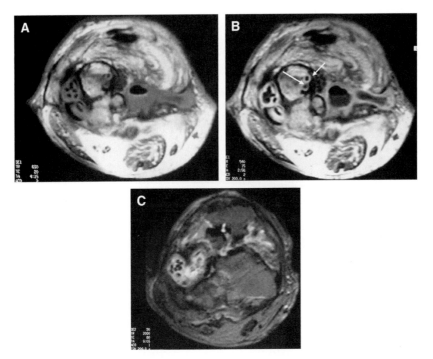

Fig. 19. MRI of chronic osteomyelitis of the femur in a patient who has diabetes. (*A*) Trans-axial T1-weighted (TR/TE 650/20) SE image demonstrates fluid collections around the femur with extensive soft tissue inflammatory changes, abscess formation, and gas collections. (*B*) Transaxial T1-weighted (TR/TE 540/80) SE images with gadolinium reveal intramedullary gas collections and subperiosteal abscess formation (*arrows*). (*C*) Transaxial T2-weighted (TR/TE 2000/80) image shows an intramedullary area of low signal intensity surrounded by alternating bands of high and low signal intensity reminiscent of target appearance.

on T1-weighted images and high signal intensity on T2-weighted images in joint and adjacent bone [93].

Tuberculous osteomyelitis is suggested by the presence of hypointense T2-weighted image (secondary to areas of caseation) associated with soft tissue abscess [131]. Spinal tuberculosis typically starts at the anteroinferior aspect of vertebral body and spreads to contiguous vertebrae along the an-terior longitudinal ligament of the spine [88,132]. Although one report has indicated the presence of high signal intensity in diseased areas on T1-weighted spin-echo MR images [133], low signal intensity on such images and high signal intensity on T2-weighted images are characteristic [134]. Typical findings are erosions of the anterior surfaces of the vertebral bodies with relative preservation of the disks and posterior elements, at least early in the course of the disease [128]. Subligamentous spread and pronounced paravertebral and epidural abscesses with tendency for distant caudal exten-sion are frequent [88]. As the disease progress, collapse of the anterior por-tion of the vertebrae can lead to a kyphotic wedging deformity of the spine,

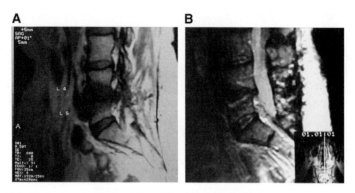

Fig. 20. Spinal infection. (*A*) Sagittal T1-weighted (TR/TE 600/25) and (*B*) proton density (TR/TE 2500/80) weighted MR images reveal abnormalities consistent with L4–L5 infection. In (*A*), abnormal regions of low signal intensity within the vertebral bodies. In (*B*), the signal intensity in these intraosseous regions is greater than that of the adjacent bone marrow.

the gibbous of Pott's disease. It has been suggested that tuberculous spondylitis has a lesser extent of marrow edema than observed in pyogenic spondylitis [130]. In almost 70% of cases it presents as a fusiform cold paraspinal abscess, with or without calcifications [135,136]. Vertebral bodies adjacent to infected disks are hypointense on T1-weighted MRI and hyperintense on T2-weighted MRI, with contrast enhancement and delineation of the extent of epidural involvement [137].

In neuropathic arthritis patients, mainly in patients who have diabetes, osteomyelitis could be a difficult diagnosis. MRI can be useful to demonstrate the presence of associated osteomyelitis (15%) or septic arthritis. Pedal osteomyelitis results almost exclusively from contiguous infection coming from the soft tissue ulceration and occurs most frequently around the fifth and first metatarsophalangeal joints. The formation of adventitious bursa or subcutaneous callus is a precursor to the ulceration that can be seen in the diabetic foot. Recognition of these bursae before onset of tissue breakdown may prevent sinus tract formation and osteomyelitis [138]. One third of patients who have advanced infection of the foot show evidence of septic arthritis on MRI [139]. Osteomyelitis in neuropathic feet of leprosy patients has similar findings to those of patients who have diabetes [140].

In children, diagnosis of a very early stage of osteomyelitis can be made with high sensitivity using the turbo inversion recovery magnitude (TIRM) with standard T1-weighted and T2-weigted MRI, with the advantage of no sedation being needed. A recognized limitation of TIRM sequences is the high signal in hematopoietic marrow of children under 3 years of age and the different degrees of marrow fat that are heterogeneous in the pediatric population [141]. MRI is especially useful for children who have pelvic [87] or vertebral osteomyelitis [2]; in the latter MRI has been found to have a sensitivity of 96% and a specificity of 93% [142].

The presence of osteomyelitis and bone infarction may coexist. Medullary infarcts might function as sequestra, predisposing to osteomyelitis and soft tissue infection [143]. The hallmark of avascular necrosis is hypointense peripheral band signal on all sequences, similar to rim sign; however, identification of a double-line sign on T2-weighted images is considered pathognomonic for osteonecrosis [144]. Gadolinium can also help to distinguish between infarction and osteomyelitis. The former shows thin, linear rim or long serpiginous central medullary enhancement, whereas osteomyelitis displays a thick, irregular peripheral enhancement around a nonenhancing center.

Patients who have rheumatoid arthritis have an increased risk for joint infection, so that in presence of a single disproportionately inflamed joint with inadequate therapy response and fever or in presence of immunosuppressive therapy, infection should be strongly considered. Osteoarticular rheumatic abnormalities in these patients might be difficult to distinguish from anatomic changes secondary to infection, however. MRI is an accurate method to evaluate the extent of the infective process; additionally, fat-suppressed gadolinium-enhanced sequences help to delineate marrow extension [145].

MRI is not useful for whole-body examinations (unlike radionuclide studies); metal implants in the region of interest may produce focal artifacts, mainly with high field systems [94].

Development of squamous cell carcinoma of the sinus tract is an uncommon, well-known complication of longstanding chronic osteomyelitis, which occurs in 0.23% to 1.6% of these patients [146,147]. MRI can identify this complication as an abnormal soft tissue mass [147–149].

Positron emission tomography and single photon emission computed tomography

The Positron Emission Tomography (PET) systems are relatively novel techniques that are being applied in several medical fields. Unfortunately there is limited availability of PET systems.

A nonspecific indicator of increased intracellular glucose metabolism, 18 fluorodeoxyglucose ([18]FDG) accumulates in infection and inflammation sites (leukocytes, granulocytes, and macrophages) [150,151]. Guhlmann and colleagues [152] were the first authors to evaluate the role of fluorodeoxyglucose PET (FDG-PET) in chronic osteomyelitis, reporting a high diagnostic accuracy of this method, especially in the axial skeleton. Further studies have deepened the diagnosis of acute and chronic osteomyelitis [153–155]. It has been demonstrated that FDG-PET has the highest diagnostic accuracy for confirming or excluding the diagnosis of chronic osteomyelitis in comparison with bone scintigraphy, MRI, or leukocyte scintigraphy; FDG-PET also is superior to leukocyte scintigraphy for detecting chronic osteomyelitis in the axial skeleton [44,156,157]. A limitation of this technique is that early bone healing involves a short inflammatory phase with highly activated metabolism and glucose consumption, which might be confused with osteomyelitis; however, this period of false positive images is smaller than with nuclear medicine modalities [158]. It is proposed, therefore, that in postsurgical and traumatic bone healing ^{18}FDG-PET should be avoided in the first 3 to 6 months to minimize the risk for false positive findings [151]. This technique also may have limited usefulness in patients who have failed joint prosthesis or a tumor [66]. FDG-PET might play a role in the future in the diagnosis of osteomyelitis, but its value currently is not well defined.

Gallium-67 (^{67}Ga) has been used successfully as an infection-detecting tracer in scintigraphy. PET imaging confirmed that the uptake of ^{68}Ga was lower than that of ^{18}FDG during normal bone healing; this fact has been proposed to play a significant role in lowering the possibility of false positive findings of osteomyelitis in postsurgical and posttraumatic bone healing. Further studies are needed to verify the value of ^{68}Ga PET for clinical purposes, however [151]. Single positron emission computed tomography (SPECT)/CT combines the functional evaluation provided by SPECT with the spatial definition of CT [159]. It can accurately identify the location of osteomyelitis foci in the appendicular and axial skeleton and differentiate between cortical, corticomedullary, and subperiosteal foci [160]. In addition, it may allow the discrimination between osteomyelitis, septic arthritis, and soft tissue infection [159]. Furthermore, this method had been suggested to be accurate for the evaluation of chronic posttraumatic osteomyelitis [159]. This claim is supported by the fact that acute fractures and postsurgical intervention of bone can increase ^{18}FDG uptake, but this phenomenon lasts a maximum of 3 months; therefore, any abnormal increased ^{18}FDG bone uptake after this period must be suspected to be secondary to infection or malignancy [161]. It has been suggested that SPECT/CT in addition to ^{67}Ga or ^{111}In WBC scintigraphy can accurately help in the precise localization and definition of the extension of infections, highlighting the potential role of combined imaging techniques [160].

Summary

Osteomyelitis frequently requires more than one imaging technique for an accurate diagnosis. Conventional radiography still remains the first imaging modality. MRI and nuclear medicine are the most sensitive and specific methods for the detection of osteomyelitis. MRI provides more accurate information regarding the extent of the infectious process. Ultrasound represents a noninvasive method to evaluate the involved soft tissues and cortical bone and may provide guidance for diagnostic or therapeutic aspiration, drainage, or tissue biopsy. CT scan can be a useful method to detect early osseous erosion and to document the presence of sequestra. PET and SPECT are highly accurate techniques for the evaluation of chronic osteomyelitis, allowing differentiation from soft tissue infection.

References

[1] Calhoun J, Manring M. Adult osteomyelitis. Infect Dis Clin N Am 2005;19:765–86.
[2] Kaplan S. Osteomyelitis in children. Infect Dis Clin N Am 2005;19:787–97.
[3] Stott NS. Review article: paediatric bone and joint infections. J Orthop Surg (Hong Kong) 2001;9:83–90.
[4] Lew DP, Waldvogel FA. Osteomyelitis. N Engl J Med 1997;336:999–1007.
[5] Cierny G III, Mader JT, Pennick JJ. A clinical staging system for adult osteomyelitis. Clin Orthop 2003;414:7–24.
[6] Patzakis M. Management of acute and chronic osteomyelitis. In: Chapman M, Szabo R, Marder R, et al, editors. Chapman's orthopaedic surgery. 3rd edition. Philadelphia: Lippincott Williams & Wilkins; 2001. p. 3523–31.
[7] Nelson JD. Acute osteomyelitis in children. Infect Dis Clin N Am 1990;4:513.
[8] Karwowska A, Davies H, Jadavji T. Epidemiology and outcome of osteomyelitis in the era of sequential intravenous-oral therapy. Pediatr Infect Dis J 1998;17:1021.
[9] Bowerman S, Green N, Menco G. Decline of bone and joint infections attributable to Haemophilus influenzae type b. Clin Orthop 1997;341:128.
[10] Christiansen P, Frederiksen B, Glazowski J, et al. Epidemiologic, bacteriologic and long-term follow up data of children with acute hematogenous osteomyelitis and septic arthritis. J Pediatr Orthop 1999;8:302.
[11] Gylys-Morin VM. MR imaging of pediatric musculoskeletal inflammatory and infectious disorders. Magn Reson Clin N Am 1998;6:537–59.
[12] Soler R, Rodríguez E, Remuiñan C, et al. MRI of musculoskeletal extraspinal tuberculosis. J Comput Assist Tomogr 2001;25:177–83.
[13] Muñoz-Sanz A, Vera A, Vidigal FR. Case 23–2000: osteomyelitis in HIV-infected patients. [letter] N Engl J Med 2001;344:67.
[14] Spencer M, Burgener FA, Hampton BA. Osteomyelitis in AIDS patients. Radiology 1991; 181(P):155–6.
[15] Steinbach L, Tehranzadeh J, Fleckenstein J, et al. Human immunodeficiency virus infection: musculoskeletal manifestations. Radiology 1993;86:833–8.
[16] Lee DL, Sartoris DJ. Musculoskeletal manifestations of human immunodeficiency virus infection: review of imaging characteristics. Radiol Clin N Am 1994;32:399–411.
[17] Major NM, Tehranzadeh J. Musculoskeletal manifestations of AIDS. Radiol Clin N Am 1997;35:1167–89.
[18] Baron AL, Steinbach LS, LeBoit PE, et al. Osteolytic lesions and bacillary angiomatosis in HIV infection: radiologic differentiation from AIDS-related Kaposi sarcoma. Radiology 1990;177:77–81.
[19] Leone A, Cerase A, Constantini A. Musculoskeletal tuberculosis. The Radiologist 2000;7: 227–37.
[20] Magid D, Fishman EK. Musculoskeletal infections in patients with AIDS: CT findings. AJR Am J Roentgenol 1992;158:603–37.
[21] Wyatt SH, Fishman EKCT. MRI of musculoskeletal complications of AIDS. Skeletal Radiol 1995;24:481–8.
[22] Resnick D, Niwayama G. Osteomyelitis, septic arthritis and soft tissue infection: mechanisms and situations. In: Resnick D, editor. Diagnosis of bone and joint disorders. 3rd edition. Philadelphia: WB Saunders; 1995. p. 2325–418.
[23] Kothari NA, Pelchovitz DP, Meyer PJ. Imaging of musculoskeletal infections. Radiol Clin N Am 2001;39:653–71.
[24] Emslie KR, Ozanne NR, Nade SM. Acute haematogenous osteomyelitis: an experimental model. J Pathol 1983;141:157–67.
[25] Lazzarini L, Mader J, Calhoun J. Osteomyelitis in long bones. J Bone and Joint Surg 2004; 86-A(10):2305–18.

[26] Waldvogel FA, Medoff G, Swartz MN. Osteomyelitis: a review of clinical features, therapeutic considerations and unusual aspects. N Engl J Med 1970;282:198–206.

[27] Dormans J, Drummond D. Pediatric hematogenous osteomyelitis: new trends in presentation, diagnosis, and treatment. J Am Acad Orthop Surg 1994;2:333–41.

[28] Nixon GW. Hematogenous osteomyelitis of metaphyseal-equivalent locations. AJR Am J Roentgenol 1978;130:123.

[29] Howard CB, Einhorn M, Dagan R, et al. Fine-needle bone biopsy to diagnose osteomyelitis. J Bone Joint Surg Br 1994;76:311.

[30] Mackowiak PA, Jones SR, Smith JW. Diagnostic value of sinus-tract cultures in chronic osteomyelitis. JAMA 1978;239:2772–5.

[31] Willis RB, Rozencwaig R. Pediatric osteomyelitis masquerading as skeletal neoplasia. Orthop Clin N Am 1996;27:625.

[32] Oudjhane K, Azouz EM. Imaging of osteomyelitis in children. Radiol Clin N Am 2001;39: 251–66.

[33] Wenaden A, Szyszko T, Saiffudin A. Imaging of periosteal reactions associated with focal lesions of bone. Clin Radiol 2005;60:439–56.

[34] Boutin R, Brossman J, Sartoris D, et al. Update on imaging of orthopedic infections. Orthop Clin N Am 1998;29:41–66.

[35] Keenan AM, Tindel NL, Alavi A. Diagnosis of pedal osteomyelitis in diabetic patients using current scintigraphic techniques. Arch Intern Med 1989;149:2262–6.

[36] Larcos G, Brown ML, Sutton RT. Diagnosis of osteomyelitis of the foot in diabetic patients: value of 111 In-leukocyte scintigraphy. AJR Am J Roentgenol 1991;157: 527–31.

[37] Yuh WTC, Corson JD, Baraniewski HM, et al. Osteomyelitis of the foot in diabetic patients: evaluation with plain film, 99Tc-MDP bone scintigraphy and MR imaging. AJR Am J Roentgenol 1989;152:795–800.

[38] Elgazzar AH, Abdel-Dayem HM, Clark JD, et al. Multimodality imaging in osteomyelitis. Eur J Nucl Med 1995;22:1043.

[39] Handmaker H, Leonards R. The bone scan in inflammatory osseous disease. Semin Nucl Med 1976;6:95–105.

[40] Maurer AH, Chen DCP, Camargo EE, et al. Utility of three-phase skeletal scintigraphy in suspected osteomyelitis: concise communication. J Nucl Med 1981;22:941–9.

[41] Alazraki N, Dries DJ, Datz F, et al. Value of a 24 hour image four phase scan in assessing osteomyelitis in patients with peripheral vascular disease. J Nucl Med 1985;26:711–7.

[42] Schauwecker DS. The scintigraphic diagnosis of osteomyelitis. AJR Am J Roentgenol 1992;158:9–18.

[43] Seldin DW, Heiken JP, Feldman F, et al. Effect of soft tissue pathology on detection of pedal osteomyelitis in diabetes. J Nucl Med 1985;26:988–93.

[44] Termaat MF, Raijmakers PG, Scholtein HJ, et al. The accuracy of diagnostic imaging for the assesment of chronic osteomyelitis: a systematic review and Meta-analysis. J Bone Joint Surg 2005;87-A(11):2464–71.

[45] Johnson JE, Kennedy EJ, Shereff MJ, et al. Prospective study of bone indium-111-labeled white blood cell, gallium-67 scanning for the evaluation osteomyelitis in diabetic foot. Foot Ankle Int 1996;17:10–6.

[46] Palestro CJ, Chun CK, Swyer AJ, et al. Radionuclide diagnosis of vertebral osteomyelitis: indium-111 leukocyte and technetium-99m-methylene diphosphonate bone scintigraphy. J Nucl Med 1991;32:1861–5.

[47] Peters AM. The use of nuclear medicine in infections. Br J Radiol 1998;71:252–61.

[48] Williamson SL, Seibert JJ, Glasier CM, et al. Ultrasound in advance pediatric osteomyelitis. Pediatr Radiol 1991;21:288–90.

[49] McCarthy K, Velchik MG, Alavi A, et al. In-111 labeled white blood cells in detection of osteomyelitis complicated by a pre-existing condition. J Nucl Med 1988;29:1015–21.

[50] Al-Sheikh W, Sfakianakis GN, Mnaymneh W, et al. Subacute and chronic bone infections: diagnosis using In-111, Ga-67 and Tc-99m MDP bone scintigraphy and radiography. Radiology 1985;155:501–6.

[51] Schauwecker DS, Burt RW, Park HW, et al. Evaluation of complicating osteomyelitis with Tc-99m MDP, In-111 granulocytes, and Ga-67 citrate. J Nucl Med 1984;25: 848–53.

[52] Tumeh SS, Aliabadi P, Weissman BN, et al. Chronic osteomyelitis: bone and gallium scan patterns associated with active disease. Radiology 1986;158:685–8.

[53] Lewin JS, Rosenfield NS, Hoffer PB, et al. Acute osteomyelitis in children: combined Tc-9m and Ga-67 imaging. Radiology 1986;158:795.

[54] Merkel KD, Brown ML, Dewanjee MK, et al. Comparison of Indium-labeled leukocyte imaging with sequential technetium–gallium scanning in diagnosis of low grade musculoskeletal sepsis. J Bone Joint Surg Am 1985;67:465–76.

[55] Galpérine T, Dutronc H, Lafarie S, et al. Cold bone defecto on granulocytes labelled with technetium-99m-HMPAO Scintigraphy: significance and usefulness for diagnosis and follow-up of osteoarticular infections. Scand J Infect Dis 2004;36:209–12.

[56] Kumar VQ. Radiolabeled white blood cells and direct targeting of micro-organisms for infection imaging. J Nucl Med Mol Imaging 2005;49:325–38.

[57] Jaramillo D, Treves ST, Kasser J, et al. Osteomyelitis and septic arthritis in children: appropriate use of imaging to guide treatment. AJR Am J Roentgenol 1995;165:399–403.

[58] Singh B, Mittal BR, Bhattacharya A, et al. Technetium-99m ciprofloxacin imaging in the diagnosis of postsurgical bony infection and evaluation and the response to antibiotic therapy: a case report. J Orthop Surg (Hong Kong) 2005;13(2):190–4.

[59] Sing AK. 99mTc-4flouroquinolone: evaluation as a specific infection imaging agent. Indian J Nucl Med 1997;12:148.

[60] Britton KE, Wareham DW, Das SS, et al. Imaging bacterial infection with ^{99m}Tc-ciprofloxacin (Infecton). J Clin Pathol 2002;55:817–23.

[61] Britton KE, Vinjamuri S, Hall AV, et al. Clinical evaluation of technetium −99m Infecton for the localization of bacterial infection. Eur J Nucl Med 1997;24:553–6.

[62] Malamitsi J, Giamarellou H, Kanellakopoulou K, et al. Infecton: a 99mTc-ciprofloxacin radiopharmaceutical for the detection of bone infection. Clin Microbiol Infect 2003;9: 101–9.

[63] Siaens RH, Rennen HJ, Boerman OC, et al. Synthesis and comparison of 99mTc-enrofloxacin and 99mTc-ciprofloxacin. J Nucl Med 2005;45(12):2088–94.

[64] Rubello D, Casara D, Maran A, Avogaro A, Tiengo A, Muzzio P. Role of antigranulocyte Fab fragment antibody scintigraphy (Leukoscan) in evaluating bone infection: acquisition protocol, interpretation criteria and clinical results. Nucl Med Commun 2004;25:39–47.

[65] Lazzeri E, Pauwels E, Erba P, et al. Clinical feasibility of two-step streptavidin/111In-biotin scintigraphy in patients with suspected vertebral osteomyelitis. Eur J Nucl Med Mol Imaging 2004;31:1505–11.

[66] Love C, Tomas M, Tronco G, et al. FDG PET of infection and inflammation. Radiographics 2005;25(5):1357–68.

[67] Vinjamuri S, Hall AV, Solanki K, et al. Comparison of Tc-99m infecton imaging with radiolabelled white-cell imaging in the evaluation of bacterial infection. Lancet 1996;347: 233–5.

[68] Aliabadi P, Nikpoor N. Imaging osteomyelitis. Arthritis Rheumatol 1994;37:617.

[69] Ram PC, Martínez S, Korobin M, et al. CT detection of intraosseous gas: a new sign of osteomyelitis. AJR Am J Roentgenol 1981;137:721–3.

[70] Gold R, Hawkins R, Katz R. Bacterial osteomyelitis: findings on plain radiography, CT MR and scintigraphy. AJR Am J Roentgenol 1991;157:365–70.

[71] Helms C, Jeffrey RB, Wing V. Computed tomography and plain film appearance of bony sequestration: significance and differential diagnosis. Skel Radiol 1987;16:117.

[72] Spaeth HJ, Chandnani VP, Beltran J, et al. Magnetic resonance imaging detection of early experimental periostitis: comparison of magnetic resonance imaging, computed tomography and plain radiography with histopathological correlation. Invest Radiol 1991;26:304–8.

[73] Bohndorf K. Infection of the appendicular skeleton. Eur Radiol 2004;14:E53–63.

[74] Cardinal E, Bureau NJ, Aubin B, et al. Role of ultrasound in musculoskeletal infections. Radiol Clin North Am 2001;39:191–201.

[75] Riebel TW, Nasir R, Nazarenko O. The value of sonography in the detection of osteomyelitis. Pediatr Radiol 1996;26:291–7.

[76] Albiri MM, Kirpekar M, Ablow RC. Osteomyelitis: detection with US. Radiology 1989; 172:509–14.

[77] Howard CB, Einhorn M, Dagan R, et al. Ultrasound diagnosis and management of acute hematogenous osteomyelitis in children. J Bone Joint Surg Br 1993;75-B:79–82.

[78] Bureau N, Chhem R, Cardinal E. Musculoskeletal infections: US manifestations. Radiographics 1999;19:1585–92.

[79] Rifai A, Nyman R. Scintigraphy and ultrasonography in differentiating osteomyelitis from bone infarction in sickle cell disease. Acta Radiol 1997;38:139.

[80] Chau CLF, Griffith JF. Musculoskeletal infections: ultrasound appearances. Clin Radiol 2005;60:149–59.

[81] Blickman JG, van Die CE, de Rooy JW. Current imaging concepts in pediatric osteomielitis. Eur Radiol 2004;14:L55–64.

[82] Venkatesh S, Riederer B, Chhem R, et al. Reactivation in post-traumatic chronic osteomyelitis: ultrasonographic findings. Can Assoc Radiol 2003;54:163–8.

[83] Chhem RK, Kaplan PA, Dussault RG. Ultrasonography of the musculoskeletal system. Radiol Clin North Am 1994;32:275–89.

[84] Kocher M, Lee B, Dolan M, et al. Pediatric orthopedic infections: early detection and treatment. Pediatr Ann 2006;35:112–22.

[85] William RR, Hussein SS, Jeans WD, et al. A prospective study of soft-tissue ultrasonography in sickle cell disease patients with suspected osteomyelitis. Clin Radiol 2000;5:307–10.

[86] Unger E, Moldofsky P, Gatenby R, et al. Diagnosis of osteomyelitis by MR imaging. AJR Am J Roentgenol 1988;150:605–10.

[87] Connolly LP, Connolly SA, Drubach LA, et al. Acute hematogenous osteomyelitis of children: assessment of skeletal scintigraphy-based diagnosis in the era of MRI. J Nucl Med 2002;43:1310–6.

[88] Jevtic V. Vertebral infection. Eur Radiol 2004;14:E43–52.

[89] Fletcher BD, Scoles PV, Nelson AD. Osteomyelitis in children: detection by magnetic resonance. Radiology 1984;150:57–60.

[90] Modic MT, Pavlicek W, Weinstein MA. Magnetic resonance imaging of intervertebral disk disease: clinical and pulse sequences considerations. Radiology 1984;152:103–11.

[91] Modic MT, Feiglin DH, Piraino DW, et al. Vertebral osteomyelitis: assessment using MR. Radiology 1985;157:157–66.

[92] Modic MT, Pflanze W, Feiglin DHI, et al. Magnetic resonance imaging of musculoskeletal infections. Radiol Clin N Am 1986;24:247–58.

[93] Theodorou DJ, Theodorou SJ, Kakitsubata Y, et al. Imaging characteristics and epidemiologic features of atypical mycobacterial infections involving the musculoskeletal system. AJR Am J Roentgenol 2001;176:341–9.

[94] Flemming D, Murphey M, McCarthy K. Imaging of the foot and ankle: summary and update. Curr Opin Orthop 2005;16:54–9.

[95] Dangman B, Hoffer F, Rand F, et al. Osteomyelitis in children: gadolinium-enhanced MR imaging. Radiology 1992;182:743.

[96] Chandnani VP, Beltran J, Morris CS, et al. Acute experimental osteomyelitis and abscesses: detection with MR imaging vs. CT. Radiology 1990;174:233–6.

[97] Towers JD. The use of intravenous contrast in MRI of extremity infection. Semin US CT Magn Reson Imaging 1997;18:269–75.

[98] Stöver B, Sigmund G, Langer M, et al. MRI in diagnostic evaluation of osteomyelitis in children. Eur Radiol 1994;4:347–52.

[99] Mandell GA. Imaging in the diagnosis of the musculoskeletal infections in children. Curr Probl Pediatr 1996;26:218–37.

[100] Baker LL, Goodman S, Perkash I. Benign versus pathologic compression fractures of vertebral bodies: assessment with conventional spin-echo, chemical shift and STIR MR imaging. Radiology 1990;174:495–502.

[101] Bobman SA, Scott A, Listerud J. Postoperative lumbar spine: contrast enhanced chemical shift MR imaging. Radiology 1991;179:557–62.

[102] Fritz RC, Stoller DW. Fat-supression MR arthrography of the shoulder. Radiology 1992; 185:614–5.

[103] Georgy A, Hesselink JR. Evaluation of fat suppression in contrast-enhanced MR of neoplastic and inflammatory spine disease. AJNR Am J Neuroradiol 1994;15: 409–17.

[104] Harned EM, Mitchell DG, Burk DL Jr, et al. Bone marrow findings on MR images of the knee: accentuation by fat suppression. J Magn Reson Imaging 1990;8:27–31.

[105] Hernandez RJ, Keim DR, Chenevert TL, et al. Fat-supressed MR imaging of myositis. Radiology 1992;182:217–9.

[106] Huang AB, Schweitzer ME, Hume E, et al. Osteomyelitis of the pelvis/hips in paralyzed patients: accuracy and clinical utility of MRI. J Comput Assist Tomogr 1998; 22:437–43.

[107] Jones KM, Schwartz B, Mantello W. Fast spin-echo MR in the detection of vertebral metastases: comparison of three sequences. AJNR Am J Neuroradiol 1994;15:401–7.

[108] Mitchell DG, Joseph PM, Fallon M, et al. Chemical shift imaging of the femoral head: an in vitro study of normal hips and hips with avascular necrosis. AJR Am J Roentgenol 1987; 148:1159–64.

[109] Morrison WB, Schweitzer ME, Bock GW, et al. Diagnosis of osteomyelitis: utility of fat suppressed contrast-enhanced MR imaging. Radiology 1993;189:251–7.

[110] Quinn SF, Sheley RC, Demlow TA, et al. Rotator cuff tendon tears: evaluation with fat-supressed MR imaging with arthroscopic correlation in 100 patients. Radiology 1995; 195:497–501.

[111] Rose PM, Demlow T, Szumowski J, et al. Chondromalacia patellae: fat suppressed MR imaging. Radiology 1994;193:437–40.

[112] Totterman S, Weiss SL, Szumowski J, et al. MR fat suppression technique in the evaluation of normal structures of the knee. J Comput Assist Tomogr 1989;13:473–9.

[113] Chung T. Magnetic resonance imaging in acute osteomyelitis in children. Pediatr Infect Dis J 2002;22:869–70.

[114] Tehranzadeh J, Wong E, Wang F, et al. Imaging of osteomyelitis in the mature skeleton. Radiol Clin N Am 2001;39:223–50.

[115] Rubin HB, Fischman AJ. The use of radiolabeled nonspecific immunoglobulin in the detection of focal inflammation. Semin Nucl Med 1994;24:169–79.

[116] Erdman WA, Tamburro F, Jayson HT, et al. Osteomyelitis: characteristics and pitfalls of diagnosis with MR imaging. Radiology 1991;180:533–9.

[117] Jones KM, Unger EC, Granstrom P, et al. Bone marrow imaging using STIR at 0.5 and 1.5 T. Magn Reson Imaging 1992;10:169–76.

[118] Davies AM, Hughes DE, Grimer RJ. Intramedullary and extramedullary fat globules on magnetic resonance imaging as a diagnostic sign for osteomyelitis. Eur Radiol 2005;15: 2194–9.

[119] Pöyhiä T, Azouz EM. MR imaging evaluation of subacute and chronic bone abscesses in children. Pediatr Radiol 2000;30:763–8.

[120] Tehranzadeh J, Wang F, Mesgarzadeh M. Magnetic resonance imaging of osteomyelitis. Crit Rev Diag Imag 1992;33:495.

[121] Berquist TH, Brown ML, Fitzgerald RH Jr, et al. Magnetic resonance imaging: application in musculoskeletal infection. Magn Reson Imaging 1985;3:219–30.

[122] Marti-Bonmati L, Aparisi F, Poyatos C, et al. Brodie abscess: MR imaging appearance in 10 patients. J Magn Reson Imag 1993;3:543.

[123] Beltran J, Noto AM, McGhee RB, et al. Infections of the musculoskeletal system: high field strength MR imaging. Radiology 1987;164:449–54.

[124] Abernathy L, Carty H. Modern approach to the diagnosis of osteomyelitis in children. Br J Hosp Med 1997;58:464.

[125] Cohen MD, Cory DA, Kleiman M, et al. Magnetic resonance differentiation of acute and chronic osteomyelitis in children. Clin Radiol 1990;41:53.

[126] Kaim A, Gross T, von Schulthess GK. Imaging of chronic posttraumatic osteomyelitis. Eur Radiol 2002;12:1193–202.

[127] Kaim A, Ledermann HP, Bongartz G, et al. Chronic post-traumatic osteomyelitis of the lower extremity: comparison of magnetic resonance imaging and combined bone scintigraphy/immunoscintigraphy with radiolabelled monoclonal antigranulocyte antibodies. Skeletal Radiol 2000;29:378–86.

[128] Lederman HP, Schweitzer ME, Morrison W, et al. MR imaging findings in spinal infections: rules or myths? Radiology 2003;228:506–14.

[129] Yao DC, Sartoris DJ. Musculoskeetal tuberculosis. Radiol Clin North Am 1995;33: 679–89.

[130] Hong S, Kim S, Ahn J, et al. Tuberculous versus pyogenic arthritis: MR imaging evaluation. Radiology 2001;218:848–53.

[131] Sharma P. MR features of tuberculous osteomyelitis. Skeletal Radiol 2003;32:279–85.

[132] Griffit JF, Kumta SM, Leung PC, et al. Imaging of musculoskeletal tuberculosis: a new look at a old disease. Clin Orthop Retal Res 2002;398:32–9.

[133] Quinn SF, Murray W, Prochaska J, et al. MRI appearance of disseminated osseous tuberculosis. Magn Reson Imaging 1987;5:493.

[134] Smith AS, Weinstein MA, Mizushima A, et al. MR imaging characteristic of tuberculous spondylitis vs vertebral osteomyelitis. AJR 1989;153:399.

[135] Hoffman EB, Crosier JH, Cremin BJ. Imaging in children with spinal tuberculosis: a comparison of radiography, computed tomography and magnetic resonance imaging. J Bone Joint Surg Br 1993;75:233–9.

[136] Gardam M, Lin S. Mycobacterial osteomyelitis and arthritis. Infect Dis Clin N Am 2005; 19:819–30.

[137] Gold GE, Suh B, Sawyer-Glover A, et al. Musculoskeletal MRI at 3.0T: initial clinical experience. AJR Am J Roentgenol 2004;183:1479–86.

[138] Jurik AG, Egund N. MRI in chronic recurrent multifocal osteomielitis. Skeletal Radiol 1997;26:230–8.

[139] Lederman HP, Morrison WB, Schweitzer ME. MR Image analysis of pedal osteomyelitis: distribution, patterns of spread, and frequency of associated ulceration and septic arthritis. Radiology 2002;223:747–55.

[140] Maas M, Slim EJ, Heoksma AF, et al. MR imaging of neuropathic feet in leprosy patients with suspected osteomyelitis. Int J Lepr 2002;70:97–103.

[141] Hauer M, Uhl M, Llaman KH, et al. Comparison of turbo inversion recovery magnitude (TIRM) with T2-weighted spin-echo MR imaging in the early diagnosis of acute osteomyelitis in children. Pediatr Radiol 1998;28:846–50.

[142] Fernández M, Carrol CL, Baker CJ. Discitis and vertebral osteomyelitis in children: an 18-year review. Pediatrics 2000;105:1299–304.

[143] Blacksin MF, Finzel KC, Benevenia J. Osteomyelitis originating in and around bone infarcts: giant sequestrum phenomena. AJR Am J Roentgenol 2001;176:387–91.

[144] Mitchel DG, Rao VM, Dalinka MK, et al. Femoral head avascular necrosis: correlation of MR imaging, radiographic staging, radionuclide imaging and clinical findings. Radiology 1987;162:709–15.

[145] Narváez JA, Narváez J, Roca Y, et al. MR imaging assessment of clinical problems in rheumatoid arthritis. Eur Radiol 2002;12:1819–28.

[146] Sedlin ED, Fleming JL. Epidermoid carcinoma arising in chronic osteomyelitis foci. J Bone Joint Surg North Am 1963;45:827–38.

[147] Sonin AH, Resnik CS, Mulligan ME, et al. General case of the day. Radiographics 1998;18: 530–2.

[148] Luchs JS, Hines J, Katz DS. MR imaging of squamous cell carcinoma complicating chronic osteomyelitis of the femur. AJR Am J Roentgenol 2002;178:512–3.

[149] McGrory JE, Pritchard DJ, Unni KK, et al. Malignant lesions arising in chronic osteomyelitis. Clin Orthop 1999;362:181–9.

[150] Keidar Z, Militianu D, Melamed E, et al. The diabetic foot: initial experience with 18F-FDG PET/CT. J Nucl Med 2005;46:444–9.

[151] Mäkinen T, Lankinen P, Pöyhönen T, et al. Comparison of ^{18}F-FDG and ^{68}Ga PET imaging in the assessment of experimental osteomyelitis due to Staphylococcus aureus. Eur J Nucl Med Mol Imaging 2005;32:1259–68.

[152] Guhlmann A, Brecht Krauss D, Suger G, et al. Fluorine-18-FDG PET and technetium-99m antigranulocyte antibody scintigraphy in chronic osteomyelitis. J Nucl Med 1998; 39:2145–52.

[153] Zhuang H, Duarte PS, Pourdehand M, et al. Exclusion of chronic osteomyelitis with F-18 fluorodeoxyglucose positron emission tomographic imaging. Clin Nucl Med 2000;25: 281–4.

[154] Kalcke T, Schmitz A, Risse JH, et al. Fluorine-18 fluorodeoxyglucose PET in infectious bone diseases: results of histologically confirmed cases. Eur J Nucl Med 2000;27:524–8.

[155] Jones-Jackson L, Walker R, Purnell G, et al. Early detection of bone infection and differentiation from post-surgical inflammation using 2-deoxy-2-[^{18}F]-fluoro-D-glucose positron emission tomography (FDG-PET) in an animal model. J Orthop Res 2005;23:1484–9.

[156] Meller J, Köster G, Liersch T, et al. Chronic bacterial osteomyelitis: prospective comparison of ^{18}F-FDG imaging with a dual-head coincidence camera and ^{111}In-labelled autologous leucocyte scintigraphy. Eur J Nucl Med 2002;29:53–60.

[157] Winter D, van der Wiele C, Vogelaers D, et al. Fluorine-18 fluorodeoxyglucose-positron emission tomography: a highly accurate imaging modality for the diagnosis of chronic musculoskeletal infections. J Bone Joint Surg 2001;83A:651–60.

[158] El-Haddad G, Zhuang H, Gupta N, et al. Evolving role of positron emission tomography in the management of patients with inflammatory and other benign disorders. Semin Nucl Med 2004;34:313–29.

[159] Horger M, Eschmann SE, Pfannenberg C, et al. The value of SPET/CT in chronic osteomyelitis. Eur J Nucl Med Mol Imaging 2003;30:1665–73.

[160] Bar-Shalom R, Yefremov N, Guralnik L, et al. SPECT/CT using 67Ga and 111In-labeled leukocyte scintigraphy for diagnosis of infection. J Nucl Med 2006;47:587–94.

[161] Zhuang H, Sam JW, Chaco TK, et al. Rapid normalization of osseous FDG uptake following traumatic or surgical fractures. Eur J Nucl Med Mol Imaging 2003;30:1096–103.

ELSEVIER
SAUNDERS

Infect Dis Clin N Am
20 (2006) 827–847

INFECTIOUS
DISEASE CLINICS
OF NORTH AMERICA

Reactive Arthritis: Defined Etiologies, Emerging Pathophysiology, and Unresolved Treatment

John D. Carter, MD

Division of Rheumatology, University of South Florida, 12901 Bruce B. Downs Boulevard,
MDC 81, Tampa, FL 33612, USA

Reactive arthritis (ReA) is an inflammatory arthritis that arises after certain types of gastrointestinal or genitourinary infections. It belongs to the group of arthritidies known as the "spondyloarthropathies." The earliest description of ReA might date back to the writings of Hippocrates: "A youth does not suffer from gout until sexual intercourse" [1]. In 1916, Hans Reiter described the clinical triad of arthritis, nongonococcal urethritis, and conjunctivitis that occurred in a German soldier after an episode of bloody diarrhea. He incorrectly assumed it was caused by a spirochete and named this triad "spirochetosis arthritica" [2]. In 1942, the symptoms were recognized as a syndrome by two Harvard researchers (Bauer and Engleman), which they dubbed Reiter syndrome.

More recently the term "reactive arthritis" has been adopted and the eponym Reiter syndrome has fallen out of favor. During World War II, Reiter authorized medical experiments on concentration camp prisoners. Because of this, some have argued against the use of the Reiter eponym [3]. Further, it is now known that most cases do not include the complete triad [4]. Because ReA is a more descriptive term and it does not rely on the clinical triad for diagnosis, it has become the appropriate terminology for this disease process. Given the bacterial persistence associated with ReA, however, which is discussed herein, yet another new name has recently been suggested: postinfectious arthritis [5]. For the purposes of this article, this disease process is referred to as "reactive arthritis."

E-mail address: jocarter@health.usf.edu

0891-5520/06/$ - see front matter © 2006 Elsevier Inc. All rights reserved.
doi:10.1016/j.idc.2006.09.004

id.theclinics.com

Epidemiology

The lack of a disease definition or specific diagnostic criteria for ReA makes epidemiologic studies problematic [6,7]. The incidence of ReA varies widely between different studies. The variability of genetic background, including different prevalence of HLA-B27 in the various communities studied, might be a partial explanation. Local environmental factors also play a role in the apparent variable attack rate of ReA. For example, infection with one of the causative organisms, *Yersinia enterocolitica*, is uncommon in the United States but more commonly reported in Europe [8]. To further complicate this, infections with the same organisms in the same community can vary over time [9,10] and it is possible that local differences in the microbes themselves may lend to a different prevalence of ReA. Increased recognition and improved treatment of the causative organisms may also alter the subsequent attack rate of ReA.

The postdysentery form of ReA affects males and females with the same frequency, whereas the postvenereal form occurs at a male to female ratio of 9:1. Adults are more likely to develop ReA than children [9,11]. The attack rate of postdysentery ReA ranges from 1.5% [12] to about 30% [13]. ReA is thought to occur in about 4% of individuals who develop an acute *Chlamydia trachomatis* (Ct) infection [14].

Bacteria that commonly cause ReA are *Salmonella*, *Shigella*, *Campylobacter*, *Yersinia*, and Ct. There is also mounting evidence that *Chlamydophila (Chlamydia) pneumoniae* (Cpn) is another etiology of ReA [15–17]. Acute Ct infections are often asymptomatic or occult [18]. Cpn is a common cause of atypical pneumonia or bronchitis and as many as 70% of infections are asymptomatic [19]. In addition, when an acute infection with Cpn is symptomatic, a definitive diagnosis of this organism is often never established.

In 1996, the Centers for Disease Control and Prevention estimated 3 million new cases of Ct infections among persons 15 to 44 years of age in the United States [20]. Assuming the published attack rate of 4.1%, this equates to an annual incidence of 123,000 cases of ReA to Ct in the United States. This estimate may actually be low because this study consisted primarily of African Americans and the prevalence of HLA-B27 in that population is known to be lower than in white Americans. This also does not include cases that are secondary to Cpn or are postdysentery in nature. As a comparison, the estimated annual incidence of rheumatoid arthritis in the United States is 44.6 per 100,000 [21]. In the 2000 United States census, the population was 281 million. This equates to about 125,000 new cases of rheumatoid arthritis in the United States every year. A 2002 study in Sweden found the annual incidence of ReA to be higher than that of rheumatoid arthritis [22]. ReA represents a considerable burden on the United States population, and around the world, which may be vastly underrecognized.

Although ReA seems to be underrecognized, there are some data to suggest that the incidence may be decreasing in recent years [23]. The reasons for this are not entirely clear, but they may relate to better prevention and treatment of acute Ct infections. After the outbreak of HIV in the 1980s, sexual education and the increased use of barrier protection may have lead to less Ct-induced ReA. There are also data to suggest that the use of antibiotics that are active against Ct when patients present for treatment of their venereal disease reduces the risk of postvenereal ReA [24].

Clinical features

The clinical features of ReA are well described and are generally congruent for the postvenereal and the postenteric forms. These include articular, tendon, mucosal, cutaneous, ocular, and occasionally cardiac manifestations (Box 1) or systemic features (fever, malaise, weight loss). These symptoms start within 1 to 4 weeks of the initial infection. As stated, however, the inciting infection could be asymptomatic; reliance on a symptomatic triggering infection results in underdiagnosis or misdiagnosis.

Generally half of the individuals afflicted with ReA experience spontaneous resolution of their symptoms within 6 months and half evolve into a chronic form of ReA. Of those who develop chronic ReA some exhibit a relapsing disease course. A large United States study demonstrated that 63% of individuals who develop ReA experience chronic symptoms [19]. Individuals with postenteric ReA may develop chronic mild diarrhea.

Triggering microbes

The triggering microbes of ReA are gram-negative bacteria with a lipopolysaccharide component of their cell walls. All of these bacteria, or their bacterial products, have been demonstrated in the synovial tissue or fluid of patients with ReA. This has been demonstrated in multiple studies involving many different laboratories [25–33]. It is apparent that the entire bacteria or bacterial components traffic to the joints of patients with ReA. Aside from the definite bacterial triggers of ReA, there are many other bacteria that have been implicated as potential causes (Box 2).

Chlamydia

Ct is a very common pathogen and believed to be the most common cause of ReA [34]. Ct has been demonstrated in 50% of patients with a preceding symptomatic urogenital infection who developed ReA [35]. The routine presence of Ct has been demonstrated by polymerase chain reaction (PCR) in the synovial tissue of patients with ReA [27,36,37]. Of special interest is the fact that these chlamydiae are viable, albeit in an aberrant state [27,36]. These persistently viable chlamydiae have been demonstrated years after the initial infection [27]. Similar PCR studies have demonstrated Cpn in the synovial tissue of patients with ReA, although it is less commonly

Box 1. Clinical manifestations of reactive arthritis

Articular
Most commonly present with oligoarthritis, but can also present
    with polyarthritis or monoarthritis
Axial
    Frequently involved
        Sacroiliac joints
        Lumbar spine
    Occasionally involved
        Thoracic spine (usually seen in chronic ReA)
        Cervical spine (usually seen in chronic ReA)
        Cartilagenous joints (symphysis pubis, sternoclavicular
            joints)
Peripheral
    Frequently involved
        Large joints of the lower extremities (especially knees)
Dactylitis (sausage digit)
    Very specific for a spondyloarthropathy

Enthesitis
Hallmark feature
Transitional zone where collagenous structures, such as tendons
    and ligaments, insert into bone
Inflammation causes collagen fibers to undergo metaplasia
    forming fibrous bone
Chronic enthesitis leads to radiographic findings
    Plantar or Achilles spurs
    Periostitis
    Nonmarginal syndesmophytes
    Syndesmoses of the sacroiliac joints

Mucosal
Oral ulcers (generally painless)
Sterile dysuria

Cutaneous
Keratoderma blennorrhagicum
    Pustular or plaquelike rash on the soles or palms
        Grossly and histologically indistinguishable from pustular
            psoriasis
    May also involve
        Nails (onycholysis, subungual keratosis, nail pits)
        Scalp
        Extremities

Circinate balanitis
Erythema or plaquelike lesions on the shaft or glans of penis

Ocular
Conjunctivitis
Typically during acute stages only
Anterior uveitis (iritis)
Often recurrent
Rarely described
Scleritis, pars planitis, iridocyclitis, and others

Cardiac
Aortic regurgitation
Pericarditis
Valvular pathologies

---

detected [28]. Both Ct and Cpn, however, have occasionally been demonstrated in the synovial tissue of patients with other types of arthritis or even asymptomatic individuals [38,39]. These findings are discussed in more detail in the pathophysiology section.

It has been suggested that individuals with postchlamydial ReA display different clinical features than those with nonchlamydial ReA. Specifically, postchlamydial individuals more often develop a monoarthritis or oligoarthritis with predominant lower extremity involvement, sacroiliitis, urethritis, a longer period between inciting infection and arthritis, and lower C-reactive protein levels [40].

Shigella

In 1944, *Shigella* was the first bacteria to be directly implicated as a cause of ReA [41]. *Shigella*, however, is the least common of the gastrointestinal-inducing organisms that are associated with ReA in developed countries [42]. This is in large part caused by the rarity of this organism in these communities. All four of the species of *Shigella* (*S flexneri, S dysenteriae, S sonnei,* and *S boydii*) can cause ReA. Previous data suggested that *S flexneri* and *S dysenteriae* are the most common causes, and *S sonnei* is a rare cause worldwide [42,43]. A study in 2005 from Finland, however, revealed cases of ReA to *S sonnei, S flexneri,* and *S dysenteriae,* with *S sonnei* being the most common cause [44]. The overall attack rate in this study was 7%.

Humans are the only known host for *Shigella,* so this makes the use of animal models impossible. Interestingly, *Shigella* is phylogenetically indistinguishable from *Escherichia coli. S flexneri* shares all but 175 of 3235 open reading frames with two strains of *E coli* [42]. Despite these similarities, they behave very differently. *Shigella* has the ability to invade human

Box 2. Triggering microbes of reactive arthritis

Definite causes
Postvenereal
Chlamydia trachomatis

Postenteric
*Salmonella (S enteritidis, S typhimurium, S bovismorbificans,
    S blockley)*
Shigella (S flexneri, S dysenteriae, S sonnei, S boydii)
Campylobacter (C jejuni, C coli)
Yersinia (Y enterocolitica, Y pseudotuberculosis)

Probable causes
Chlamydophila (Chlamydia) pneumoniae
Ureaplasma urealyticum
Bacille Calmette-Guérin (intravesicular)

Possible causes
Bacillus cereus
Brucella abortis
Clostridium difficile
Escherichia coli
Helicobacter pylori
Hafnia alvei
Lactobacillus
Neisseria meningitidis serogroup B
Pseudomona
Intestinal parasites (*Strongyloides stercolis, Taenia saginata,
    Giardia lamblia, Ascaris lumbricoides, Filariasis*, and
    Cryptosporidium)

*Other types of inflammatory arthritis in which bacteria may
    play a causative role*
Borrelia burgdorferi (Lyme disease)
Propionbacterium acnes (SAPHO)
Streptococcus sp (poststreptococcal ReA)
Tropheryma whippelii (Whipple's disease)

enterocytes, lyse intracellular vacuoles to enter the cytoplasm, and move from cell to cell. *E coli* can do none of these [42]. These capabilities are likely critical to the causation of ReA. Similar to Ct and Cpn, bacterial DNA from *Shigella* has been demonstrated in the synovial tissue of patients with ReA. In contrast, there have been no studies to detect viable organisms, only bacterial fragments [25,29].

Salmonella

Salmonella is a rod-shaped, motile bacterium (with two nonmotile exceptions that are not thought to cause human disease: *S gallinarum* and *S pullorum*). It is widespread in animals and environmental sources, and is one of the most common enteric infections in the United States. *Salmonella* is the most frequently studied enteric bacteria associated with ReA. After salmonellosis, individuals of white descent may be more likely than those of Asian descent to develop ReA [45], and children may be less susceptible than adults [11]. The attack rate of *Salmonella*-induced ReA has ranged between 6% and 30% [13,46]. As with the other causative organisms, efforts have been made to detect *Salmonella* in synovial tissue or fluid. *Salmonella* bacterial degradation products, but not bacterial DNA, have been detected in the synovial fluid from patients with *Salmonella*-induced ReA [31].

There have been large outbreaks of *Salmonella typhimurium* and *Salmonella enteritidis* with rheumatologic follow-up of affected individuals. Regarding the outbreaks of *S typhimurium*, these occurred in three different countries and the attack rate of ReA ranged from 6% to 14.6% with the HLA-B27 prevalence ranging from 17% to 50% of these individuals [46–49]. The attack rate of ReA ranged from 6.9% to 29% with four different outbreaks of *S enteritidis* in four different countries [13,50,51]. A HLA-B27 prevalence of 33% affected individuals was reported in one of these outbreaks [51]. There has also been one outbreak of *Salmonella bovismorbificans* that resulted in 12% of individuals developing ReA, of whom 45% were HLA-B27 positive [52].

Campylobacter

Campylobacter jejuni infections are now the leading cause of bacterial gastroenteritis reported in the United States [53]. In 1996, 46% of laboratory-confirmed cases of bacterial gastroenteritis reported to the Centers for Disease Control and Prevention were caused by *Campylobacter* species. This was followed in prevalence by salmonellosis (28%) and shigellosis (17%) [53]. It is estimated that 2.1 to 2.4 million cases of human campylobacter infections occur in the United States each year [53].

A study in Finland in 2002 of 870 patients with *Campylobacter*-positive stool cultures found that 7% of these individuals developed ReA [54]. Interestingly, the development of ReA was not associated with HLA-B27 in this study. Fourteen percent of affected individuals were HLA-B27 positive. This is similar to the background prevalence in Finland. Most of the cases were associated with *C jejuni*, but *Campylobacter coli* were also a cause. Other studies suggest a lower attack rate (1%–3%) of ReA after a *Campylobacter* infection with a possible slight increased risk in HLA-B27–positive individuals [12,55].

Yersinia

There are three species in the genus *Yersinia*, but only *Y enterocolitica* and *Y pseudotuberculosis* cause gastroenteritis. Both *Y enterocolitica* and *Y pseudotuberculosis* have been associated with ReA. In 1998, two different outbreaks of *Y pseudotuberculosis* were reported [56,57]. One occurred in Finland (serotype O:3) and resulted in 12% of affected individuals developing ReA [56]. The other occurred in Canada (serotype Ib) and 12% reported "joint pain" after their infection [57].

As with most of the other known triggering microbes, attempts have been made to localize *Yersinia* in the synovial tissue or fluid of affected individuals. Two studies have shown that *Yersinia* does indeed traffic to the joints, as is the case with the other organisms [26,30]. One of these studies suggested that these *Yerisinae* are metabolically active [26]. Conversely, the other only demonstrated bacterial degradation products [30].

Other possible triggering microbes

Many other organisms have been implicated as potential causes of ReA (see Box 2). Most of these reports exist in the form of case reports and the pathophysiology is not studied with these other organisms.

Intravesicular instillation of bacillus Calmette-Guérin is successfully used as a treatment for intermediate- and high-risk superficial bladder carcinoma. It has also been reported as a rare cause of ReA. A recent review found 48 papers reporting this complication of intravesicular bacillus Calmette-Guérin therapy [58]. This form of ReA generally responds to discontinuation of bacillus Calmette-Guérin therapy or nonsteroidal anti-inflammatory drugs; however, it rarely can evolve into a chronic process.

Poststreptococcal ReA, Lyme disease, and Whipple's disease are all caused by bacterial infections. Their clinical symptoms include inflammatory arthritis but they all have enough different features that are not part of traditional ReA that they should be considered separate. Poststreptococcal ReA includes small joint involvement, vasculitis, glomerulonephritis, and increased prevalence of HLA-DRB1*01 [59]. A migratory arthritis with central nervous system involvement is typical of Whipple's disease. Lyme disease includes a characteristic rash (erythema migrans) with central nervous system symptoms.

Pathophysiology

Triggering microbes persist

PCR technology has occasionally demonstrated the presence of chromosomal DNA from the known triggers in the synovial tissue of patients with the postdysentery form of ReA [30,31,33]. This same technology has demonstrated the routine presence of both Ct and Cpn in the synovial tissue of patients with the postchlamydial arthritis [27,28,36,37]. One important difference is that these chlamydiae exist in a persistent metabolically active state, whereas the postenteric organisms do not, with the possible exception of *Yersinia* [26]. The causative bacteria (or bacterial fragments) of ReA have occasionally been demonstrated in the synovial tissue of patients with various types of arthritis [60–62], so the importance of this finding has been questioned. Further, bacterial DNA from various bacteria not associated with ReA has been discovered in synovial tissue [38]. Conversely, the well-documented finding of viable *Chlamydia* highlights an important potential difference in the pathophysiology of postvenereal versus postenteric ReA.

The pattern of gene expression associated with persistently viable *Chlamydia* is significantly different than that seen during normal active infections. For example, during the persistent state expression of the major outer membrane protein (*omp1*) gene and several genes required for the cell division process are severely down-regulated. This is coupled with differential regulation of the three paralog genes specifying Ct heat shock proteins (HSP)-60 (Ct110, Ct604, and Ct755) [37].

It is important to remember that the findings regarding these specific HSP paralog genes apply only to Ct and not Cpn. There are differences even within the *Chlamydia* genus. There have also been differences in cytokine and chemokine mRNA profiles demonstrated in human synovial tissue chronically infected with Ct versus Cpn [36]. Further, a detailed gene expression profile of intracellular viable Ct and Cpn revealed different transcriptional response, which was no longer present when the organisms were UV-inactivated [63]. These differences suggest more than innate immunity is involved and may explain the apparent higher risk of ReA with Ct as opposed to Cpn.

Although there are differences in the HSP paralog genes between Ct and Cpn, HSPs in general are paramount to the persistent state of both Ct and Cpn. They provide many functions involved with cell survival. HSPs are conserved molecules synthesized by both prokaryotic and eukaryotic cells, and they are known to play an essential role in protein folding, assembly, and translocation. Under stressful conditions, HSPs allow cells to survive lethal assaults by preventing protein denaturation [64,65]. The HSP-60 molecule has many functions that seem to be important to the pathophysiology of ReA. HSP-60 has been shown to be pivotal in the inability of *Chlamydia*-infected cells to undergo apoptosis [66,67]. These same molecules are also thought to play a role in antibiotic resistance [64,68] and be potentially immunogenic [69]. Elimination of the HSPs is likely to be important in abrogating the pathogenic sequelae of *Chlamydia*-induced ReA or ReA in general. Such an act either eliminates the immunogenic nidus itself or renders the infected cell more susceptible to apoptosis or therapy.

Host response

Although the presence of viable *Chlamydia* or postenteric bacterial DNA in the synovium of patients with ReA has been demonstrated, many questions remain. It is clear that the entire *Chlamydia* organism is incorporated intracellularly. The same might also be true for *Yersinia*. It is also apparent that bacterial fragments of the postenteric organisms are incorporated into the cell. These intracellular bacteria or bacterial products are then trafficked to the synovium. What governs this process is not yet evident. It is also not clear if their presence in the affected organs represents a trigger for an autoimmune response, or if these organisms are the source for the inflammatory process. As this mystery unravels, it seems that this phenomenon of host tolerance is multifactorial in nature.

HLA-B27

Because HLA-B27 is a class I histocompatibility antigen, it has been postulated that HLA-B27 presents arthritogenic microbial peptides to T cells stimulating an autoimmune response, so called "molecular mimicry." A previous study has shown a high degree of conservation in the T-cell responses obtained from the synovial fluid of patients with recent ReA irrespective of the triggering organism [70].

Conversely, B27 itself may serve as the autoantigen that is targeted by the immune system. It is possible that exposure to the triggering bacteria may alter tolerance to the B27 antigen. Animal data exist to support this theory. Unlike their wild-type counterparts, HLA-B27 transgenic rats are tolerant of B27 immunization using B27-positive splenocytes or plasmid DNA. If these same splenocytes are exposed to *Chlamydia* in vitro, however, a cytotoxic response is generated [71]. No such response was generated with targets transfected with control B7, B14, B40, B44, or HLA-A2. Self-tolerance to B27 may be subverted by *Chlamydia* and possibly by the other gram-negative–triggering bacteria.

The role of HLA-B27 may, at least in part, function outside of antigen presentation. It has been suggested that HLA-B27 enhances the invasion of *Salmonella* into human intestinal epithelial cells [72]. It has also been suggested that *Salmonella* invasion leads to significant recognizable changes in the B27-bound peptide repertoire [73]. A similar study, however, found only minimal changes in the peptide repertoire [74]. Invasion of *Chlamydia* may not be altered by HLA-B27, but intracellular replication and formation of inclusion bodies might be suppressed by the cytoplasmic tail of this antigen [75]. If true, this could predispose the cell to chlamydial persistence. Conversely, it has been suggested that HLA-B27 has no influence on invasion or replication of Ct serovar L2 within cell lines [76].

Recent data suggest that HLA-B27 restricted epitopes derived from proteoglycans, specifically human aggrecan, serve as autoantigens, and are involved in the inflammation that is characteristic of the spondyloarthropathies and

ReA [77]. Perhaps the only clarity of HLA-B27's role in the pathophysiology of ReA is that its exact role is still undefined and it is not the sole determinant of disease predilection.

Cellular uptake

It is clear that the causative organisms of ReA are incorporated into peripheral blood mononuclear cells. These same organisms or bacterial products persist intracellularly in synovial cells (primarily macrophages). How this process of intracellular uptake occurs is less apparent. Chlamydial infection, specifically, is initiated when the elementary body binds to the target eukaryotic cell. There are some data that suggest that the elementary body of both Ct and Cpn interact with host cell surface glycosaminoglycans during cellular uptake [78]. Following invasion, however, the Ct was confined to distinct vacuoles that did not develop into characteristic inclusion bodies. Intriguing recent evidence suggests that apolipoprotein E, which is adherent to the surface of Ct and Cpn elementary bodies, attaches to the host cell LDL receptor family carrying the elementary body with it [79]. This could represent a truly remarkable adaptation of *Chlamydia* using a basic cellular function involving cell homeostasis as its pathway to host cell attachment and uptake.

Toll-like receptors

The Toll-like receptors (TLRs) recognize extracellular pathogens and activate immune cell responses as part of the innate immune system. TLR-4 recognizes lipopolysaccharide, thereby potentially playing a role in the pathophysiology of ReA. Recent mice data have shown that effective host clearance of Ct depends on appropriate TLR-4 expression by neutrophils [80]. TLR-4–deficient mice exposed to *Salmonella* demonstrate dramatically increased bacterial growth and increased demise [81]. Certain polymorphisms of TLR-4 have been associated with gram-negative infections and Crohn's disease and ulcerative colitis, two inflammatory conditions related with the spondyloarthropathies [82–84]. These same polymorphisms, however, seem not to confer risk of ReA [85].

Peripheral blood mononuclear cells from eight patients with *Salmonella* infections (four with ReA and four without) have been analyzed in both the acute and recovery phase of the infection [86]. All patients revealed high levels of activation and adhesion molecules and increased inflammatory and anti-inflammatory cytokine levels. During the recovery phase, the patients with ReA demonstrated completed down-regulation of CD14, whereas it was similar to healthy controls in those without ReA. Interestingly, CD14 is expressed in particularly high levels on macrophages. It functions as a coreceptor with TLR-4 for the detection of bacterial lipopolysaccharide [87].

Chemokine involvement

After an acute infection with the causative bacteria, these organisms are trafficked to the synovial tissue and other target organs. It is possible that chemokines guide this process for it is known that chemokines and chemokine receptors regulate leukocyte recruitment into inflamed tissues. CCR1 and CCR5 are known to play a role recruiting Th1-type T cells under inflammatory conditions [88]. It has been demonstrated that there is increased expression of CCR1, CXCR4, and CCR5 in the synovial tissue of patients with several types of arthritis including ReA [89]. There was no apparent unique chemokine profile related to ReA, however, compared with the other types of arthritis studied.

Th1 versus Th2/Th3 response

Although the Th1 cytokines play a role in the clinical manifestations of ReA, their importance seems to be less than that in other types of inflammatory arthritis. This might be particularly true for chronic ReA. Tumor necrosis factor (TNF)-α has been measured in the peripheral blood of patients with ReA. Compared with patients with rheumatoid arthritis, ReA patients demonstrated significantly lower levels of TNF-α [90]. Further, patients who were HLA-B27 positive or had disease duration of greater than 6 months secreted significantly less TNF-α in their peripheral blood. Similar findings have been demonstrated in the joints of patients with ReA (ie, higher levels of interleukin-10 and lower levels of TNF-α and interferon-γ, favoring a Th2 profile) [91,92].

Temporal relationships of these different Th1 and Th2 cytokines may also be important in disease manifestations and maintenance. Slight changes in the Th1-Th2 balance may explain the relapsing course that is frequently seen with ReA. Alterations in the initial Th1-Th2 balance may also predispose to disease initiation. A *Chlamydia*-induced arthritis rat model demonstrated that susceptible rats mounted a lesser initial TNF-α, interferon-γ, and interleukin-4 response to their *Chlamydia* infection [93]. Lower initial responses of these Th1 cytokines may increase the likelihood of developing ReA compared with those patients who are exposed to the causative organism but do not develop ReA.

Other data suggest a role for the Th3 response. Gammadelta-positive synovial-based T cells from patients with ReA predominantly express transforming growth factor-β_2 and granulocyte-monocyte–colony stimulating factor [94]. Compared with CD4$^+$ and CD8$^+$ T cells from the same patients, they expressed a more heterogeneous cytokine profile that favored that of the Th3 response.

Finally, background cytokine levels favoring a Th2 response might contribute to bacterial persistence. In vitro data have shown that low levels of TNF-α and interferon-γ help to promote the persistent state of both Ct and

Cpn [95–99]. Indeed, if the levels of these cytokines are low enough this may stimulate increased metabolic activity of the organism.

Diagnostic tests

Unfortunately, there is not a diagnostic test for ReA. During the acute stage, individuals often display elevated acute phase reactants, such as an elevated sedimentation rate or C-reactive protein. Conversely, patients with chronic ReA typically display normal levels. HLA-B27 is generally increased in ReA, although rates have varied from 0% to 88% [100,101]. Most of the data regarding ReA suggest an HLA-B27 prevalence of 30% to 50% [44,48,51,52,54,55,102,103]. There may be an overreliance on this HLA type for diagnostic purposes. Isolation of the triggering infection is helpful, but this is usually not possible with routine cultures after the onset of arthritis. It has been suggested that chlamydial IgG or IgA titers are useful at diagnosing patients with persistent *Chlamydia* infections [104–107]. Most of these data, however, apply only to Cpn in disease states other than ReA. There is also cross-reactivity between chlamydial serotypes, so their use has been questioned. PCR analysis of synovial tissue or fluid for the causative organisms or degradation products is useful but not readily available to most practitioners.

The radiographic features of ReA include sacroiliitis, periostitis, nonmarginal syndesmophytes, periosteal new bone formation, joint erosions, and joint space narrowing. These findings, however, are only apparent on plain radiographs with chronic disease. There may be a role for MRI or ultrasound (of the sacroiliac or other joints) to detect earlier changes, but they have not been formally studied in ReA.

Treatment

Traditional therapies for ReA include nonsteroidal anti-inflammatory drugs, corticosteroids, and disease-modifying antirheumatic drugs. Nonsteroidal anti-inflammatory drugs have been used to treat the joint inflammation associated with ReA. Although they seem to improve the articular symptoms of ReA, they are not thought to have any impact on the associated extra-articular symptoms. Although a breadth of clinical experience suggests that they help with the inflammatory arthritis associated with ReA, there are no well-designed prospective trials analyzing their efficacy for this indication.

Corticosteroids have limited benefit for the axial symptoms and may be more effective for the peripheral arthritis of ReA [9]. Local corticosteroid injections into affected joints may provide short-term relief. Corticosteroids also seem to be helpful at treating some of the extra-articular manifestations, such as iritis. Topical corticosteroids may also be useful for circinate balanitis (CB) and keratoderma blennorrhagicum (KB).

Traditional disease-modifying antirheumatic drugs have also been used for patients with chronic ReA because these patients can develop radiographic abnormalities with subsequent joint deformities if left untreated. The best studied disease-modifying antirheumatic drug in the setting of ReA is sulfasalazine. A prospective trial of 134 subjects designed to assess the efficacy of sulfasalazine in ReA [108]. In this trial there was a trend favoring sulfasalazine compared with placebo, because improvement was documented in 62% of the participants on sulfasalazine and 47% on placebo ($P = .089$). There were no significant improvements in any of the clinical measures followed compared with placebo, however, including swollen and tender joint counts. Methotrexate, azathioprine, and cyclosporine have been advocated as potential treatments but never formally evaluated in a prospective trial.

The TNF-α antagonists have demonstrated great success in the treatment of other types of spondyloarthropathies. There are potential theoretical concerns, however, regarding TNF-α antagonism in ReA. Lower levels of TNF-α have been demonstrated in ReA compared with other types of inflammatory arthritis, and ReA is believed to be more of a Th2-driven disease [90–92]. Also, in vitro data suggest that persistent Ct and Cpn levels are inversely associated with TNF-α levels [95–99]. There are no randomized trials in ReA to assess accurately their efficacy in this setting. There have, however, been a small open label study and case reports suggesting clinical benefit with these drugs in the treatment of ReA [109–111]. In an open label study with etanercept, there were five patients who were PCR positive for *Chlamydia* at some time during the observation period. Of the five, three were PCR positive in the synovium for Ct before treatment. Of these three, two of the patients were PCR negative on therapy and one remained positive. Two patients, however, with negative PCR results at baseline became PCR positive for Cpn while on etanercept [109]. These equivocal results do not dissuade the theoretical concerns that exist regarding the use of these drugs in ReA. Conversely, patients with ReA do exhibit higher serum levels of TNF-α levels compared with normal controls [94], so this might suggest that these patients would benefit from TNF-α antagonists. The use of TNF-α antagonists in the treatment of ReA is unanswered.

The exact role of antibiotics as a treatment for ReA has yet to be fully defined. A trial assessing 3 months of treatment with lymecycline showed no benefit to patients with postdysentery ReA, whereas there was improvement in patients with *Chlamydia*-induced ReA [112]. A subgroup analysis of another previous trial studying ciprofloxacin as a treatment for ReA suggested benefit in postchlamydial patients with no such improvement in the other patients [113]. Other studies assessing doxycycline, ciprofloxacin, and azithromycin in ReA failed to show benefit, but there was no effort to separate postchlamydial patients [103,114–116]. Interestingly, a follow-up of one of the aforementioned ciprofloxacin trials suggested that this antibiotic significantly improved long-term prognosis [117]. Finally, another study suggested significant improvement in patients with postchlamydial ReA with a combination of knee synovectomy and 3 months of azithromycin [118]. It seems that there may be benefit in the postchlamydial form but not ReA that is secondary to the postdysentery organisms. The observation of viable *Chlamydia*, and the general lack of viable postdysentery organisms, in the synovial tissue of patients with ReA support this finding.

The complexity of antibiotics as a potential treatment for *Chlamydia*-induced ReA runs even deeper. In vitro data have shown that intracellular chlamydiae are driven into a persistent state when exposed to chronic monotherapy with several antibiotics including doxycycline, azithromycin, rifampin, and ciprofloxacin [119–122]. These data suggest that chronic monotherapy with the aforementioned antibiotics is unlikely to eradicate the persistent infection. Interesting in vitro data suggest successful synergistic eradication of cells infected with persistent *Chlamydia* with a combination rifampin and azithromycin [120]. In this same study, monotherapy with both of these same antibiotics did not eradicate the persistent infection. A 2004 study revealed significant improvement in patients with presumed *Chlamydia*-induced ReA after 9 months of a combination of rifampin and doxycycline compared with doxycycline monotherapy [102]. It is possible that a prolonged combination of antibiotics may eradicate the persistent state of *Chlamydia* along with its pathogenic sequelae. As is the case with TNF-α antagonists, the exact role of antibiotics in ReA is still not clear. It seems, however, that their only potential role relates to the treatment of *Chlamydia*-induced ReA and not to the postenteric form.

Summary

ReA is unique in that it is one of the few disease states of which there is a known trigger. This insight into disease initiation has led to great advances in the pathophysiology. Despite this detailed knowledge, the proper treatment remains elusive. In the years to come it is possible that the specific treatment will be dictated by the triggering microbe.

References

[1] Amor B. Reiter's syndrome: diagnosis and clinical features. Rheum Dis Clin North Am 1998;24:677–95.

[2] Reiter H. Uber eine bisher unerkannate spirochateninfektion (Spirochetosis arthritica). Dtsch Med Wochenschr 1916;42:1535–6.

[3] Lu DW, Katz KA. Declining use of the eponym "Reiter's syndrome" in the medical literature, 1998–2003. J Am Acad Dermatol 2005;53:720–3.

[4] Parker CT, Thomas D. Reiter's syndrome and reactive arthritis. J Am Osteopath Assoc 2000;100:101–4.

[5] Hannu T, Inman R, Granfors K, et al. Reactive arthritis or post-infectious arthritis? Best Pract Res Clin Rheumatol 2006;20:419–33.

[6] Braun J, Kingsley G, van der Heijde D, et al. On the difficulties of establishing a consensus on the definition of and diagnostic investigations of reactive arthritis. Results and

discussion of a questionnaire prepared for the 4th International Workshop on Reactive Arthritis, Berlin, Germany, July 3–6, 1999. J Rheumatol 2000;27:2185–92.

[7] Michet CJ, Machado EBV, Ballard DJ, et al. Epidemiology of Reiter's syndrome in Rochester, Minnesota 1950–1980. Arthritis Rheum 1988;31:428–32.

[8] Leirisalo-Repo M, Suoranta H. Ten-year follow-up study on patients with *Yersinia* arthritis. Arthritis Rheum 1988;31:533–7.

[9] Flores D, Marquez J, Garza M, et al. Reactive arthritis: newer developments. Rheum Dis Clin North Am 2003;29:37–59.

[10] Leirisalo-Repo M. Treatment of reactive arthritis. Rheumatol Eur 1995;24:20–2.

[11] Rudwaleit M, Richter S, Braun J, et al. Low incidence of reactive arthritis in children following a salmonella outbreak. Ann Rheum Dis 2001;60:1055–7.

[12] Eastmond CJ, Rennie JA, Reid TM. An outbreak of *Campylobacter* enteritis: a rheumatological followup survey. J Rheumatol 1983;10:107–8.

[13] Dworkin MS, Shoemaker PC, Goldoft MJ, et al. Reactive arthritis and Reiter's syndrome following and outbreak of gastroenteritis caused by *Salmonella enteritidis*. Clin Infect Dis 2001;33:1010–4.

[14] Rich E, Hook EW III, Alarcon GS, et al. Reactive arthritis in patients attending and urban sexually transmitted disease clinic. Arthritis Rheum 1996;39:1172–7.

[15] Braun J, Laitko S, Treharne J, et al. *Chlamydia pneumoniae*: a new causative agent of reactive arthritis and undifferentiated oligoarthritis. Ann Rheum Dis 1994;53:100–5.

[16] Hannu T, Puolakkainen M, Leirisalo-Repo M. *Chlamydia pneumoniae* as a triggering infection in reactive arthritis. Rheumatology (Oxford) 1999;38:411–4.

[17] Saario R, Toivanen A. *Chlamydia pneumonia* as a cause of reactive arthritis. Br J Rheumatol 1993;32:1112.

[18] Stamm WE. *Chlamydia trachomatis* infections: progress and problems. J Infect Dis 1999; 179(Suppl 2):380–3.

[19] Miyashita N, Niki Y, Nakajima M, et al. Prevalence of asymptomatic infection with *Chlamydia pneumoniae* in subjectively healthy adults. Chest 2001;119:1416–9.

[20] Groseclose SL, Zaidi AA, Delisle SJ, et al. Estimated incidence and prevalence of genital *Chlamydia trachomatis* infections in the United States, 1996. Sex Transm Dis 1999;26: 339–44.

[21] Doran MF, Pond GR, Crowson CS, et al. Trends in incidence and mortality in rheumatoid arthritis in Rochester, Minnesota, over a forty-year period. Arthritis Rheum 2002;46: 625–31.

[22] Soderlin MK, Borjesson O, Kautiainen H, et al. Annual incidence of inflammatory joint disease in a population based study in southern Sweden. Ann Rheum Dis 2002;61:911–5.

[23] Iliopoulos A, Karras D, Ioakimidis D, et al. Change in the epidemiology of Reiter's syndrome (reactive arthritis) in the post-AIDS era? An analysis of cases appearing in the Greek Army. J Rheumatol 1995;22:252–4.

[24] Bardin T, Enel C, Cornelis F, et al. Antibiotic treatment of venereal disease and Reiter's syndrome in a Greenland population. Arthritis Rheum 1992;35:190–4.

[25] Braun J, Tuszewski M, Ehlers S, et al. Nested polymerase chain reaction strategy simultaneously targeting DNA sequences of multiple bacterial species in inflammatory joint diseases. II. Examination of sacroiliac and knee joint biopsies of patients with spondyloarthropathies and other arthritides. J Rheumatol 1997;24:1101–5.

[26] Gaston JS, Cox C, Granfors K. Clinical and experimental evidence for persistent *Yersinia* infection in reactive arthritis. Arthritis Rheum 1999;42:2239–42.

[27] Gerard HC, Branigan PJ, Schumacher HR Jr, et al. Synovial *Chlamydia trachomatis* in patients with reactive arthritis/Reiter's syndrome are viable but show aberrant gene expression. J Rheumatol 1998;25:734–42.

[28] Gerard HC, Schumacher HR, El-Gabalawy H, et al. *Chlamydia pneumoniae* present in the human synovium are viable and metabolically active. Microb Pathog 2000;29:17–24.

[29] Granfors K, Jalkanen S, Toivancn P, et al. Bacterial lipopolysaccharide in synovial fluid cells in *Shigella* triggered reactive arthritis. J Rheumatol 1992;19:500.

[30] Nikkari S, Merilahti-Palo R, Saario R, et al. *Yersinia*-triggered reactive arthritis. Use of polymerase chain reaction and immunocytochemical in the detection of bacterial components from synovial specimens. Arthritis Rheum 1992;35:682–7.

[31] Nikkari S, Rantakokko K, Ekman P, et al. Salmonella-triggered reactive arthritis: use of polymerase chain reaction, immunocytochemical staining, and gas-chromatography-mass spectrometry in the detection of bacterial components from synovial fluid. Arthritis Rheum 1999;42:84–9.

[32] Taylor-Robinson D, Gilroy CB, Thomas BJ, et al. Detection of *Chlamydia trachomatis* DNA in joints of reactive arthritis patients by polymerase chain reaction. Lancet 1992; 340:81–2.

[33] Viitanen AM, Arstila TP, Lahesmaa R, et al. Application of the polymerase chain reaction and immunoflourescence to the detection of bacteria in *Yersinia*-triggered reactive arthritis. Arthritis Rheum 1991;34:89–96.

[34] Barth WF, Segal K. Reactive arthritis (Reiter's syndrome). Am Fam Physician 1999;60: 499–503, 507.

[35] Rahman MU, Hudson AP, Schumacher HR. *Chlamydia* and Reiter's syndrome (reactive arthritis). Rheum Dis Clin North Am 1992;18:67–79.

[36] Gerard HC, Wang Z, Whittum-Hudson JA, et al. Cytokine and chemokine mRNA produced in synvovial tissue chronically infected with *Chlamydia trachomatis* and *C. pneumoniae*. J Rheumatol 2002;29:1827–35.

[37] Gerard HC, Whittum-Hudson JA, Schumacher HR, et al. Differential expression of three *Chlamydia trachomatis* hsp60-encoding genes in active vs. persistent infections. Microb Pathog 2004;36:35–9.

[38] Gerard HC, Wang Z, Wang GF, et al. Chromosomal DNA from a variety of bacterial species is present in synovial tissue from patients with various forms of arthritis. Arthritis Rheum 2001;44:1689–97.

[39] Schumacher HR Jr, Arayssi T, Crane M, et al. *Chlamydia trachomatis* nucleic acids can be found in the synovium of some asymptomatic subjects. Arthritis Rheum 1999;42: 1281–4.

[40] Ozgul A, Dede I, Taskaynatan MA, et al. Clinical presentations of chlamydial and non-chlamydial reactive arthritis. Rheumatol Int 2006;26:879–85.

[41] Paronen J. Reiter's disease: a study of 344 cases observed in Finland. Acta Med Scand 1948; 131(Suppl 212):1–112.

[42] Gaston JS. *Shigella* induced reactive arthritis. Ann Rheum Dis 2005;64:517–8.

[43] Barrett-Connor E, Connor JD. Extra-intestinal manifestations of shigellosis. Am J Gastroenterol 1970;52:234–45.

[44] Hannu T, Mattila L, Siitonen A, et al. Reactive arthritis attributable to *Shigella* infection: a clinical and epidemiological nationwide study. Ann Rheum Dis 2005;64:594–8.

[45] McColl GJ, Diviney MB, Holdswaorth RF, et al. HLA-B27 expression and reactive arthritis susceptibility in two patient cohorts infected with *Salmonella typhimurium*. Aust N Z J Med 2000;30:28–32.

[46] Buxton JA, Fyfe M, Berger S, et al. Reactive arthritis and other sequelae following sporadic *Salmonella typhimurium* infection in British Columbia, Canada: a case control study. J Rheumatol 2002;29:2154–8.

[47] Hannu T, Mattila L, Siitonen A, et al. Reactive arthritis following an outbreak of *Salmonella typhimuriom* phage type 193 infection. Ann Rheum Dis 2002;61:264–6.

[48] Inman RD, Johnston ME, Hodge M, et al. Postdysenteric reactive arthritis: a clinical and immunogenetic study following an outbreak of salmonellosis. Arthritis Rheum 1988;31: 1377–83.

[49] Lee AT, Hall RG, Pile KD. Reactive joint symptoms following an outbreak of *Salmonella typhimurium* phage type 135a. J Rheumatol 2005;32:524–7.

[50] Locht H, Kihlstrom E, Lindstrom FD. Reactive arthritis after *Salmonella* among medical doctors: study of an outbreak. J Rheumatol 1993;20:845–8.

[51] Mattila L, Leirisalo-Repo M, Koskimies S, et al. Reactive arthritis following an outbreak of *Salmonella* infection in Finland. Br J Rheumatol 1994;33:1136–41.

[52] Mattila L, Leirisalo-Repo M, Pelkonene P, et al. Reactive arthritis following an outbreak of *Salmonella bovismorbificans* infection. J Infect 1998;36:289–95.

[53] Altekruse SF, Stern NJ, Fields PI, et al. *Campylobacter jejuni*: an emerging foodborne pathogen. Emerg Infect Dis 1999;5:28–35.

[54] Hannu T, Mattila L, Rautelin H, et al. *Campylobacter*-triggered reactive arthritis: a population-based study. Rheumatology 2002;41:312–8.

[55] Hannu T, Kauppi M, Tuomala M, et al. Reactive arthritis following an outbreak of *Campylobacter jejuni* infection. J Rheumatol 2004;31:528–30.

[56] Hannu T, Mattila L, Nuorti JP, et al. Reactive arthritis after an outbreak of *Yersinia* pseudotuberculosis serotype O:3 infection. Ann Rheum Dis 2003;62:866–9.

[57] Press N, Fyfe M, Bowie W, et al. Clinical and microbiological follow-up of an outbreak of *Yersinia* pseudotuberculosis serotype Ib. Scand J Infect Dis 2001;33:523–6.

[58] Tinazzi E, Ficarra V, Simeoni S, et al. Reactive arthritis following BCG immunotherapy for urinary bladder carcinoma: a systematic review. Rheumatol Int 2006;26:481–8.

[59] Ahmed S, Ayoub EM, Scornik JC, et al. Poststreptococcal reactive arthritis: clinical characteristics and associations with HLA-DR alleles. Arthritis Rheum 1998;41:1096–102.

[60] Cox CJ, Kempsell KE, Gaston JS. Investigation of infectious agents associated with arthritis by reverse transcription PCR of bacterial rRNA. Arthritis Res Ther 2003;5:R1–8.

[61] Cuchacovich R, Japa S, Huang WQ, et al. Detection of bacterial DNA in Latin American patients with reactive arthritis by polymerase chain reaction and sequencing analysis. J Rheumatol 2002;29:1426–9.

[62] Wilkinson NZ, Kingsley GH, Jones HW, et al. The detection of DNA from a range of bacterial species in the joints of patients with a variety of arthritidies using a nested, broad-range polymerase chain reaction. Rheumatology 1999;38:260–6.

[63] Hess S, Peters J, Bartling G, et al. More than just innate immunity: comparative analysis of *Chlamydophila pneumoniae* and *Chlamydia trachomatis* effects on host-cell gene regulation. Cell Microbiol 2003;5:785–95.

[64] Zugel U, Kaufmann SH. Role of heat shock proteins in protection from and pathogenesis of infectious diseases. Clin Microbiol Rev 1999;12:19–39.

[65] Zugel U, Kaufmann SH. Immune response against heat shock proteins in infectious diseases. Immunobiology 1999;201:22–35.

[66] Airenne S, Surcel HM, Tuukkanen J, et al. *Chlamydia pneumoniae* inhibits apoptosis in human epithelial and monocyte cell lines. Scand J Immunol 2002;55:390–8.

[67] Dean D, Powers VC. Persistent *Chlamydia trachomatis* infections resist apoptotic stimuli. Infect Immun 2001;69:2442–7.

[68] Qoronfleh MW, Gustafson JE, Wilkinson BJ. Conditions that induce *Staphylococcus* heat shock proteins also inhibit autolysis. FEMS Microbiol Lett 1998;166:103–7.

[69] Curry AJ, Portig I, Goodall JC, et al. T lymphocyte lines isolated from atheromatous plaque contain cells capable of responding to *Chlamydia* antigens. Clin Exp Immunol 2000;121:261–9.

[70] Dulphy N, Peyrat MA, Tieng V, et al. Common intra-articular T cell expansions in patients with reactive arthritis: identical beta-chain junctional sequences and cytotoxicity toward HLA-B27. J Immunol 1999;162:3830–9.

[71] Popov I, Dela Cruz CS, Barber BH, et al. Breakdown of CTL tolerance to self HLA-B*2705 induced by exposure to *Chlamydia trachomatis*. J Immunol 2002;169:4033–8.

[72] Saarinen M, Ekman P, Ikeda M, et al. Invasion of *Salmonella* into human intestinal epithelial cells is modulated by HLA-B27. Rheumatology (Oxford) 2002;41:651–7.

[73] Maksymowych WP, Ikawa T, Yamaguchi A, et al. Invasion by *Salmonella typhimurium* induces increased expression of the LMP, MECL, and PA28 proteasome genes and changes in the peptide repertoire of HLA-B27. Infect Immun 1998;66:4624–32.

[74] Ramos M, Alvarez I, Garcia-del-Portillo F, et al. Minimal alterations in the HLA-B27-bound peptide repertoire induced upon infection of lymphoid cells with *Salmonella typhimurium*. Arthritis Rheum 2001;44:1677–88.

[75] Kuipers JG, Bialowons A, Dollmann P, et al. The modulation of chlamydial replication by HLA-B27 depends on the cytoplasmic domain of HLA-B27. Clin Exp Rheumatol 2001;19:47–52.

[76] Young JL, Smith L, Matyszak MK, et al. HLA-B27 expression does not modulate intracellular *Chlamydia trachomatis* infection of cell lines. Infect Immun 2001;69:6670–5.

[77] Kuon W, Kuhne M, Busch DH, et al. Identification of novel human aggrecan T cell epitopes in HLA-B27 transgenic mice associated with spondyloarthropathy. J Immunol 2004; 173:4859–66.

[78] Matyszak MK, Young JL, Gaston JS. Uptake and processing of *Chlamydia trachomatis* by human dendritic cells. Eur J Immunol 2002;32:742–51.

[79] Hudson AP, Whittum-Hudson JA, Gérard HO. *C trachomatis* utilizes the LDL receptor family for host cell attachment. Arthritis Rheum 2006;54(9 Suppl):S783.

[80] Zhang X, Glogauer M, Zhu F, et al. Innate immunity and arthritis: neutrophil Rac and toll-like receptor 4 expression define outcomes in infection-triggered arthritis. Arthritis Rheum 2005;52:1297–304.

[81] Vazquez-Torres A, Vallance BA, Bergman MA, et al. Toll-like receptor 4 dependence of innate and adaptive immunity to *Salmonella*: importance of the Kupffer cell network. J Immunol 2004;172:6202–8.

[82] Agnese DM, Calvano JE, Hahm SJ, et al. Human toll-like receptor 4 mutations but not CD14 polymorphisms are associated with an increased risk of gram-negative infections. J Infect Dis 2002;186:1522–5.

[83] Brand S, Staudinger T, Schnitzler F, et al. The roll of Toll-like receptor 4 Asp299Gly and Thr399Ile polymorphisms and CARD15/NOD2 mutations in the susceptibility and phenotype of Crohn's disease. Inflamm Bowel Dis 2005;11:645–52.

[84] Torok HP, Glas J, Tonenchi L, et al. Polymorphisms of the lipopolysaccharide-signaling complex in inflammatory bowel disease: association of a mutation in the Toll-like receptor 4 gene with ulcerative colitis. Clin Immunol 2004;112:85–91.

[85] Gergely P Jr, Blazsek A, Weiszhar Z, et al. Lack of genetic association of the Toll-like receptor 4 (TLR4) Asp299Gly and THR399Ile polymorphisms with spondyloarthropathies in Hungarian population. Rheumatology (Oxford) 2006;45(10):1194–6.

[86] Kirveskari J, He Q, Holmstrom T, et al. Modulation of peripheral blood mononuclear cell activation status during *Salmonella*-triggered reactive arthritis. Arthritis Rheum 1999;42: 2045–54.

[87] Rallabhandi P, Bell J, Boukhvalova MS, et al. Analysis of TLR4 polymorphic variants: new insights into TLR4/MD-2/CD14 stoichiometry, structure, and signaling. J Immunol 2006; 177:322–32.

[88] Weber C, Weber KS, Klier C, et al. Specialized roles of the chemokine receptors CCR1 and CCR5 in the recruitment of monocytes and T(H)1-like/CD45RO(+) T cells. Blood 2001;97: 1144–6.

[89] Haringman JJ, Smeets TJ, Reinders-Blankert P, et al. Chemokine and chemokine receptor expression in paired peripheral blood mononuclear cells and synovial tissue of patients with rheumatoid arthritis, osteoarthritis, and reactive arthritis. Ann Rheum Dis 2006;65: 294–300.

[90] Braun J, Yin Z, Spiller I, et al. Low secretion of tumor necrosis factor alpha, but no other Th1 or Th2 cytokines, by peripheral blood mononuclear cells correlates with chronicity in reactive arthritis. Arthritis Rheum 1999;42:2039–44.

[91] Thiel A, Wu P, Lauster R, et al. Analysis of the antigen-specific T cell response in reactive arthritis by flow cytometry. Arthritis Rheum 2000;43:2834–42.

[92] Yin Z, Braun J, Neure L, et al. Crucial role of interleukin-10/interleukin-12 balance in the regulation of the type 2 T helper cytokine response in reactive arthritis. Arthritis Rheum 1997;40:1788–97.

[93] Inman RD, Chiu B. Early cytokine profiles in the joint define pathogen clearance and severity of arthritis in *Chlamydia*-induced arthritis in rats. Arthritis Rheum 2006;54: 499–507.

[94] Rihl M, Gu J, Baeten D, et al. Alpha beta but not gamma delta T cell clones in synovial fluids of patients with reactive arthritis show active transcription of tumour necrosis factor alpha and interferon gamma. Ann Rheum Dis 2004;63:1673–6.

[95] Ishihara T, Aga M, Hino K, et al. Inhibition of *Chlamydia trachomatis* growth by human interferon-alpha: mechanisms and synergistic effect with interferon-gamma and tumor necrosis factor-alpha. Biomed Res 2005;26:179–85.

[96] Perry LL, Feilzer K, Caldwell HD. Immunity to *Chlamydia trachomatis* is mediated by T helper 1 cells through IFN-gamma-dependent and –independent pathways. J Immunol 1997;158:3344–52.

[97] Quinn TC, Gaydos CA. In vitro infection and pathogenesis of *Chlamydia pneumoniae* in endovascular cells. Am Heart J 1999;138(5 Pt 2):S507–11.

[98] Takano R, Yamaguchi H, Sugimoto S, et al. Cytokine response of lymphocytes persistent infected with *Chlamydia pneumoniae*. Curr Microbiol 2005;50:160–6.

[99] Yang X, Gartner J, Zhu L, et al. IL-10 knockout mice show enhanced Th1-like protective immunity and absent granulomas formation following *Chlamydia trachomatis* lung infection. J Immunol 1999;162:1010–7.

[100] Leirisalo-Repo M, Helenius P, Hannu T, et al. Long-term prognosis of reactive salmonella arthritis. Ann Rheum Dis 1997;56:516–20.

[101] Thomson GT, Chiu B, De Rubeis D, et al. Immunoepidemiology of post-*Salmonella* reactive arthritis in a cohort of women. Clin Immunol Immunopathol 1992;64:227–32.

[102] Carter JD, Valeriano J, Vasey FB. A prospective, randomized 9-month comparison of doxycycline vs. doxycycline and rifampin in undifferentiated spondyloarthritis with special reference to *Chlamydia*-induced arthritis. J Rheumatol 2004;31:1973–80.

[103] Kvien TK, Gaston JS, Bardin T, et al. Three-month treatment of reactive arthritis with azithromycin: a EULAR double-blind, placebo-controlled study. Ann Rheum Dis 2004;63: 1113–9.

[104] den Hartog JE, Land JA, Stassen FR, et al. Serological markers of persistent *C. trachomatis* infections in women with tubal factor subfertility. Hum Reprod 2005;20:986–90.

[105] Falck G, Gnarpe J, Hansson LO, et al. Comparison of individuals with and without specific IgA antibodies to *Chlamydia pneumoniae*: respiratory morbidity and the metabolic syndrome. Chest 2002;122:1587–93.

[106] Huittinen T, Leinonen M, Tenkanen L, et al. Synergistic effect of persistent *Chlamydia pneumoniae* infection, autoimmunity, and inflammation on coronary risk. Circulation 2003;107:2566–70.

[107] Schumacher A, Seljeflot I, Lerkerod AB, et al. *Chlamydia* LPS and MOMP seropositivity are associated with different cytokine profiles in patients with coronary heart disease. Eur J Clin Invest 2005;35:431–7.

[108] Clegg DO, Reda DJ, Weisman MH, et al. Comparison of sulfasalazine and placebo in the treatment of reactive arthritis (Reiter's syndrome). A Department of Veterans Affairs Cooperative Study. Arthritis Rheum 1996;39:2021–7.

[109] Flagg SD, Meador R, Hsia E, et al. Decreased pain and synovial inflammation after therapy in patients with reactive and undifferentiated arthritis: an open-label trial. Arthritis Rheum 2005;53:613–7.

[110] Oili KS, Niinisalo H, Korpilahde T, et al. Treatment of reactive arthritis with infliximab. Scand J Rheumatol 2003;32:122–4.

[111] Haibel H, Brandt J, Rudawaleit M, et al. Therapy of chronic enteral reactive arthritis with infliximab [abstract]. Ann Rheum Dis 2003;62:AB0380.

[112] Lauhio A, Leirisalo-Repo M, Lahdevirta J, et al. Double-blind, placebo-controlled study of three-month treatment with lymecycline in reactive arthritis, with special reference to *Chlamydia* arthritis. Arthritis Rheum 1991;34:6–14.

[113] Sieper J, Fendler C, Laitko S, et al. No benefit of long-term ciprofloxacin in patients with reactive arthritis and undifferentiated oligoarthritis: a three-month, multicenter, double-blind, randomized, placebo-controlled study. Arthritis Rheum 1999;42:1386–96.

[114] Smieja M, MacPherson DW, Kean W, et al. Randomised, blinded, placebo controlled trial of doxycycline for chronic seronegative arthritis. Ann Rheum Dis 2001;60:1088–94.

[115] Wakefield D, McCluskey P, Verma M, et al. Ciprofloxacin treatment does not influence course or relapse rate of reactive arthritis and anterior uveitis. Arthritis Rheum 1999;42: 1894–7.

[116] Yli-Kerttula T, Luukkainen R, Yli-Kerttula U, et al. Effect of a three month course of ciprofloxacin on the outcome of reactive arthritis. Ann Rheum Dis 2000;59:565–70.

[117] Yli-Kerttula T, Luukkainen R, Yli-Kerttula U, et al. Effect of three month course of ciprofloxacin on the late prognosis of reactive arthritis. Ann Rheum Dis 2003;62:880–4.

[118] Pavlica L, Nikolic D, Magic Z, et al. Successful treatment of postvenereal reactive arthritis with synovectomy and 3 months' azithromycin. J Clin Rheumatol 2005;11:257–63.

[119 Dreses-Werringloer U, Padubrin I, Jurgens-Saathoff B, et al. Persistence of *Chlamydia trachomatis* is induced by ciprofloxacin and ofloxacin in vitro. Antimicrob Agents Chemother 2000;44:3288–97.

[120] Dreses-Werringloer U, Padubrin I, Zeidler H, et al. Effects of azithromycin and rifampin on *Chlamydia trachomatis* infection in vitro. Antimicrob Agents Chemother 2001;45:3001–8.

[121] Morrissey I, Salman H, Bakker S, et al. Serial passage of *Chlamydia* spp. In sub-inhibitory fluoroquinolone concentrations. J Antimicrob Chemother 2002;49:757–61.

[122] Suchland RJ, Geisler WM, Stamm WE. Methodologies and cell lines used for antimicrobial susceptibility testing of *Chlamydia* spp. Antimicrob Agents Chemother 2003;47:636–42.

ELSEVIER
SAUNDERS

Infect Dis Clin N Am
20 (2006) 849–875

INFECTIOUS
DISEASE CLINICS
OF NORTH AMERICA

Infections in Systemic Connective Tissue Diseases: Systemic Lupus Erythematosus, Scleroderma, and Polymyositis/Dermatomyositis

Graciela S. Alarcón, MD, MPH

Division of Clinical Immunology and Rheumatology,
Department of Medicine, The University of Alabama at Birmingham,
Faculty Office Tower, 510 20th Street South, Birmingham,
AL 35294-3408, USA

Systemic lupus erythematosus (SLE), scleroderma, and polymyositis/dermatomyositis (PM/DM) are autoimmune diseases with high morbidity and mortality [1]. The important role infections play in these diseases has been documented in the literature over the years [2–17]. This article reviews the role of infections in these three disorders, emphasizing in each (1) the predisposing factors for the development of infections, (2) the effect of infections on mortality, and (3) the most common microorganisms involved in these infectious processes.

Infections in systemic lupus erythematosus

Infections are responsible for 30% to 50% of the morbidity and mortality in children and adults who have SLE [2,3,5,11–13,17–24]. These infectious processes usually result from common microorganisms [2,11,14,16,17,20,25–28], but opportunistic infections also may occur and are important causes of death in patients who receive corticosteroid and immunosuppressive therapy [9,18–20,25,29–32].

Portions of this article originally appeared in Juárez M, Misischia R, Alarcón GS. Infections in systemic connective tissue diseases: systemic lupus erythematosus, scleroderma, and polymyositis/dermatomyositis. Rheumatic Disease Clinics of North America 2003;29(1):163–84.

Supported by MCRC grant M01-RR00032 from the National Institute of Arthritis and Musculoskeletal and Skin Disorders.

E-mail address: graciela.alarcon@ccc.uab.edu

id.theclinics.com

Predisposing factors

Genetic predisposition to immune dysfunction

Patients who have SLE with inherited complement deficiencies may present abnormalities of all complement proteins, particularly those of the early classic pathway [33]. Patients who have SLE with early complement deficiencies have a higher risk for infections caused mainly by *Streptococcus pneumoniae*, whereas patients who have SLE with late complement deficiencies show a greater susceptibility to infections by *Neisseria meningitidis* and *N gonorrhoeae* [33,34].

Variant alleles in the coding portion of the mannose binding lectin (*MBL*) gene have been associated with lower levels of MBL, a protein that plays an important role in the phagocytosis of microorganisms and has a function similar to C1q [35]. Patients who have SLE homozygous for *MBL* variant alleles also have a significantly higher risk for developing infections, such as pneumonia by *S pneumoniae*. It has been demonstrated, for example, that the annual incidence of infections requiring hospitalization is four times higher in these patients who have SLE than in those heterozygous for the variant allele or homozygous for the normal allele [35,36].

Abnormalities in the immune system

Patients who have SLE have lower levels of complement proteins and a reduced number of cellular complement receptors (CR1, CR2, CR3) [37,38]; this is particularly the case for B cells and polymorphonuclear leukocytes (PMNs) [39]. These abnormalities may increase the risk for infections [34]. Petri and colleagues [13] described lower C3 levels 1 year later among patients who had lupus who required hospitalization for infection, and Kim and coworkers [40] reported reduced complement levels among those patients who died of infection.

SLE can affect various cell functions, and PMNs show many abnormalities. Chemotaxis, recognition of microorganisms, phagocytosis, and oxidative metabolism usually are altered [37,38]. In active SLE, a decreased production of interleukin 8 (IL-8) by PMNs resulting in an altered acute inflammatory response has been described [41]; finally, elevated levels of granulocyte macrophage-colony stimulating factor have also been described in SLE [24]. These PMN abnormalities predispose patients who have SLE to the development of infections [37,38,41].

Several macrophage and monocyte functions, including phagocytosis and oxidative metabolism, also are impaired in patients who have SLE, thus increasing the risk for infections [38]. These abnormalities result from the presence of autoantibodies directed against all three types of Fc gamma receptors (FcγR) [38,42] and from a decrease in the production of tumor necrosis factor alpha (TNFα) [38,42].

During exacerbations of SLE, patients present with decreased levels of T cells and diminished activity of T-helper cells against viral antigens, toxoids, and alloantigens [38,43]. Prolonged corticosteroid therapy also impairs T-cell immunity producing redistribution of T cells, lymphopenia, and inhibition of T-cell activation and proliferation [44]. These T-cell abnormalities result in a higher risk for infections particularly by intracellular microorganisms [19,43–47]. The spleen, through its system of macrophages, is involved in the clearance of microorganisms, thus preventing them from dissemination [45]. When splenic function is impaired, as it is in some SLE patients, the risk for developing severe infections caused by encapsulated microorganisms, such as *S pneumoniae, N meningitidis,* and *N gonorrhoeae* increases [34,45,48].

Disease activity

Disease activity (quantified by validated activity scores) has been found to be an independent risk factor for the occurrence of infections [12,13,17,49–51]. Immune abnormalities, such as decreased complement levels and dysfunction of PMNs, macrophages, monocytes, and T cells, seem to be more pronounced during periods of SLE activity [37,38,41,43]. Duffy and colleagues [49] found that disease activity (quantified by the SLE disease activity index [SLEDAI]) is associated with infections independent of the duration of SLE and the dose of prednisone used. Petri and coworkers [13] demonstrated that SLE activity (quantified by the lupus activity index and the SLEDAI) is a predictive factor for hospitalization because of infections, even after carrying out statistical adjustment for corticosteroid use [13]. Chen and colleagues also have shown that disease activity is a risk factor for the occurrence of infections in hospitalized children who have SLE [23]. Finally, Wu and coworkers have shown that disease activity as measured by the SLEDAI is a risk factor for the occurrence of salmonella osteomyelitis in patients who have SLE [52]. There are, however, studies that dispute this association [26,53] and others in which disease activity has not been found to be a risk factor for the occurrence of infections after carrying out adequate multivariable analyses [5,11,29,54].

Corticosteroids and other immunosuppressive drugs

The use of corticosteroids has been associated with increased occurrence of infections in patients who have SLE [5,11,13,19,29,49–51,55]; it is not clear, however, whether this risk relates to doses larger than 10 mg per day [13], incremental doses of corticosteroids [29], or the use of the intravenous route [12,13]. Probable reasons underlying this risk include decreased production of cytokines by suppression of nuclear factor kappa B (NFkB) [56] and the inhibition of different PMN, monocyte, and T-lymphocyte functions [44].

Cyclophosphamide is now commonly used for the treatment of diffuse proliferative glomerulonephritis and other serious manifestations of SLE otherwise unresponsive to high doses of corticosteroids [57]. Unfortunately, the use of cyclophosphamide increases the risk for severe infections in patients who have SLE [11,31,58]. Risk factors strongly associated with infections in SLE patients who receive cyclophosphamide are the sequential use of intravenous and oral cyclophosphamide and a leukocyte count less than 3000 cells/mL^3 [58]. These patients have an increased risk for developing fatal opportunistic infections [19,58]. This risk is greater when patients also are receiving high doses of corticosteroids [21,58].

Although less long-term data and overall experience are available with mycophenolate mofetil, the data from some but not all of the randomized clinical trials support the fact than infections are much less common with this agent than with cyclophosphamide or even azathioprine [59–61].

Procedures

Certain procedures have been associated with increased risk for infections in patients who have SLE. Patients who receive both plasmapheresis and pulses of cyclophosphamide are at greater risk for developing severe and fatal bacterial and viral infections than patients who have comparable clinical features receiving cyclophosphamide alone [62]. The risk is increased because the levels of B cells, T cells, and immunoglobulins, and consequently their functions, are markedly decreased as a result of plasmapheresis, particularly when this therapy is combined with immunosuppressive therapy [62]. Patients who have SLE receiving chronic peritoneal dialysis have a greater risk for peritonitis or catheter-related infections than patients who do not have SLE (or diabetes) who have comparable clinical characteristics [63]. Immunoablation, with or without autologous stem cell transplantation, has emerged as an alternative treatment of patients who have SLE not responding to other treatment modalities [64]. Data are scarce, and follow-up is still short, but some severe infections, such as herpes zoster (HZ), herpes simplex, and *Pneumocystis carinii* pneumonia (PCP) have been reported in these patients, most likely resulting from profound immunosuppression [64].

Infections as a cause of death

Infection is the primary cause of death in patients who have SLE in developing countries [20,65–72]. In a Chinese cohort of patients who had SLE followed from 1992 to 1996, 66% of deaths were caused by infections [70]. In a series of autopsies performed in SLE patients from Brazil, infections were responsible for 58% of all deaths; 34% of deaths were attributed to active SLE [20]. In developed countries, infection also is one of the most important causes of death among SLE patients and is considered the first or second most common cause of mortality in several studies [2,3,11,16,18,19,40,73,74]. In the multicenter European study of 1000 patients followed for more than 5 years, infections and disease activity were found to be responsible for more than half of all deaths [3]. Similar data come from a study performed in France between 1960 and 1997; in this study active SLE and infections were responsible for 28% and 20% of deaths, respectively [11]. This high rate of mortality from infections is probably the result of the more aggressive use of corticosteroids, immunosuppressive drugs, and support therapy (including dialysis and critical care) in controlling the activity and complications of SLE.

Opportunistic infections are emerging as important causes of death in patients who have SLE in both developed and developing countries. These infections frequently are associated with the increased use of high doses of corticosteroids and immunosuppressants and often are diagnosed only post mortem [9,18–23,58]. Table 1 summarizes the published data regarding infections as a cause of death in SLE; however, the different studies summarized in this table are not directly comparable because their methodologies vary significantly.

Types of infections occurring in systemic lupus erythematosus

Infections cause 25% to 50% of morbidity in patients who have SLE, and major infections are important causes of hospitalization. These infections have been described in different studies that are summarized in Table 2. The most frequent infection sites and most common microorganisms affecting SLE patients are presented in Table 3. Like the studies summarized in Table 1, the studies presented in these tables are not directly comparable because their methodologies vary substantially.

Bacterial infections

Common bacteria are responsible for most infections in patients who have SLE [3,5,9–11,13,16,17,20,50,53,58]. The most frequently described bacteria are Gram-negative bacilli [5,9,17,18,40] and Gram-positive cocci [5,10,16]. Among the Gram-positive bacteria, *Staphylococcus aureus* is a common pathogen that often gains entry through injured skin [10,11]. Infections with *S aureus* may be localized to the integument [10], bones, and joints [55]; however, severe and fatal infections, such as bacteremia [16,18,19,23,58], pneumonia [14], and catheter-related infections [11], also may occur.

S pneumoniae in patients who have SLE typically causes pneumonia [11,16,17]; however, meningitis [16], sepsis, [16,66,75], and cutaneous infections also have been described [76]. The more severe presentations occur in those patients who either have associated inherited deficiencies of the early complement pathway or splenic dysfunction [33,34,38,45,48].

Infections with *Listeria monocytogenes* are rare, but meningitis and sepsis have been reported in patients receiving high doses of corticosteroids or immunosuppressive therapy [58,77] and in those who have active SLE [77]. Listeriosis therefore should be ruled out in critically ill patients who have SLE who present with infections of the central nervous system (CNS) [77].

Table 1
Mortality from infections in patients who have systemic lupus erythematosus

Author/year	Study characteristics[a]	Place	Total patients	Ethnicity	Deaths (all causes) %	n	Deaths (infection) %	(%)	Causal microorganism (%) Common/Unidentified	Opportunistic	5-Year survival (%)
Hellmann/1987 [19]	Chart review (1969–1985[b]) (deceased patients)	United States	44 (33 autopsies)	Caucasian / Black / Other	57 / 14 / 29	44	100	30	53	47	NA
de Luis/1990 [18]	Chart review (1979–1987)	Spain	96	White[c]	100	12	13	50	50	50	NA
Massardo/1991 [9]	Chart review (1978–1990)	Chile	159	Hispanic[c]	100	30	19	63	89	11	NA
Ward/1995 [16, 170]	Cohort (1969–1983) Follow-up: ~11 years	United States	408	White[d] / African American[d]	51 / 49	144	35	22	75	25	82[d]
Huicochea/1996 [68]	Chart review (1970–1993)	Mexico	65 (2–18 years of age)	Hispanic[c]	100	14	22	29	NA	NA	60[e]
Kim/1999 [40]	Chart review (1993–1997)	Korea	544	Asian[c]	100	43	8	33	69	31	94

Reference	Study design	Location	No.	Ethnic group	%						
Cervera/1999 [3]	Multinational cohort (1990) Follow-up: 5 years	Europe	1000	White Black Other	97 2 1	45	5	29	85	15	95
Jacobsen/1999 [73]	Cohort (1975–1995) Follow-up: ~8 years	Denmark	513	White[c]	100	122	24	21	88	12	91
Mok/2000 [70]	Cohort (1992–1999) Follow-up: variable	China (Hong Kong)	186	Asian[c]	100	9	5	67	50	50	93
Bellomio/2000 [65]	Chart review (1990–1998)	Argentina	366	Hispanic[c]	100	44	12	54	100	0	91
Jindal/2000 [69]	Chart review (1984–1998) (deceased patients)	India	25 (all autopsies)	Asian (Indian)[c]	100	25	100	40	67	33	NA
Rodriguez/2000 [71]	Chart review (1960–1994)	Puerto Rico	662	Hispanic[c]	100	161	24	27	82	18	95[f]
Hernandez-Cruz/2001 [67]	Case control autopsy study (1958–1994)	Mexico	152	Hispanic[c]	100	76 (all autopsies)	50	42	59	41	NA
Alarcón/2001 [2]	Cohort (1993–1999) Follow-up: variable	United States	288	Hispanic African American White	28 41 31	34	12	32	NA	NA	86
Iriya/2001 [20,171]	Chart review (1981–1994) (deceased patients)	Brazil	113 (all autopsies)	Multiethnic[c]	100	113	100	58	77	23	NA

(continued on next page)

Table 1 (*continued*)

Author/year	Study characteristics[a]	Place	Total patients	Ethnicity	Deaths (all causes) %	Deaths (all causes) n	Deaths (infection) %	Deaths (infection) (%)	Causal microorganism (%) Common/ Unidentified	Causal microorganism (%) Opportunistic	5-Year survival (%)
Nöel/2001 [11]	Chart review (1960–1997)	France	87	White[c]	100	10	12	20	100	0	NA
Chen/2004 [23]	Chart review (1991–2000)	Taiwan (children)	125	Asian[c] (Chinese)	100	4	3	4	3	NA	NA
Opastirakul/ 2005 [21]	Chart review	Thailand	11	Asian[c] (Chinese)	100	2	18	2	18	NA	NA
Bernatski/2006 [22]	Multisite International cohort (1970–2001[g])	Multinational (Europe, Asia and North America)	9547	Multiethnic[h]	100	1255	13	64	5	NA	NA

Abbreviation: NA, not available or not applicable.
a Length of follow up noted only for cohort studies.
b Closing date inferred.
c Inferred based on country origin.
d Inferred based on characteristics of cohort.
e At 5–10 years.
f Patients without renal involvement.
g The bulk of these patients entered the cohort during this period.
h Precise breakdown by ethnic group is not available, but Caucasians, African Americans, Afro-Carribbeans, Asians, Hispanics and patients of mixed ethnicity included.

Gram-negative bacilli (*Escherichia coli*, *Klebsiella* spp, *Pseudomonas* spp, among others) are often the cause of urinary tract infections [17,18,27,58], lower respiratory tract infections [16,17,58], and severe and lethal bacteremias [16,18,19,40,58].

Infections by Salmonella occur mainly in patients who have SLE who have lower levels of complement or splenic dysfunction or who are receiving immunosuppressive therapy or ingesting desiccated rattlesnake [78–82]. The typical presentation is bacteremia [11,18,78,79], and the most commonly isolated species are *Salmonella choleraesuis*, *Salmonella enteritidis*, *Salmonella typhimurium*, and *Salmonella arizona* [78–80,83]. Localized infections also have been described, however [52,84]. In fact, SLE is the most frequent underlying disease in patients who present with salmonella bacteremia [78,79]. Infections with encapsulated organisms, such as *N gonorrhoeae* and *N meningitides*, are infrequent in patients who have SLE unless there is an underlying complement deficiency or splenic dysfunction [33,34,85].

Other less common bacteria also result in infection in patients who have SLE. Pelvic actinomycosis has been reported in an immunocompromised woman [86]. Nocardiosis is a rare and fatal opportunistic infection that involves mainly the lungs and the CNS [58,81,87,88]. The mortality rate in nocardial infections is 35%, but that rate doubles when there is CNS involvement [87].

Mycobacterial infections, mainly *Mycobacterium tuberculosis*, are important opportunistic infections in these patients, particularly in developing countries [20,28,72,89]. It is thus important to suspect and rule out tuberculosis in patients who have SLE living in or coming from areas of the world where tuberculosis is endemic. Pulmonary tuberculosis is the most common presentation [11,16,18,89], but cases of miliary, urinary, osteoarticular, soft tissue, and CNS tuberculosis also have been described [17,89,90].

Infections caused by atypical mycobacteria have been reported in patients who have SLE who are receiving immunosuppressive therapy [58]. These infections are usually insidious rather than acute and often are localized in the musculoskeletal and integument systems [91–93]; occasionally, they may produce the hemophagocytic syndrome [94]. The author has had the opportunity to diagnose and treat two patients who had SLE with atypical mycobacterial infections. The first patient developed osteomyelitis of the thoracic vertebrae but presented only with mild pleuritic chest pain (believed to be related to lupus activity); chest and thoracic spine radiographs were not informative at that time. A few months later she was found to have *M avium intracellulare* on biopsy material obtained when thoracic spine radiographs (Fig. 1) and MR imaging studies clearly demonstrated vertebral and disc space involvement (Fig. 2). The second patient presented with an extremely large and deep cutaneous ulceration of the left lower extremity, initially believed to be related to active disease; deep tissue biopsies were taken from which *M chelonae* was isolated. These cases illustrate the difficulties usually encountered in diagnosing infections in the immunocompromised patient who has SLE.

Table 2
Morbidity from infections in patients with SLE

Author/year	Study characteristics[a]	Country	No. of patients	Ethnicity	%	Patients infected %	Episodes of infections
De Luis/1990 [18]	Chart review (1979–1987)	Spain	96	White[b]	100	55	102
Massardo/1991 [9]	Chart review (1972–1990)	Chile	159	Hispanic[c]	100	49	155
Petri/1992 [13,172]	Cohort (1989–1990) Follow-up: 2 years	United States	261[d]	African American[c] White Other	51 48 1	14[d]	51
Oh/1993 [26]	Chart review (1988–1989)	Singapore	28	Asian (Chinese) Asian (Malay) Asian (Indian or other)	78 11 11	100	38
Shyam/1996 [72]	Chart review (1989–1994)	India	309	Asian (Indian)[b]	100	27	NA
Paton/1996 [12]	Chart review (1978–1993)	Malaysia	102	Asian (Chinese) Asian (Malay) Asian (Indian)	47 46 7	NA	240
Cervera/1999 [3]	Multinational cohort (1990) Follow-up: 5 years	Europe	1000	White Black Other	97 2 1	27	389
Zonana-Nacach/2001 [17]	Cohort (1990–1996) Follow-up: 2 years	Mexico	200	Hispanic[b]	100	32	65
Al-Mayouf/2001 [53]	Chart review (1990–1998)	Saudi Arabia	70 (children)	Arab[b]	100	41	NA
Nöel/2001 [11]	Chart review (1960–1997)	France	87	White[b]	100	40	57
Gladman/2002 [5,173]	Cohort (1987–1992) Follow-up: 5 years	Canada	363	White[c] African American Asian Other	86 7 6 1	26	148

Study	Type (period)	Country	N	Ethnicity			
Wongchinsri/2002 [174]	Chart review (1994–1999)	Thailand	488	Asian (Chinese)	100	39	191
Pope/2004 [175]	Case-control (undetermined)	Canada	61 (173 controls)	White[b]	100	19[e]	12[e]
Hidalgo-Tenorio/2004 [27]	Case-control 12 months	Spain	81 (86 controls)	White[b]	100	36[g]	NA
Chen/2004 [23]	Chart review (1991–2001)	Taiwan	125 (children)	Asian[b] (Chinese)	100	31	72
Sayartioglu/2004 [28]	Chart review (1978–2001)	Turkey	556	Indo European[b]	100	4[h]	NA
Galindo/2005 [55]	Cohort (1979–2003)	Spain	315	White[b]	100	1[f]	NA
Ng/2006 [54]	Chart review (12 months)	Hong Kong	91	Asian	100	30[i]	48
				(Chinese)		41[i]	62

Abbreviation: NA, not available.

[a] Length of follow up noted only for cohort studies.
[b] Inferred based on country of origin.
[c] Inferred based on characteristics of cohort.
[d] 354 hospitalizations (number used as denominator).
[e] Only zoster infections included (frequency in controls: 7%).
[f] Only polyorticular septic arthritis included.
[g] Only urinary tract infections included (frequency in control: 10%).
[h] Only tuberculosis infections included.
[i] Major and minor infections, respectively.

Table 3
Sites of infection and infectious organisms in patients who have systemic lupus erythematosus

Author/year	Site of infections (%)						Causal microorganisms			
	Respiratory	Skin	Urinary tract	CNS	Blood	Other	Bacteria	Virus	Fungus	Parasites
de Luis/1990 [18]	26	18	31	0	17	8	90[a]	9	1	0
Massardo/1991 [9]	30	17	23	1	NA	29	74[a]	8	15	3
Petri/1992 [13]	NA	NA	NA	NA	NA	NA	88[a]	4[a]	8[a]	0
Oh/1993 [26]	29	32	8	0	13	18	86[a]	11	3	0
Shyam/1996 [72]	54	5	17	0	0	24	82[a,b]	7	11	0
Paton/1996 [12]	28	19	10	2	13	28	97[a,c]	0[c]	3[c]	0[c]
Cervera/1999 [3]	19	20	29	1	6	25	NA	NA	NA	NA
Zonana-Nacach/2001 [17]	12	23	26	0	0	39	71[a]	13	16	0
Al-Mayouf/2001 [53]	NA	NA	28	NA	14	NA	NA	NA	NA	NA
Nöel/2001 [11]	40	NA	NA	NA	29	NA	82	16	2	0
Gladman/2002 [5]	29	23	18	3	5	22	65[a]	27	6	2
Wongchinsri/2002 [174]	25	16	16	0	14	29	100	0	0	0
Pope/2004 [175]	NA	NA	NA	100	NA	NA	0	100	0	0
Hidalgo-Tenorio/2004 [27]	NA	NA	100	NA	NA	NA	100	0	0	0
Chen/2004	NA	5	45	0	50	NA	100	0	0	0
Sayarlioglu/2004 [28]	55	0	0	10	NA	35	100	0	0	0
Galindo/2005 [55]	NA	NA	NA	NA	NA	100	100	NA	NA	NA
Ng/2006 [54]	40	10	27	2	10	17	100[d]	0	0	0

Abbreviation: NA, not available.
[a] Inferred from data presented; includes patients in whom no pathogen was isolated but who responded to antibiotic treatment.
[b] Mycobacterium tuberculosis is the most frequent isolate.
[c] Only major infections included.
[d] Minor and major infections included.

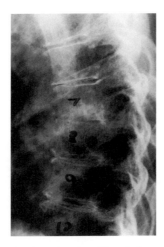

Fig. 1. Lateral radiograph of the thoracic spine. There is loss of intervertebral disc space at T7–8 with loss of the endplate cortex anteriorly and little reactive bone formation (*Courtesy of* Robert López-Ben, Division of Diagnostic Radiology, Department of Radiology, The University of Alabama at Birmingham, Birmingham, Alabama).

Viral infections

Herpes zoster is the most frequent viral infection [5,11,13,17,58,62], occurring mainly in patients who have SLE with previous histories of nephritis, hemolytic anemia, thrombocytopenia, and previous use of cyclophosphamide [95]. Localized HZ is the most common clinical presentation and generally occurs during periods of disease quiescence and in patients receiving 20 mg or less of prednisone per day [95]. Disseminated HZ and bacterial superinfection also may occur and usually are related to the use of high doses of corticosteroids (prednisone $\geq$ 60 mg/d) or immunosuppressants [58,95].

Cytomegalovirus (CMV) is another opportunistic infection occurring in patients who have SLE, especially in those receiving cyclophosphamide or high doses of corticosteroids [16,18,96–98] or in patients receiving plasmapheresis [62]. Pneumonia and encephalitis produced by CMV are fatal in most cases [16,19]. Risk behaviors leading to infection by retroviruses are not believed to be increased in SLE patients [99]; thus, retroviral infections have not been described with increased frequency. Case reports, however, are emerging [100,101]. Nevertheless, infections with the human immunodeficiency virus need to be distinguished from SLE, because the illnesses share some clinical characteristics and some of the same autoantibodies [102,103].

Human parvovirus B19 DNA has been detected in patients who have SLE, but its clinical relevance is unclear to date [104].

Fungal infections

Fungal infections can occur frequently in patients who have SLE who are receiving high doses of corticosteroids or immunosuppressive therapy

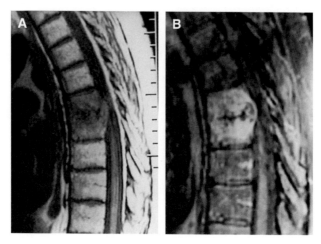

Fig. 2. Magnetic resonance image of the thoracic spine. (*A*) Sagittal T1-weighted MR image of the thoracic spine. There is marked marrow edema in T7 and T8 vertebral bodies. An epidural mass bulges the posterior longitudinal ligament and compresses the spinal cord at this level. (*B*) Sagittal T1-weighted MR image of the thoracic spine with fat suppression after intravenous administration of gadolinium contrast. There is marked contrast enhancement of the vertebral bodies of T7 and T8. There is rim enhancement of the epidural mass and the contiguous posterior disc space is better appreciated (*Courtesy of* Robert López-Ben, Division of Diagnostic Radiology, Department of Radiology, The University of Alabama at Birmingham, Birmingham, Alabama).

[16,19,58]. The most common fungal infections are produced by *P carinii* and *Candida* spp. The risk factors for developing PCP are the use of high doses of corticosteroids or of immunosuppressive drugs, and lymphopenia [58,105–110]. Although PCP occurs infrequently, it has a high mortality rate [19,58,106,107]; therefore, PCP prophylaxis may be indicated in patients who have SLE who have these risk factors. Infections by *Candida* spp (mainly *Candida albicans*) are common in patients who have SLE [11,17,19,20,58]. The clinical spectrum includes oral and esophageal mucosa infections and infections of the genitourinary tract [17]. Disseminated candidiasis, which is frequently fatal, occurs less often [16,18–20,58]. Cryptococcal infection has been described in 10 of 17 patients who had CNS involvement observed over a 20-year period [31]. A case of disseminated cutaneous eumycotic mycetoma secondary to *Cladophialophora bantiana* has been described in a woman who had lupus and was receiving corticosteroids [111].

Disease flares, immunosuppressive therapy, leukopenia, and associated bacterial infections are risk factors for the development of aspergillosis in patients who have SLE [112,113]. There are only a few reported cases of aspergillosis; however, most of them have been lethal [16,112].

Parasitic infections

Disseminated strongyloidiasis with massive pulmonary hemorrhage was reported in a patient from Japan who had SLE [114]. Visceral leishmaniasis was reported in a German patient [115]. A case of *Trypanosoma cruzi* infection with high degree of parasitemia was reported in a Brazilian patient [116]. Encephalitis caused by *Toxoplasma gondii* has been described in patients who have SLE [117]. The cases of strongyloidiasis and leishmaniasis did not occur in areas where these infections are endemic, and it is unclear how these patients became infected with these pathogens. It is important to take appropriate diagnostic measures, because these parasitic infections can simulate clinical presentations of active SLE when they include neurologic, pulmonary, and gastrointestinal manifestations.

Infections in scleroderma

Predisposing factors

Risk factors associated with infections in patients who have scleroderma include esophageal and pulmonary involvement, severe Raynaud's phenomenon or calcinosis, and the use of specific treatments for the management of the disease. Scleroderma patients who have smooth muscle involvement of the esophagus are at increased risk for aspiration pneumonia, because these patients usually have lower esophageal sphincter dysfunction and severe gastroesophageal reflux [14,118–120]. To avoid postoperative infections, esophageal involvement should be considered and ruled out in patients who have scleroderma with lung involvement selected to receive lung transplants [119,121]. Pneumonia has been described in patients who have scleroderma with pulmonary involvement, particularly in those who have interstitial lung disease [6], suggesting that pulmonary fibrosis may be a predisposing factor for the development of pulmonary infections. Oftentimes, bronchoalveolar lavage is necessary to determine if there is a concomitant infection [122].

In patients who have scleroderma, severe Raynaud's phenomenon with digital ischemia and ulcerations increases the risk for localized superinfections, which may be complicated by gangrene [119]. Severe calcinosis also has been associated with bacterial infections, especially in the soft tissues around the calcific lesions [123]. Although there are no large studies from which to draw conclusive data, some reported cases show that the risk for infection relates to specific treatments. For example, the aggressive use of immunosuppression and autologous stem cell transplantation resulted in a lethal infection in a neutropenic patient who had scleroderma [124]. Pneumonia has been reported with cyclophosphamide and corticosteroid use [125], and local infections have been reported in 10% of patients receiving subcutaneous relaxin [126].

Infections as a cause of death

In patients who have scleroderma, pulmonary complications cause 17% to 24% of the mortality [127,128]. Pneumonia has been described in patients who had scleroderma who died of pulmonary involvement [6]. In the

Swedish scleroderma cohort studied by Hesselstrand and colleagues [6], approximately 12% of deaths were caused by pneumonia and severe lung fibrosis occurring simultaneously. Aspiration pneumonia also has been described as a cause of death in patients who have scleroderma with esophageal involvement, often producing adult respiratory distress syndrome [14,120]. A fatal case of myocardial necrosis has been reported recently in which *Staphylococcus lugdunensis* and CMV were identified at necropsy [129]. Unlike SLE, however, there are no conclusive data regarding infections as a predictive factor of mortality in scleroderma [6,73,127,128,130].

Types of infections occurring in scleroderma

Bacterial infections

Data about common bacterial infections in patients who have scleroderma are limited to case reports. Group G streptococcus pyomyositis was described in a patient who had scleroderma who was receiving chlorambucil [131], and soft tissue *S aureus* infection around multiple calcific lesions was reported in a patient who had scleroderma and a long history of Raynaud's phenomenon [123]. Another patient who had scleroderma with lower gastrointestinal tract involvement was reported to have developed bacterial peritonitis secondary to colon perforation [132].

M avium intracellulare, an opportunistic infection, was the cause of septic arthritis in another patient who had scleroderma; he did not respond to medical treatment, refused surgical intervention, and went on to develop osteomyelitis and subsequently Charcot's arthropathy [133]. *M kansasii* was the cause of tenosynovitis in a woman who had scleroderma receiving corticosteroids [134]. An ocular infection secondary to nocardia was described in a patient who had scleroderma who was receiving a moderate dose of corticosteroids [135].

A report from Japan describes an increased frequency of *Helicobacter pylori* infection in patients who have scleroderma; a possible role of this infection in esophageal dysfunction has been suggested but remains unproven for now [136].

Viral and fungal infections

There has been only one case report of viral infections complicating the course of scleroderma. This patient was a 40-year-old who had limited scleroderma and developed a flu-like illness followed by acute heart failure and high IgM anti-adenovirus titer; as serologic conversion to IgG occurred, heart failure resolved [137]. Nevertheless, Epstein-Barr virus and CMV have been described as triggering the onset of scleroderma, particularly in pediatric patients [138,139], and parvovirus B19 DNA has been detected in patients who have scleroderma, but the clinical correlate of this finding is unclear at the present [140]. *P carinii* pneumonia has been reported in some patients who have scleroderma. This infection is rare but has a rapid and usually fatal course. An early diagnosis in patients who have respiratory failure is important if the survival rate is to be improved [141].

Esophageal fungal infections have been described with the same frequency in patients who have scleroderma with and without esophageal involvement [142]; treatment of these fungal infections, however, is not followed by improvement of esophageal motility.

Infections in polymyositis/dermatomyositis

Predisposing factors

Patients PM/DM have a host of predisposing factors placing them at risk for developing infections. These factors include upper esophageal involvement, thoracic muscle myopathy, calcinosis cutis, and the use of immunosuppressive drugs.

Some patients who have PM/DM have involvement of the striated muscle of the hypopharynx and the upper third of the esophagus resulting in altered swallowing, gastroesophageal reflux, and aspiration, and a greater risk for developing aspiration pneumonia [7,8,14,118,143,144]. Likewise, the myopathy affecting the thoracic muscles, present in less than 5% to 10% of PM/DM patients, creates difficulty in handling bronchial secretions [7,8,143]. This difficulty may lead to the development of atelectasis and ventilatory insufficiency [8,144]. This ventilatory compromise can worsen the course of aspiration pneumonia, thereby increasing the risk for death from this complication [8,144].

Calcinosis cutis, frequently described in patients who have juvenile dermatomyositis [7,143], is a known risk factor for the development of staphylococcal soft tissue and dermal infections around calcinotic lesions [145–147]. This risk probably results from the decreased granulocyte chemotaxis to S aureus that has been described in these patients [147]. These infections may cause severe growth retardation of the extremities and significant functional impairment, thus worsening the course of the disease [146].

To date, there are no large-scale studies comparing the use of immunosuppressive drugs and the incidence of infections. Reported case studies, however, suggest that the simultaneous use of corticosteroids and immunosuppressive drugs in the treatment of PM/DM could increase the risk for infections [148]. For example, a patient who had PM/DM who was treated with methotrexate (22.5 mg/wk) and prednisone (50 mg/d) developed PCP [148], and a pediatric patient who had severe dermatomyositis treated with methotrexate (25 mg/wk) and prednisone (150 mg/d) (extremely high dose verified) developed disseminated nocardiosis [149].

Infections as a cause of death

Malignancy [7,8,143,150] and pulmonary complications [7,8,143,150,151] are the main causes of death among patients who have PM/DM. Aspiration pneumonia is one of the most common pulmonary complications [7,8,14,143,144,150,151] and causes of death in patients who have PM/DM [8,144]. In the study published by Marie and coworkers [8], aspiration pneumonia was reported in 17% of all patients who had PM/DM and was \responsible for 30% of the mortality. Aspiration pneumonia has emerged as an independent predictive factor for PM/DM deterioration and as a risk factor for death in patients who have PM/DM. Patients who have esophageal and respiratory compromise should be diagnosed and treated early to decrease the probability of a fatal outcome [7,8,14,118,143,144].

Types of infections occurring in polymyositis/dermatomyositis

Bacterial infections

Aspiration pneumonia, produced by Gram-positive and anaerobic bacteria, is the most common infection, occurring in 15% to 20% of patients who have PM/DM [8,144].

S aureus infections involving the soft tissue and skin around calcinotic lesions are described frequently in patients who have juvenile dermatomyositis and calcinosis cutis [145,147]. Other bacterial infections in dermatomyositis constitute only isolated reported cases. For example *Streptococcus pyogenes* myositis has been described in patients who have juvenile and adult DM with or without calcinosis; in these patients the myopathy probably favored the bacterial colonization of muscle from bacteremia originating in dermal lesions [152,153]. Recently the case of a patient who had polymyositis and severe gastric symptoms was reported in which these symptoms resolved after triple therapy to eradicate *H heilmanii* [154].

Opportunistic infections have been described in about 12% of patients who have PM/DM, being fatal in nearly 28% of these patients in a study from France [155]. Among the opportunistic infections, disseminated *Nocardia brasiliensis* involving the skin and the lungs has been reported in both children and adults who have myositis receiving corticosteroids and immunosuppressive therapy [149,156], and extrapulmonary infections produced by *M tuberculosis* and generalized *M avium intracellulare* have been described in patients who have PM/DM [157,158]. Other atypical mycobacterial infections also have been described [156]. Although opportunistic infections in these patients are uncommon, early diagnosis and adequate treatment are essential to improve survival.

Viral infections

HZ is a common viral infection in patients who have PM/DM and usually occurs during periods of disease inactivity [159]. CMV is an uncommon opportunistic viral infection in patients who have PM/DM; however, some cases of severe and fatal infection, such as interstitial pneumonia, have been noted in patients receiving corticosteroid or immunosuppressive therapy [160–163]. Some studies have demonstrated a temporal relationship between coxsackievirus, parvovirus B19, hepatitis C, and other enterovirus infections and the onset of PM/DM; however, the role of these pathogens in the cause of PM/DM remains speculative [164–166].

Fungal infections

PCP is frequently fatal in patients who have PM/DM. This infection has a rapid and severe course, and most patients require critical care support [105,110,167]. Known risk factors for the development of PCP are interstitial pulmonary disease [106], lymphopenia [105,106,167], and the use of corticosteroids [105,167] and immunosuppressive drugs [105]. Based on the often fatal course of PCP, patients who have these risk factors can benefit from the initiation of PCP prophylaxis, although there are no definite published guidelines.

Candidiasis is another fungal infection occurring in patients who have dermatomyositis. In a large study of more than 40,000 patients who had various skin disorders, the frequency of mucocutaneous candidiasis was three times higher in patients who had dermatomyositis, bullous pemphigoid, tinea inguinalis, or condylomata acuminata than in the general population, suggesting that preexisting dermal involvement may increase the susceptibility of patients who have dermatomyositis to this infection [168].

Finally, disseminated histoplasmosis involving the muscles and fascia has been reported in a patient who had dermatomyositis being treated with corticosteroids and methotrexate, who was initially believed to have a disease flare [169].

Summary

In SLE, scleroderma, and PM/DM, infections are important causes of morbidity and mortality. This increased risk for developing infections is the result of immune abnormalities and of organ system manifestations associated with these diseases and their treatments. Common bacteria are responsible for most mild and lethal infections; however, opportunistic microorganisms cause death in some patients, particularly in those receiving high doses of corticosteroid and immunosuppressive therapy. Various viral and fungal infections also contribute to the morbidity and mortality associated with these diseases. Regardless of the cause of infections, adequate and prompt recognition and proper treatment of the infected patient are imperative. Patients who have these diseases, especially when receiving high doses of corticosteroids and immunosuppressive therapy, need to be monitored closely for these infections. This care and concern is necessary to ensure optimal patient outcomes, both in morbidity and mortality.

References

[1] Juárez M, Misischia R, Alarcón GS. Infections in systemic connective tissue diseases: systemic lupus erythematosus, scleroderma, and polymyositis/dermatomyositis. Rheum Dis Clin North Am 2003;29:163–84.

[2] Alarcón GS, McGwin G Jr, Bastian HM, et al. Systemic lupus erythematosus in three eth-nic group VII: predictors of early mortality in the LUMINA cohort. Arthritis Rheum 2001; 45:191–202 [Arthritis Care Res].

[3] Cervera R, Khamashta MA, Font J, et al. Morbidity and mortality in systemic lupus eryth-ematosus during a 5-year period. A multicenter prospective study of 1,000 patients. Euro-pean Working Party on Systemic Lupus Erythematosus. Medicine 1999;78:167–75.

[4] Fessler BJ. Infectious diseases in systemic lupus erythematosus: risk factors, management and prophylaxis. Best Pract Res Clin Rheumatol 2002;16:281–91.

[5] Gladman DD, Hussian F, Ibanez D, et al. The nature and outcome of infection in systemic lupus erythematosus. Lupus 2002;11:234–9.

[6] Hesselstrand R, Scheja A, Akesson A. Mortality and causes of death in a Swedish series of systemic sclerosis patients. Ann Rheum Dis 1998;57:682–6.

[7] Koler RA, Motemarano A. Dermatomyositis. Am Fam Physician 2001;64:1565–72.

[8] Marie I, Hachulla E, Hatron PY, et al. Polymyositis and dermatomyositis: short term and longterm outcome, and predictive factors of prognosis. J Rheumatol 2001;28:2230–7.

[9] Massardo L, Martinez ME, Baro M, et al. Infections in systemic lupus erythematosus. [Infecciones en lupus eritematoso sistémico] Rev Med Chil 1991;119:1115–22.

[10] Nived O, Sturfelt G, Wollheim F. Systemic lupus erythematosus and infection: a controlled and prospective study including an epidemiological group. QJM 1985;55:271–87.

[11] Noel V, Lortholary O, Casassus P, et al. Risk factors and prognostic influence of infection in a single cohort of 87 adults with systemic lupus erythematosus. Ann Rheum Dis 2001;60: 1141–4.

[12] Paton NI, Cheong IK, Kong NC, et al. Risk factors for infection in Malaysian patients with systemic lupus erythematosus. QJM 1996;89:531–8.

[13] Petri M, Genovese M. Incidence of and risk factors for hospitalizations in systemic lupus erythematosus: A prospective study of the Hopkins lupus cohort. J Rheumatol 1992;19: 1559–65.

[14] Prakash UBS. Thoracic manifestations of the systemic autoimmune diseases. Respiratory complications in mixed connective tissue disease. Clin Chest Med 1998;19:733–46.

[15] Rahman P, Gladman DD, Urowitz MB, et al. Early damage as measured by the SLICC/ ACR damage index is a predictor of mortality in systemic lupus erythematosus. Lupus 2001;10:93–6.

[16] Ward MM, Pyun E, Studenski S. Causes of death in systemic lupus erythematosus: long-term followup of an inception cohort. Arthritis Rheum 1995;38:1492–9.

[17] Zonana-Nacach A, Camargo-Coronel A, Yañez P, et al. Infections in outpatients with systemic lupus erythematosus: a prospective study. Lupus 2001;10:505–10.

[18] de Luis A, Pigrau C, Pahissa A, et al. Infections in 96 cases of systemic lupus erythematosus. [Infecciones en 96 casos de lupus eritematoso sistémico] Med Clin (Barc) 1990;94:607–10.

[19] Hellmann DB, Petri M, Whiting-O'Keefe Q. Fatal infections in systemic lupus erythema-tosus: the role of opportunistic organisms. Medicine 1987;66:341–8.

[20] Iriya SM, Capelozzi VL, Calich I, et al. Causes of death in patients with systemic lupus er-ythematosus in Sao Paulo, Brazil: a study of 113 autopsies. Arch Intern Med 2001;161: 1557–61.

[21] Opastirakul S, Chartapisak W. Infection in children with lupus nephritis receiving pulse and oral cyclophosphamide therapy. Pediatr Nephrol 2005;20:1750–5.

[22] Bernatsky S, Boivin JF, Joseph L, et al. Mortality in systemic lupus erythematosus. Arthri-tis Rheum 2006;54:2550–7.

[23] Chen YS, Yang YH, Lin YT, et al. Risk of infection in hospitalised children with systemic lupus erythematosus: a 10-year follow-up. Clin Rheumatol 2004;23:235–8.

[24] Zandman-Goddard G, Shoenfeld Y. Infections and SLE. Autoimmunity 2005;38:473–85.

[25] Le Moing V, Leport C. Infections et lupus (Infections and lupus). Rev Prat 1998;48:637–42.

[26] Oh HM, Chng HH, Boey ML, et al. Infections in systemic lupus erythematosus. Singapore Med J 1993;34:406–8.

[27] Hidalgo-Tenorio C, Jimenez-Alonso J, de Dios LJ, et al. Urinary tract infections and lupus erythematosus. Ann Rheum Dis 2004;63:431–7.

[28] Sayarlioglu M, Inanc M, Kamali S, et al. Tuberculosis in Turkish patients with systemic lupus erythematosus: increased frequency of extrapulmonary localization. Lupus 2004;13: 274–8.

[29] Ginzler E, Diamond H, Kaplan D, et al. Computer analysis of factors influencing frequency of infection in systemic lupus erythematosus. Arthritis Rheum 1978;21:37–44.

[30] Garcia C, Ugalde E, Campo AB, et al. Fatal case of community-acquired pneumonia caused by Legionella longbeachae in a patient with systemic lupus erythematosus. Eur J Clin Microbiol Infect Dis 2004;23:116–8.

[31] Hung JJ, Ou LS, Lee WI, et al. Central nervous system infections in patients with systemic lupus erythematosus. J Rheumatol 2005;32:40–3.

[32] Kiertiburanakul S, Wirojtananugoon S, Pracharktam R, et al. Cryptococcosis in human immunodeficiency virus-negative patients. Int J Infect Dis 2006;10:72–8.

[33] Ross SC, Densen P. Complement deficiency states and infection: epidemiology, pathogenesis and consequences of neisserial and other infections in an immune deficiency. Medicine 1984;63:243–73.

[34] Mitchell SR, Nguyen PQ, Katz P. Increased risk of neisserial infections in systemic lupus erythematosus. Sem Arthritis Rheum 1990;20:174–84.

[35] Garred P, Madsen HO, Halberg P, et al. Mannose-binding lectin polymorphisms and susceptibility to infection in systemic lupus erythematosus. Arthritis Rheum 1999;42: 2145–52.

[36] Garred P, Voss A, Madsen HO, et al. Association of mannose-binding lectin gene variation with disease severity and infections in a population-based cohort of systemic lupus erythematosus patients. Genes Immun 2001;2:442–50.

[37] Bouza E, Moya JG-L, Munoz P. Infections in systemic lupus erythematosus and rheumatoid arthritis. Infect Dis Clin North Am 2001;15:335–61.

[38] Petri M. Infection in systemic lupus erythematosus. Rheum Dis Clin North Am 1998;24: 423–56.

[39] Wilson JG, Ratnoff WD, Schur PH, et al. Decreased expression of the C3b/C4b receptor (CR1) and the C3d receptor (CR2) on B lymphocytes and of CR1 on neutrophils of patients with systemic lupus erythematosus. Arthritis Rheum 1986;29:739–47.

[40] Kim WU, Min JK, Lee SH, et al. Causes of death in Korean patients with systemic lupus erythematosus: a single center retrospective study. Clin Exp Rheumatol 1999;17:539–45.

[41] Hsieh SC, Tsai CY, Sun KH, et al. Decreased spontaneous and lipopolysaccharide stimulated production of interleukin 8 by polymorphonuclear neutrophils of patients with active systemic lupus erythematosus. Clin Exp Rheumatol 1994;12:627–33.

[42] Boros P, Muryoi T, Spiera H, et al. Autoantibodies directed against different classes of Fc gamma R are found in sera of autoimmune patients. J Immunol 1993;150:2018–24.

[43] Bermas BL, Petri M, Goldman D, et al. T helper cell dysfunction in systemic lupus erythematosus (SLE). Relation to disease activity. J Clin Immunol 1994;14:169–77.

[44] Boumpas DT, Chrousos GP, Wilder RL, et al. Glucocorticoid therapy for immune-mediated disease: Basic and clinical correlates. Ann Intern Med 1993;119:1198–208.

[45] Cunha BA. Infections in nonleukopenic compromised hosts (diabetes mellitus, SLE, steroids, and asplenia) in critical care. Crit Care Clin 1998;14:264–82.

[46] Hrycek A, Kusmierz D, Mazurek U, et al. Human cytomegalovirus in patients with systemic lupus erythematosus. Autoimmunity 2005;38:487–91.

[47] Kang I, Quan T, Nolasco H, et al. Defective control of latent Epstein-Barr virus infection in systemic lupus erythematosus. J Immunol 2004;172:1287–94.

[48] Huhn R, Schmeling H, Kunze C, et al. Pneumococcal sepsis after autosplenectomy in a girl with systemic lupus erythematosus. Rheumatology (Oxford) 2005;44:1586–8.

[49] Duffy KN, Duffy CM, Gladman DD. Infection and disease activity in systemic lupus erythematosus: a review of hospitalized patients. J Rheumatol 1991;18:1180–4.

[50] Iliopoulos AG, Tsokos GC. Immunopathogenesis and spectrum of infections in systemic lupus erythematosus. Semin Arthritis Rheum 1996;25:318–36.

[51] Suh C-H, Jeong Y-S, Park H-C, et al. Risk factors for infection and role of C-reactive protein in Korean patients with systemic lupus erythematosus. Clin Expr Rheumatol 2001;19: 191–4.

[52] Wu KC, Yao TC, Yeh KW, et al. Osteomyelitis in patients with systemic lupus erythematosus. J Rheumatol 2004;31:1340–3.

[53] Al-Mayouf SM, Al-Jumaah S, Bahabri S, et al. Infections associated with juvenile systemic lupus erythematosus. Clin Exp Rheumatol 2001;19:748–50.

[54] Ng WL, Chu CM, Wu AK, et al. Lymphopenia at presentation is associated with increased risk of infections in patients with systemic lupus erythematosus. QJM 2006;99:37–47.

[55] Galindo M, Mateo I, Pablos JL. Multiple avascular necrosis of bone and polyarticular septic arthritis in patients with systemic lupus erythematosus. Rheumatol Int 2005;25: 72–6.

[56] Auphan N, DiDonato JA, Rosette C, et al. Immunosuppression by glucocorticoids: inhibition of NF-kappa B activity through induction of I kappa B synthesis. Science 1995;270: 286–90.

[57] Ortmann RA, Klippel JH. Update on cyclophosphamide for systemic lupus erythematosus. Rheum Dis Clin North Am 2000;26:363–75.

[58] Pryor BD, Bologna SG, Kahl LE. Risk factors for serious infection during treatment with cyclophosphamide and high-dose corticosteroids for systemic lupus erythematosus. Arthritis Rheum 1996;39:1475–82.

[59] Ginzler EM, Dooley MA, Aranow C, et al. Mycophenolate mofetil or intravenous cyclophosphamide for lupus nephritis. N Engl J Med 2005;353:2219–28.

[60] Contreras G, Pardo V, Leclercq B, et al. Sequential therapies for proliferative lupus nephritis. N Engl J Med 2004;350:971–80.

[61] Ong LM, Hooi LS, Lim TO, et al. Randomized controlled trial of pulse intravenous cyclophosphamide versus mycophenolate mofetil in the induction therapy of proliferative lupus nephritis. Nephrology (Carlton) 2005;10:504–10.

[62] Aringer M, Smolen JS, Graninger WB. Severe infections in plasmapheresis-treated systemic lupus erythematosus. Arthritis Rheum 1998;41:414–20.

[63] Huang JW, Hung KY, Yen CJ, et al. Systemic lupus erythematosus and peritoneal dialysis: outcomes and infectious complications. Peritoneal Dial Internl 2001;21:143–7.

[64] Traynor AE, Schroeder J, Rosa RM, et al. Treatment of severe systemic lupus erythematosus with high-dose chemotherapy and haemopoietic stem-cell transplantation: a phase I study. Lancet 2000;356:701–7.

[65] Bellomio V, Spindler A, Lucero E, et al. Systemic lupus erythematosus: mortality and survival in Argentina. A multicenter study. Lupus 2000;9:377–81.

[66] Harris EN, Williams E, Shah DJ, et al. Mortality of Jamaican patients with systemic lupus erythematosus. Br J Rheumatol 1989;28:113–7.

[67] Hernández-Cruz B, Tapia N, Villa-Romero AR, et al. Risk factors associated with mortality in systemic lupus erythematosus. A case-control study in a tertiary care center in Mexico City. Clin Exp Rheumatol 2001;19:395–401.

[68] Huicochea Grobet ZL, Berron R, Ortega Martell JA, et al. Survival up to 5 and 10 years of Mexican pediatric patients with systemic lupus erythematosus. Overhaul of 23 years experience. Allergol Immunopathol (Madr) 1996;24:36–8.

[69] Jindal B, Joshi K, Radotra BD, et al. Fatal complications of systemic lupus erythematosus-An autopsy study from North India. Indian J Pathol Microbiol 2000;43:311–7.

[70] Mok CC, Lee KW, Ho CT, et al. A prospective study of survival and prognostic indicators of systemic lupus erythematosus in a southern Chinese population. Rheumatol 2000;39: 399–406.

[71] Rodríguez VE, González-Parés EN. Mortality study in Puerto Ricans with systemic lupus erythematosus. PRHSJ 2000;19:335–9.

[72] Shyam C, Malaviya AN. Infection-related morbidity in systemic lupus erythematosus: a clinico-epidemiological study from northern India. Rheumatol Int 1996;16:1–3.

[73] Jacobsen S, Halberg P, Ullman S. Mortality and causes of death of 344 Danish patients with systemic sclerosis (scleroderma). BJR 1998;37:750–5.

[74] Rosner S, Ginzler EM, Diamond HS, et al. A multicenter study of outcome in systemic lupus erythematosus. II. Causes of death. Arthritis Rheum 1982;25:612–7.

[75] La Spina M, Russo G. Pneumococcal sepsis in a girl with systemic lupus erythematosus. Br J Haematol 2003;122:172.

[76] Chiu WJ, Kao HT, Huang JL. Necrotizing pneumonia caused by Streptococcus pneumoniae in a child with systemic lupus erythematosus. Acta Paediatr Taiwan 2002;43:291–4.

[77] Kraus A, Cabral AR, Sifuentes-Osornio J, et al. Listeriosis in patients with connective tissue diseases. J Rheumatol 1994;21:635–8.

[78] Abramson S, Kramer SB, Radin A, et al. Salmonella bacteremia in systemic lupus erythematosus. Eight year experience at a municipal hospital. Arthritis Rheum 1985;28:75–9.

[79] Chen YH, Chen TP, Lu PL, et al. Salmonella choleraesuis bacteremia in southern Taiwan. Kaohsiung J Med Sci 1999;15:202–8.

[80] Kraus A, Guerra-Bautista G, Alarcón-Segovia D. Salmonella arizona arthritis and septicemia associated with rattlesnake ingestion by patients with connective tissue diseases. A dangerous complication of folk medicine. J Rheumatol 1991;18:1328–31.

[81] Mc-Nab P, Fuentealba C, Ballesteros F, et al. Nocardia asteroides infection in a patient with systemic lupus erythematosus. [Infección por Nocardia asteroides en un paciente con lupus eritematoso sistémico] Rev Med Chil 2000;128:526–8.

[82] Tsao CH, Chen CY, Ou LS, et al. Risk factors of mortality for salmonella infection in systemic lupus erythematosus. J Rheumatol 2002;29:1214–8.

[83] Wang TK, Ho PL, Wong SS. Recurrent bacteraemia caused by different Salmonella species in a systemic lupus erythematosus patient. New Microbiol 2005;28:151–6.

[84] Joshua F, Riordan J, Sturgess A. Salmonella typhimurium mediastinal abscess in a patient with systemic lupus erythematosus. Lupus 2003;12:710–3.

[85] Betrosian AP, Balla M, Papanikolaou M, et al. Meningococcal purpura fulminans in a patient with systemic lupus erythematosus: a mimic for catastrophic antiphospholipid antibody syndrome? Am J Med Sci 2004;327:373–5.

[86] Oztekin K, Akercan F, Yucebilgin MS, et al. Pelvic actinomycosis in a postmenopausal patient with systemic lupus erythematosus mimicking ovarian malignancy: case report and review of the literature. Clin Exp Obstet Gynecol 2004;31:154–7.

[87] Mok CC, Yuen KY, Lau CS. Nocardiosis in systemic lupus erythematosus. Sem Arthritis Rheum 1997;26:675–83.

[88] Pelayes DE, Colombero D, Gioino JM, et al. [Endogenous Nocardia asteroides endophthalmitis in a patient with systemic lupus erythematosus] Medicina (B Aires) 2004;64:146–8.

[89] Victorio-Navarra ST, Dy EE, Arroyo CG, et al. Tuberculosis among Filipino patients with systemic lupus erythematosus. Sem Arthritis Rheum 1996;26:628–34.

[90] Duzgun N, Peksari Y, Sonel B, et al. Localization of extrapulmonary tuberculosis in the synovial membrane, skin, and meninges in a patient with systemic lupus erythematosus and IgG deficiency. Rheumatol Int 2002;22:41–4.

[91] Hoffman GS, Myers RL, Stark FR, et al. Septic arthritis associated with mycobacterium avium: a case report and literature review. J Rheumatol 1978;5:199–209.

[92] Zvetina JR, Demos TC, Rubinstein H. Mycobacterium intracellulare infection of the shoulder and spine in a patient with steroid-treated systemic lupus erythematosus. Skeletal Radiol 1982;8:111–3.

[93] Hsu PY, Yang YH, Hsiao CH, et al. Mycobacterium kansasii infection presenting as cellulitis in a patient with systemic lupus erythematosus. J Formos Med Assoc 2002;101:581–4.

[94] Yang WK, Fu LS, Lan JL, et al. Mycobacterium avium complex-associated hemophagocytic syndrome in systemic lupus erythematosus patient: report of one case. Lupus 2003;12:312–6.

[95] Kahl LE. Herpes zoster infections in systemic lupus erythematosus: Risk factors and outcome. J Rheumatol 1994;21:84–6.

[96] Bang S, Park YB, Kang BS, et al. CMV enteritis causing ileal perforation in underlying lupus enteritis. Clin Rheumatol 2004;23:69–72.

[97] Tokunaga N, Sadahiro S, Kise Y, et al. Gastrointestinal cytomegalovirus infection in collagen diseases. Tokai J Exp Clin Med 2003;28:35–8.

[98] Ohashi N, Isozaki T, Shirakawa K, et al. Cytomegalovirus colitis following immunosuppressive therapy for lupus peritonitis and lupus nephritis. Intern Med 2003;42:362–6.

[99] Drevlow BE, Schilling EM, Khabbaz RF, et al. Retroviral risk factors in patients with autoimmune disease. J Rheumatol 1996;23:428–31.

[100] Hazarika I, Chakravarty BP, Dutta S, et al. Emergence of manifestations of HIV infection in a case of systemic lupus erythematosus following treatment with IV cyclophosphamide. Clin Rheumatol 2006;25:98–100.

[101] Wanchu A, Sud A, Singh S, et al. Human immunodeficiency virus infection in a patient with systemic lupus erythematosus. J Assoc Physicians India 2003;51:1102–4.

[102] Kopelman RG, Zolla-Pazner S. Association of human immunodeficiency virus infection and autoimmune phenomena. Am J Med 1988;84:82–8.

[103] Chowdhry IA, Tan IJ, Mian N, et al. Systemic lupus erythematosus presenting with features suggestive of human immunodeficiency virus infection. J Rheumatol 2005;32: 1365–8.

[104] Hsu T-C, Tsay GJ. Human parvovirus B19 infection in patients with systemic lupus erythematosus. Rheumatol 2001;40:152–7.

[105] Godeau B, Coutant-Perronne V, Le Thi Huong D, et al. Pneumocystis carinii pneumonia in the course of connective tissue disease: report of 34 cases. J Rheumatol 1994;21:246–51.

[106] Kadoya A, Okada J, Iikuni Y, et al. Risk factors for Pneumocystis carinii pneumonia in patients with polymyositis/dermatomyositis or systemic lupus erythematosus. J Rheumatol 1996;23:1186–8.

[107] Liam CK, Wang F. Pneumocystis carinii pneumonia in patients with systemic lupus erythematosus. Lupus 1992;1:379–85.

[108] Porges AJ, Beattie SL, Ritchlin C, et al. Patients with systemic lupus erythematosus at risk for Pneumocystis carinii pneumonia. J Rheumatol 1992;19:1191–4.

[109] Wainstein E, Neira O, Guzman L. Lupus erythematosus disseminatus and Pneumocystis carinii pneumonia. [Lupus eritematoso diseminado y pneumonía a Pneumocystis carinii] Rev Med Chil 1993;121:1422–5.

[110] Li J, Huang XM, Fang WG, et al. Pneumocystis carinii pneumonia in patients with connective tissue disease. J Clin Rheumatol 2006;12:114–7.

[111] Werlinger KD, Yen MA. Eumycotic mycetoma caused by Cladophialophora bantiana in a patient with systemic lupus erythematosus. J Am Acad Dermatol 2005;52:S114–7.

[112] Katz A, Ehrenfeld M, Livneh A, et al. Aspergillosis in systemic lupus erythematosus. Sem Arthritis Rheum 1996;26:635–40.

[113] Canova EG, Rosa DC, Vallada MG, et al. Invasive aspergillosis in juvenile systemic lupus erythematosus. A clinico-pathologic case. Clin Exp Rheumatol 2002;20:736.

[114] Setoyama M, Fukumaru S, Takasaki T, et al. SLE with death from acute massive pulmonary hemorrhage cause by disseminated strongyloidiasis. Scand J Rheumatol 1997;26: 389–91.

[115] Braun J, Sieper J, Schulte KL, et al. Visceral leishmaniasis mimicking a flare of systemic lupus erythematosus. Clin Rheumatol 1991;10:445–8.

[116] dos Santos-Neto LL, Polcheira MF, Castro C, et al. [Trypanosoma cruzi high parasitemia in patient with systemic lupus erythematosus] Rev Soc Bras Med Trop 2003;36:613–5.

[117] Deleze M, Mintz G, del Carmen Mejia M. Toxoplasma gondii encephalitis in systemic lupus erythematosus. A neglected cause of treatable nervous system infection. J Rheumatol 1985;12:994–6.

[118] Domenech E, Kelly J. Swallowing disorders. Med Clin North Am 1999;83:97–113.

[119] Mitchell H, Bolster MB, Leroy EC. Scleroderma and related conditions. Med Clin North Am 1997;81:129–49.

[120] Rajapakse CN, Bancewicz J, Jones CJ, et al. Pharyngo-oesophageal dysphagia in systemic sclerosis. Ann Rheum Dis 1981;40:612–4.

[121] Rosas V, Conte JV, Yang SC, et al. Lung transplantation and systemic sclerosis. Ann Transplant 2000;5:38–43.

[122] De Santis M, Bosello S, La Torre G, et al. Functional, radiological and biological markers of alveolitis and infections of the lower respiratory tract in patients with systemic sclerosis. Respir Res 2005;6:96.

[123] Pando J, Nashel DJ. Clinical images: progressive calcifications and draining lesions following staphylococcal infection in a patient with limited scleroderma. Arthritis Rheum 1998; 41:373.

[124] Binks M, Passweg JR, Furst D, et al. Phase I/II trial of autologous stem cell transplantation in systemic sclerosis: procedure related mortality and impact on skin disease. Ann Rheum Dis 2001;60:577–84.

[125] Silver RM, Warrick JH, Kinsella MB, et al. Cyclophosphamide and low-dose prednisone therapy in patients with systemic sclerosis (Scleroderma) with interstitial lung disease. J Rheumatol 1993;20:838–44.

[126] Seibold JR, Korn JH, Simms R, et al. Recombinant human relaxin in the treatment of scleroderma. A randomized, double-blind, placebo-controlled trial. Ann Intern Med 2000;132:871–9.

[127] Ferri C, Valentini G, Cozzi F, et al. Systemic sclerosis. Demographic, clinical, and serologic features and survival in 1,012 Italian patients. Medicine 2002;81:139–53.

[128] Scussel-Lonzetti L, Joyal F, Raynauld JP, et al. Predicting mortality in systemic sclerosis. Analysis of a cohort of 309 French Canadian patients with emphasis on features at diagnosis as predictive factors for survival. Medicine 2002;81:154–67.

[129] Pirila L, Soderstrom KO, Hietarinta M, et al. Fatal myocardial necrosis caused by Staphylococcus lugdunensis and cytomegalovirus in a patient with scleroderma. J Clin Microbiol 2006;44:2295–7.

[130] Nishioka K, Katayama I, Kondo H, et al. Epidemiological analysis of prognosis of 496 Japanese patients with progressive systemic sclerosis (SSc). Scleroderma Research Committee Japan. J Dermatol 1996;23:677–82.

[131] Minor RL Jr, Baum S, Schulze-Delrieu KS. Pyomyositis in a patient with progressive systemic sclerosis. Case report and review of the literature. Arch Intern Med 1988;148: 1453–5.

[132] Pialoux G, Mouly F, Cadranel JF, et al. Infection of ascitic fluid by perforation of a sclerodermic colon. [Infection d'ascite par perforation sur colon sclerodermique] Gastroenterol Clin Bio 1992;16:705–7.

[133] Walz BH, Crosby LA. Mycobacterium avium-intracellulare infection of the knee joint. Case report. Am J Knee Surg 1995;8:35–7.

[134] Gerster JC, Duvoisin B, Dudler J, et al. Tenosynovitis of the hands caused by mycobacterium kansasii in a patient with scleroderma. J Rheumatol 2004;31:2523–5.

[135] Ferry AP, Font RL, Weinberg RS, et al. Nocardial endophthalmitis: report of two cases studied histopathologically. Br J Ophthal 1988;72:55–61.

[136] Yazawa N, Fujimoto M, Kikuchi K, et al. High seroprevalence of helicobacter pylori infection in patients with systemic sclerosis: association with esophageal involvement. J Rheumatol 2000;27:1568–9.

[137] Dziadzio M, Giovagnoni A, Pomponio G, et al. Acute myocarditis associated with adenoviral infection in a patient with scleroderma. Clin Rheumatol 2003;22:487–90.

[138] Kahaleh MB, Leroy EC. Autoimmunity and vascular involvement in systemic sclerosis (SSc). Autoimmunity 1999;31:195–214.

[139] Longo F, Saletta S, Lepore L, et al. Localized scleroderma after infection with Epstein-Barr virus. Clin Exp Rheumatol 1993;11:681–3.

[140] Ferri C, Zakrzewska K, Longombardo G, et al. Parvovirus B19 infection of bone marrow in systemic sclerosis patients. Clin Exp Rheumatol 1999;17:718–20.

[141] Ward MM, Donald F. Pneumocystis carinii pneumonia in patients with connective tissue diseases: the role of hospital experience in diagnosis and mortality. Arthritis Rheum 1999; 42:780–9.

[142] Zamost BJ, Hirschberg J, Ippoliti AF, et al. Esophagitis in scleroderma. Prevalence and risk factors. Gastroenterol 1987;92:421–8.

[143] Kovacs SO, Kovacs SC. Dermatomyositis. J Am Acad Dermatol 1998;39:899–921.

[144] Schwarz MI. Thoracic manifestations of the systemic autoimmune diseases. The lung in polymyositis. Clin Chest Med 1998;19:701–12.

[145] Bahner D, Meller J, Stiefel M, et al. Juvenile dermatomyositis–acute recidivism or sepsis. [Juvenile dermatomyositis–akutes Rezidiv oder Sepsis] Nervenarzt 1999;70:547–51.

[146] Eisenstein D, Paller AS, Pachman LM. Juvenile dermatomyositis. Pediatrics 1999;103:195.

[147] Moore EC, Cohen F, Douglas SD, et al. Staphylococcal infections in childhood dermatomyositis–association with the development of calcinosis, raised IgE concentrations and granulocyte chemotactic defect. Ann Rheum Dis 1992;51:378–83.

[148] Kanik KS, Cash JM. Methotrexate. Does methotrexate increase the risk of infection or malignancy? Rheum Dis Clin North Am 1997;23:955–67.

[149] Klein-Gitelman MS, Szer IS. Disseminated nocardia brasiliensis infection: an unusual complication of immunosuppressive treatment for childhood dermatomyositis. J Rheumatol 1991;18:1243–6.

[150] Xue L, Chen X, Chen S. Prognostic factors of dermatomyositis: analysis of 119 cases. [Chinese] Zhonghua Nei Ke Za Zhi 1997;36:32–5.

[151] Amano K, Maruyama H, Mori S, et al. [Respiratory failure in polymyositis and dermatomyositis: differential diagnosis between pulmonary infection and interstitial pneumonitis] [Japanese] Kansenshogaku Zasshi 1998;72:517–25.

[152] Casademont J, Roger N, Pedrol E, et al. Streptococcal myositis as a complication of juvenile dermatomyositis. Neuromuscular Disor 1991;1:375–7.

[153] Soriano ER, Barcan L, Clara L, et al. Streptococcus pyomyositis occurring in a patient with dermatomyositis in a country with temperate climate. J Rheumatol 1992;19:1305–7.

[154] Marie I, Herve F, Kerleau JM, et al. Helicobacter heilmanii gastritis in polymyositis. Eur J Intern Med 2006;17:213–4.

[155] Marie I, Hachulla E, Cherin P, et al. Opportunistic infections in polymyositis and dermatomyositis. Arthritis Rheum 2005;53:155–65.

[156] Kofteridis D, Mantadakis E, Mixaki I, et al. Primary cutaneous nocardiosis in 2 patients on immunosuppressants. Scand J Infect Dis 2005;37:507–10.

[157] Hernandez-Cruz B, Cardiel MH, Villa AR, et al. Development, recurrence, and severity of infections in Mexican patients with RA: a nested case-control study. J Rheumatol 1999;25: 1900–7.

[158] Schaller M, Korting HC, Meurer M, et al. Generalized mycobacterium avium-intracellulare infection due to immunosuppressive therapy of paraneoplastic dermatomyositis. [Generalisierte mycobacterium avium-intracellulare infektion immun suppressiver therapie einer paraneoplastischer dermatomyositis] Hautarzt 1997;48:118–21.

[159] Nagaoka S, Tani K, Ishigatsubo Y, et al. [Herpes zoster in patients with polymyositis and dermatomyositis]. [Japanese] Kansenshogaku Zasshi 1990;64:1394–9.

[160] Nishi K, Myoh S, Bandoh T, et al. [An autopsy case of dermatomyositis associated with interstitial pneumonia probably due to cytomegalovirus infection]. [Japanese] Nihon Kyobu Shikkan Gakkai Zasshi 1992;30:1975–80.

[161] Yoshihara S, Fukuma N, Masago R. [Cytomegalovirus infection associated with immunosuppressive therapy in collagen vascular diseases]. [Japanese] Ryumachi 1999;39:740–8.

[162] Yoda Y, Hanaoka R, Ide H, et al. Clinical evaluation of patients with inflammatory connective tissue diseases complicated by cytomegalovirus antigenemia. Mod Rheumatol 2006;16:137–42.

[163] Kasifoglu T, Korkmaz C, Ozkan R. Cytomegalovirus-induced interstitial pneumonitis in a patient with dermatomyositis. Clin Rheumatol 2006;25:731–3.

[164] Crowson AN, Magro CM, Dawood MR. A causal role for parvovirus B19 infection in adult dermatomyositis and other autoimmune syndromes. J Cutan Pathol 2000;27:505–15.

[165] Fiore G, Giacovazzo F, Giacovazzo M. HCV and dermatomyositis: report of 5 cases of dermatomyositis in patients with HCV infection. Riv Eur Sci Med Farmacol 1996;18:197–201.

[166] Lewkonia RM, Horne D, Dawood MR. Juvenile dermatomyositis in a child infected with human parvovirus B19. Clin Infect Dis 1995;21:430–2.

[167] Bachelez H, Schremmer B, Cadranel J, et al. Fulminant Pneumocystis carinii pneumonia in 4 patients with dermatomyositis (Clinical observation). Arch Intern Med 1997;157:1501–3.

[168] Henseler T. [Mucocutaneous candidiasis in patients with skin diseases]. [German] Mycoses 1995;1:7–13.

[169] Voloshin DK, Lacomis D, McMahon D. Disseminated histoplasmosis presenting as myositis and fasciitis in a patient with dermatomyositis. Muscle Nerve 1995;18:531–5.

[170] Ward MM, Pyun E, Studenski S. Long-term survival in systemic lupus erythematosus. Patient characteristics associated with poorer outcomes. Arthritis Rheum 1995;38:274–83.

[171] Jacobsen S, Petersen J, Ullman S, et al. A multicentre study of 513 Danish patients with systemic lupus erythematosus. I. Disease manifestations and analyses of clinical subsets. Clin Rheumatol 1998;17:468–77.

[172] Petri M. Musculoskeletal complications of systemidc lupus erythematosus in the Hopkins Lupus Cohort: an update. Arthritis Care Res 1995;8:137–45.

[173] Abu-Shakra M, Urowitz MB, Gladman DD, et al. Mortality studies in systemic lupus erythematosus. Results from a single center. I. Causes of death. J Rheumatol 1995;22:1259–64.

[174] Wongchinsri J, Tantawichien T, Osiri M, et al. Infection in Thai patients with systemic lupus erythematosus: a review of hospitalized patients. J Med Assoc Thai 2002;85(Suppl 1):S34–9.

[175] Pope JE, Krizova A, Ouimet JM, et al. Close association of herpes zoster reactivation and systemic lupus erythematosus (SLE) diagnosis: case-control study of patients with SLE or noninflammatory nusculoskeletal disorders. J Rheumatol 2004;31:274–9.

ELSEVIER
SAUNDERS

Infect Dis Clin N Am
20 (2006) 877–889

INFECTIOUS
DISEASE CLINICS
OF NORTH AMERICA

Hepatitis C and Arthritis: An Update

Aja M. Sanzone, MD[a], Rodolfo E. Bégué, MD[b],*

[a]Pediatric Infectious Diseases, Combined Fellowship Training Program of Tulane
University and Louisiana State University Health Sciences Center,
1430 Tulane Avenue, New Orleans, LA 70112, USA
[b]Division of Infectious Diseases, Department of Pediatrics, Louisiana State University Health
Sciences Center, Children's Hospital, 200 Henry Clay Avenue, New Orleans, LA 70118, USA

Hepatitis C virus (HCV) infects approximately 3% of the world's population or 170 million people. In the United States, HCV represents the most common blood-borne chronic infection and is a leading cause of chronic liver disease. It is estimated that the overall prevalence of HCV in the United States is 1.8% or 3.9 million people with approximately 2.7 million people chronically infected [1,2]. These figures likely are an underestimate of the true incidence of the disease, however, because the infection may be clinically silent.

The main target of the virus is the hepatocyte and thus HCV primarily causes liver disease with cirrhosis and hepatocellular carcinoma being the most devastating consequence of long-term infection. In addition, HCV infection frequently is associated with various extrahepatic manifestations, such as arthritis and arthralgias, vasculitis, mixed cryoglobulinemia, glomerulonephritis, lichen planus, porphyria cutanea tarda, and B cell lymphomas [3]. Depending on the population studied, some form of extrahepatic manifestation is observed in 24% to 74% of the patients [4–6] and they usually are seen during the chronic phase of the infection. Cacoub and colleagues [5] undertook a large, single-center evaluation of 1202 patients who had chronic HCV infection and described that 74% of them manifested extrahepatic symptoms, the risk factors being female sex, increasing age, and extensive liver fibrosis (suggesting that duration of infection or infecting genotype 1 also may represent risk factors, although these factors were not reported specifically). The mechanisms involved in extrahepatic manifestations are complex; HCV is known to be lymphotropic also [7] and persistent activation of immune cells leads to production of HCV-specific immunoglobulins with potential formation of immune complexes that may contribute to the various autoimmune and rheumatologic manifestations observed [8]. Special

---

* Corresponding author.
E-mail address: rbegue@lsuhsc.edu (R.E. Bégué).

consideration in this respect should be given to cryoglobulins. Cryoglobulins are immunoglobulins of different isotypes that precipitate at temperatures less than 37°C and when deposited in small vessels can lead to vasculitis. There are three types of cryoglobulinemias: type I—monoclonal immuno-globulin IgG; type II (mixed)—polyclonal immunoglobulins IgG plus monoclonal immunoglobulins IgM, IgG, or IgA; and type III (mixed)—polyclonal IgG plus polyclonal IgM [9]. Type II mixed cryoglobulinemia is the most common type seen in chronic HCV infection [8] and the immune complexes are composed of monoclonal IgM rheumatoid factor, polyclonal anti-HCV IgG, and HCV virions [9–11].

Although there are well-established extrahepatic immune and autoim-mune manifestations of chronic HCV infection, including arthritis, it is un-clear whether there is an arthritic syndrome particular to HCV infection. As far back as 1967, Pachas and Pinals [12] already described a nonerosive sym-metrical polyarthritis seen in patients who had cirrhosis; it is unknown whether those patients indeed had HCV infection because the antibody as-say would not be available for another two decades. Since then, several re-ports on the association of HCV and arthritis have been published, primarily in the rheumatology literature [13,14]; the interested reader is re-ferred to those review articles. Here, we update and critically review the most recent literature to make the infectious diseases community aware of the issue and try to answer two important practical questions: (1) Is there a relationship between HCV infection and arthritis? (2) Does the co-occur-rence of HCV infection and arthritis require modification of the treatment of either disease process?

Is there an association between hepatitis C virus infection and arthritis?

Prevalence data

The topic of HCV infection and arthritis has attracted more attention from the rheumatologists than the infectious diseases specialists, yet the prevalence of HCV among patients who have arthritis is comparatively low, whereas the prevalence of arthritis among patients who have HCV in-fection is comparatively high. Data on the first topic is scant. Maillefert and colleagues [15] in France found that of 309 patients who had rheumatoid ar-thritis according to criteria by the American College of Rheumatology (ACR) (formerly the American Rheumatism Association [ARA]), 2 had anti-HCV antibodies and only 1 of them was HCV-RNA positive. Subse-quent data by the same group [16] again showed that of 232 patients seen for initial evaluation of various recent-onset inflammatory arthritides only 6 had anti-HCV antibodies detected. Interestingly, despite this relatively low prevalence, the authors found that it is not infrequent for rheumatolo-gists to screen their patients for HCV [17]. Conversely, data on the preva-lence of arthritis among patients who had HCV infection is more abundant but varies widely from 2% to 27% [13]. This wide range is because of important differences in study designs and by itself makes estimation of the true prevalence of HCV arthritis difficult. Rosner and coworkers [14] underscore these limitations and note that many published studies do not specify the types of arthritis, whether joint involvement is acute or chronic, and whether arthritis is associated with cryoglobulinemia. They also noted that only three of seven studies reviewed by them were prospective and only two of them had a pre-investigation definition of arthritis. In addition, selection bias may be a major problem because most studies include patients selected by attending rheumatology clinics and in that regard they may not be representative of the overall population of HCV-infected subjects. In support of this notion, the prevalence of arthritis in a group of patients who had HCV selected at a unit of infectious diseases was much lower—only 2.2% [4]. Most of these observational studies are not standardized and have flawed study designs, limitations that make generalizations and comparisons difficult. If the true prevalence of arthritis in HCV infection is not well defined or depends on too many extraneous factors, an association of these two variables is even more difficult to measure.

Data from case-control studies

Are arthritic disorders more frequent among patients who have HCV than among comparable noninfected individuals? This case-control approach requires standardized definition of cases and the use of well-matched controls. Because of convenience many studies have used this approach yet few meet these criteria. Recent publications highlight the uncertainties. In 2005, Giordano and colleagues [4] retrospectively analyzed a cohort of 265 patients who had chronic HCV infection admitted to a unit of infectious diseases over a 3-year period and investigated the prevalence of immune and autoimmune disorders. All patients met diagnostic criteria for chronic HCV infection (ie, positive anti-HCV antibodies, presence of HCV-RNA, and inflammation on liver biopsy). The prevalence of arthritis was 4% in subjects who did not have cirrhosis and 2% in patients who had cirrhosis. The study had no control group but the authors indicated that the prevalence of rheumatoid arthritis (diagnosed by criteria of the ARA, 1987) in their study group (2.2%) was similar to the prevalence of rheumatoid arthritis (0.5%–3%) found in the general population. Barbosa and coworkers [18] looked at the issue from the opposite side. They prospectively analyzed a cohort of 367 patients who had rheumatic diseases, seen in a rheumatology clinic in Brazil, and assessed the seroprevalence of HCV infection. Systemic lupus erythematosus was seen in 47% of their patients, rheumatoid arthritis in 24.2%, and other diagnoses in 28.1%. The overall seroprevalence of HCV in the total cohort was 1.9%, which was similar to the background rate (2.2%, 95% CI: 1.6%–2.8%) illustrated in a previous study performed in blood donors in the same geographic area [19]; again, no concurrent control group was similarly evaluated. When analysis was restricted to patients who had a diagnosis of rheumatoid arthritis, the concurrent HCV infection increased slightly to 3 of 89 (3.4%, 95% CI: 0.7%–9.5%)—higher, but not enough for a statistically significant difference. Finally, Ramos-Casals and colleagues [20] in a multicenter study evaluated two groups of patients who had systemic autoimmune diseases, one with and the other without HCV infection. Compared with the HCV-negative group, those who had HCV were older and more likely to be male. They also had more frequent vasculitis, cryoglobulinemia, and neoplasia, but their frequency of articular symptoms (84 of 180 [47%] versus 97 of 180 [54%]) was not different.

Data from interventional studies

Does treatment of HCV infection improve the associated arthritis? Antiviral treatment of HCV is relatively new and consequently the available information is scarce. Information comes mostly from anecdotal reports or small series of retrospective, nonrandomized interventions with limited follow-up and sometimes concomitant use of antirheumatic medications [21,22], all limitations that make interpretation of results difficult. Zuckerman and coworkers [23] described a favorable response to antiviral therapy. They reported that of 25 patients who had HCV arthritis unresponsive to various antiinflammatory medications, including nonsteroidal antiinflammatory drugs (NSAIDs) and corticosteroids, 17 (67%) had complete (44%) or partial response (32%) of arthritis symptoms following therapy with interferon (IFN)-α for a median duration of 12 months. Although clinical improvement was noted in most of the patients studied, the role of antiviral therapy is unclear because a virologic remission and normalization of transaminases was seen in only 13 of 28 (46%) patients. Nissen and coworkers [24] recently reported a less favorable response, however. The investigators retrospectively evaluated 21 patients who had known chronic HCV infection followed in a rheumatology department. Nineteen of the patients had arthritis and 13 of them had received IFN-α either as monotherapy or combined with ribavirin. Following therapy, 4 had no change in the rheumatologic manifestation, 6 had deterioration, and only 2 had improvement.

Clinical data: specificity of the syndrome

Even if difficult to detect on epidemiologic studies, is there a type of arthritis specific to HCV infection? The rheumatologic literature seems to agree on two main types of presentation [13,14]. The first, less common (seen in one third of cases) is associated with cryoglobulinemia and described as asymmetrical pauciarticular typically involving the medium-sized and large joints [13]. Cryoglobulinemia is not seen only with HCV infection and not all patients who have HCV have cryoglobulins, but there is a strong association between the two entities. Mixed cryoglobulinemia can be observed in up to half of HCV infected patients and—depending on the geographic location—40% to 100% of people who have cryoglobulinemia may have HCV [25,26]. Most patients who have mixed cryoglobulinemia are asymptomatic and only 10% may have symptoms, such as cutaneous manifestations (vasculitis), peripheral neuropathy, liver involvement, renal involvement, sicca syndrome, and B-cell lymphoproliferative disorders. Polyarthralgias and myalgias are frequent in cryoglobulinemia syndrome but arthritis is relatively rare [27].

The second, more common type of arthritis (two thirds of cases) closely resembles rheumatoid arthritis. It is described as polyarticular symmetrical primarily involving small joints, and usually is positive for rheumatoid factor; as such many of these cases fulfill the ACR criteria for rheumatoid arthritis [28]. It differs from rheumatoid arthritis, however, in that it affects a different population (older, higher proportion male), it does not progress to erosion or destruction of the joint, there are no subcutaneous nodules, and only half of them show elevation of the erythrocyte sedimentation rate [23]. Because both HCV-related arthritis and rheumatoid arthritis can be positive for rheumatoid factor, to try to distinguish them several studies have evaluated the use of other antibodies, such as anti-cyclic citrullinated peptide antibodies (anti-CCP) and antikeratin antibodies (AKA). Van Boekel and colleagues [29] in 2002 reviewed the pertinent literature and concluded that anti-CPP had the most value for the diagnosis of rheumatoid arthritis. This conclusion was supported by Bombardieri and coworkers [30] who specifically evaluated the value of anti-CCP antibodies to distinguish between a cohort of patients who had HCV arthritis and patients who had rheumatoid arthritis. Although rheumatoid factor was present in 37.5% of 8 and 90% of 30 patients who had HCV arthritis or rheumatoid arthritis, respectively, anti-CCP antibodies were not detected in any of the 8 patients who had HCV arthritis (although 3 of them had chronic polyarthritis indistinguishable from rheumatoid arthritis), whereas it was found in 23 of the 30 patients (77%) who fulfilled ACR criteria for rheumatoid arthritis. In addition, the investigators retrospectively analyzed the sera of 10 patients who had chronic HCV infection who presented with symmetric polyarticular involvement who later developed an erosive pattern consistent with rheumatoid arthritis, and found that 60% of them had anti-CCP antibodies; these patients were believed to have a concomitant diagnosis of chronic hepatitis C and rheumatoid arthritis. Similarly, Girelli and colleagues [31] reported that rheumatoid factor was seen in 32 (91%) of 35 patients who had rheumatoid arthritis and 12 (86%) of 14 patients who had HCV-related arthritis, whereas anti-CPP was seen in 12 (71%) and none, respectively. Cojocaru and coworkers [32] evaluated AKA and found that these antibodies were more prevalent in a cohort of patients diagnosed with probable rheumatoid arthritis (64% or 18 of 28) compared with another group of patients diagnosed with symmetric polyarthritis or polyarthralgia associated with HCV infection (9% or 3 of 31); both groups of patients were rheumatoid factor positive. These data provide evidence supporting the concept that HCV arthritis is distinct from rheumatoid arthritis and that both entities can be differentiated based on a combination of serologic markers; further large-scale studies are warranted, however.

Biologic evidence: plausibility

What could be the mechanisms behind HCV arthritis and is there any evidence to support them? Olivieri and coworkers [13] proposed three potential mechanisms for the occurrence of HCV-associated arthritis: (1) direct synovial tissue invasion by HCV, (2) autoimmune synovial response to HCV, and, (3) immune complex deposition/mixed cryoglobulinemia. They suggest these factors may not be mutually exclusive but rather act synergistically to the overall effect of arthritic syndromes observed in HCV. Regarding viral tissue invasion, the limited data available show that HCV-RNA has been detected, but only in few of the evaluated patients, and only in synovial fluid but not in synovial membrane [33,34]. It is not clear whether this represents free virus, infected tissue, or infected lymphocytes in transit in the affected joint. Serum autoantibodies have been reported extensively in chronic HCV infection [13,35–38]. The HCV core antigen is known to carry domains that mimic self-antigens [39], a fact that could explain the high prevalence of autoantibodies in chronic HCV infection. It is unknown, however, whether these autoantibodies play any role in the pathogenesis of HCV arthritis. The syndrome with the strongest link to chronic HCV infection is mixed cryoglobulinemia [9,40]. Cryoglobulins are more likely to cause polyarthralgias than frank arthritis [7], however, and as common as cryoglobulins are in HCV infection they cannot explain the pathogenesis of most cases because patients who have HCV arthritis usually do not have serum cryoglobulins. The literature to support cryoglobulin deposition in the synovium is scant and aspirated joint fluid from patients who have arthralgias or arthritis and cryoglobulinemia is typically inflammatory and sterile [41].

Summary

Extrahepatic symptoms during chronic HCV infection are common and varied. Arthritis can be seen either as part of autoimmune processes (eg, associated with cryoglobulinemia) or independently. Whether there is a type of arthritis particular to HCV is not clear from epidemiologic studies but, in our judgment, is best suggested by description of a syndrome similar to rheumatoid arthritis but less aggressive that can be differentiated by serologic markers. Whether the manifestation is specifically attributable to HCV infection or rather is the nonspecific result of a chronic inflammatory process is not clear at all. Better designed studies are needed. In particular there is a need for large, collaborative, prospective studies, with standardized definitions and appropriately matched controls, that look at the frequency and type of arthritic complaints among patients who have HCV infection.

Considerations in the management of patients who have hepatitis C virus infection and arthritis

Management of hepatitis C virus infection

Guidelines for the treatment of HCV infection have been published and include weekly subcutaneous peginterferon-α (either 2a at 180 μg or 2b at 1.5 μg/kg body weight per dose) plus twice daily oral ribavirin (either at 1000 or 1200 mg daily for those that weigh either <75 kg or ≥75 kg, respectively) for 48 months [42]. Exceptional cases may respond to lower doses of ribavirin (800 mg daily) for shorter periods (24 weeks). Initiation of treatment must be individualized for each patient but is dictated mainly by persistence of viremia and evidence of progressive liver disease documented on biopsy. The same guidelines indicate that for patients who have significant extrahepatic manifestations, including cryoglobulinemia, antiviral therapy may result in improvement of the symptoms, and hence should be considered. For the most common rheumatoid arthritis type, however, antiviral treatment would be less imperative because the arthritis tends to be nondestructive to the joint and the treatment of HCV does not consistently lead to symptomatic improvement. In addition there are significant side effects associated with the use of antivirals. Of concern, because use of IFN-α has been associated with worsening of autoimmune disorders [43–45], depending on the mechanisms involved there is a possibility that arthritis may develop or deteriorate during therapy, a notion supported by some anecdotal reports [46,47]. Recent treatment trials have investigated this issue specifically. Nissen and colleagues [24] reviewed the cases of 40 patients who had chronic HCV infection and arthritis who had received IFN-α, either as monotherapy or combined with ribavirin, and noted that 12 of them had no change in the rheumatologic manifestation, whereas 17 had deterioration and only 8 had improvement. It is not clear whether the deterioration of the arthritic symptoms was attributable to the therapy or to natural progression of the disease. Zuckerman and coworkers [23] had a different experience: they reported 25 patients who had HCV arthritis who had received IFN-α therapy and 17 of them showed complete or partial response of the symptoms (no deterioration was reported). From the information provided in the articles it is not possible to speculate why the two studies may have had such differing findings. Other authors have assessed antiviral treatment of patients who have HCV infection and mixed cryoglobulinemia (some of whom had arthritis). Cacoub and colleagues [48] reported 19 such patients (5 of whom had arthralgia) treated with peginterferon-α 2b (1.5 μg/kg/wk) plus ribavirin (800–1200 mg daily) for at least 6 months and found good tolerability of the treatment (specifically, no hepatotoxicity was reported). Mazzaro and colleagues [49] treated 18 patients with a lower dose of peginterferon-α 2b (1 μg/kg/wk) plus ribavirin (1000 mg daily) for 48 weeks, and again found good tolerability of the treatment.

Management of arthritis

Regardless of the cause of the arthritis (coincidental or related to HCV) and regardless of the indications for antiviral treatment, the arthritic symptoms may need to be addressed, with the goal of therapy being to control joint inflammation without causing an exacerbation or worsening of liver disease. Arthritis is treated most commonly with NSAIDs, corticosteroids, or hydroxychloroquine. NSAIDs must be used with caution because they can cause hepatotoxicity [50]. In particular, NSAIDs are contraindicated in patients who have cirrhosis because they have been associated with variceal bleeding [51]. Rostom and coworkers [52] recently reviewed the literature on this topic and found that in patients who have arthritis (and no liver disease) elevation of transaminases three times greater than the upper limit of normal was seen more frequently in those receiving diclofenac (3.6%) or rofecoxib (1.80%) than placebo (0.29%); for other NSAIDs (naproxen, ibuprofen, celecoxib, valdecoxib, meloxicam) the frequency ($\leq 0.43\%$) was not significantly elevated. Riley and Smith [53] and Andrade and colleagues [54] have described three patients and one patient, respectively, who had HCV infection who developed marked increase in transaminases while receiving ibuprofen. Causality is difficult to infer from these few cases, but is highly suggested by recurrence of the complication on re-challenge in one of the cases. Corticosteroids are not hepatotoxic but have a relative contraindication in patients who have HCV infection because of the theoretical adverse effect they may have on the immune response to the infection. A review by the Cochrane Collaboration group [55] found insufficient evidence in favor or against the use of corticosteroids for chronic HCV or associated autoimmune processes. For hydroxychloroquine, there are limited data available. Although Lovy and coworkers [56] reported good tolerability and clinical response to hydroxychloroquine (and low-dose prednisone) in 19 patients who had HCV and arthritis, Mok and colleagues [57] noted transaminase elevation in 9 of 17 (53%) courses of treatment with hydroxychloroquine (and other antirheumatics) given to patients who had chronic viral hepatitis (hepatitis C or hepatitis B).

For arthritis unresponsive to the above medications, agents that block tumor necrosis factor (TNF)-α have been evaluated, mainly in anecdotal reports or small series, as reviewed by Khanna and colleagues [58]. Peterson and coworkers [59] recently described 24 patients who received either etanercept or infliximab for 1 to 34 months without liver toxicity or increase in viremia. Similarly, Parke and Reveille [60] found anti-TNF therapy safe for treatment of rheumatoid arthritis in 5 patients for a mean of 41 months. In 2006, Marotte and colleagues [61] described 9 patients who received etanercept (at 25 mg twice a week for 3 months) for the treatment of HCV-related arthritis. The authors concluded that etanercept was safe to use in the treatment of rheumatologic manifestations of HCV infection because they saw no increase in viremia or liver inflammation during the period of treatment (but they did not see any clear improvement in the symptoms of arthritis, either). Additional observational studies have confirmed the finding that etanercept seems safe in patients who have chronic HCV infection and various rheumatologic diseases. Magliocco and Gottlieb [62] and Rokhsar and coworkers [63] described three patients and one patient, respectively, who had psoriatic arthritis who received etanercept (25–50 mg twice weekly for 3–12 months) without deterioration of the concomitant HCV infection (stable viral load and transaminases) and improvement of psoriatic symptoms (including arthritis). In a large retrospective safety trial [64] assessing the safety of anti-TNF-α therapy, 480 patients who had rheumatoid arthritis and spondylarthropathies were identified, 6 of whom had concurrent chronic viral hepatitis: 3 with hepatitis B and 3 with hepatitis C. The authors noted that the therapy appeared to be safe in these 6 patients, with no worsening of the viral load or hepatitis. Still, caution should be used because not all patients may tolerate the therapy well. In one case reported by Pritchard and colleagues [65] worsening or exacerbation of HCV infection was noted by clinical symptoms, increase in transaminases, and viral load following the use of etanercept for rheumatoid arthritis.

Methotrexate, a disease-modifying antirheumatic drug, is used commonly in autoimmune disorders and rheumatoid arthritis. Because it can cause liver toxicity, the ACR has advised caution in its use; in particular the guidelines recommend testing the patients for hepatitis B or C infection and monitoring transaminases during therapy [66]. In addition, methotrexate may have an immunosuppressive effect. Still, few reports have suggested that methotrexate may be used safely under controlled conditions. Mok and coworkers [57] described two patients who had chronic viral hepatitis who received methotrexate without elevation in their transaminases, and Kujawska and colleagues [67] described five patients who had HCV infection and rheumatoid arthritis who tolerated methotrexate. More recently, Nissen and coworkers [24] evaluated the effects of methotrexate in a retrospective study; seven of their patients had received methotrexate (at 7.5–15 mg/wk for 5–28 weeks); six had no progression of HCV disease in viremia or liver enzyme elevations, and one demonstrated viral reactivation, which was subsequently controlled with ribavirin. Despite these encouraging small studies, experts recommend extreme caution and Palazzi and colleagues [68] have advised against the routine use of methotrexate in HCV-related arthritis until further studies can better assess its safety.

Summary

The literature available at this time is insufficient to guide the most appropriate course of treatment of HCV arthritis. Arthritis in HCV per se is not an indication for antiviral treatment but it may be considered, especially when associated with cryoglobulinemia, because mixed cryoglobulinemia may be a risk factor for the development of cirrhosis in chronic HCV infection [27,69]. Treatment of HCV viremia does not seem to improve—and some treatments (eg, IFN-α) may exacerbate—the arthritic symptoms, so it should not be undertaken routinely. Standard antirheumatic treatment can be considered (eg, NSAIDs, corticosteroids, and others), but with caution, because some of these medications occasionally may be hepatotoxic and response to therapy seems variable. Treatment decisions should be determined on a case-by-case basis.

References

[1] Thomas DL, Lemon SM, Hepatitis C. In: Mandell Gl, Bennett JE, Dolin R, editors. Principles and practice of infectious diseases. 6th edition. Philadelphia: Churchill Livingstone; 2005. p. 1950–81.
[2] Centers for Disease Control and Prevention. Sexually transmitted diseases treatment guidelines. MMWR 2006;55(No. RR-11):1–94.
[3] Sterling RK, Bralow S. Extrahepatic manifestations of hepatitis C virus. Curr Gastroenterol Rep 2006;8(1):53–9.
[4] Giordano N, Amendola A, Papakostas P, et al. Immune and autoimmune disorders in HCV chronic liver disease: personal experience and commentary on literature. New Microbiol 2005;28(4):311–7.
[5] Cacoub P, Poynard T, Ghillani P, et al. Extrahepatic manifestations of chronic hepatitis C. The MULTIVIRC group. Multidepartment virus C. Arthritis Rheum 1999;42(10): 2204–12.
[6] Zignego AL, Macchia D, Monti M, et al. Infection of peripheral mononuclear cells by hepatitis C virus. J Hepatol 1992;15:382–6.
[7] Cacoub P, Renou C, Rosental E, et al. Extrahepatic manifestations associated with hepatitis C virus infection: a prospective multicenter study of 321 patients. Medicine (Baltimore) 2000; 79(1):47–56.
[8] Starkebaum G, Sasso EH. Hepatitis C and B cells: induction of autoimmunity and lymphoproliferation may reflect chronic stimulation through cell-surface receptors. J Rheumatol 2004;31(3):416–8.
[9] Ali A, Zein NN. Hepatitis C infection: a systemic disease with extrahepatic manifestations. Cleve Clin J Med 2005;72(11):1005–8, 1010–4, 1016, 1019.
[10] Vassilopoulos D, Calabrese LH. Hepatitis C virus infection and vasculitis: implications of antiviral and immunosuppressive therapies. Arthritis Rheum 2002;46(3):585–97.
[11] Sansonno D, Dammacco F. Hepatitis C virus, cryoglobulinaemia, and vasculitis: immune complex relations. Lancet Infect Dis 2005;5(4):227–36.
[12] Pachas WN, Pinals RS. A rheumatic syndrome with Laennec's cirrhosis. Arthritis Rheum 1967;10(4):343–7.
[13] Olivieri I, Palazzi C, Padula A. Hepatitis C virus and arthritis. Rheum Dis Clin North Am 2003;29(1):111–22.
[14] Rosner I, Rozenbaum M, Toubi E, et al. The case for hepatitis C arthritis. Semin Arthritis Rheum 2004;33(6):375–87.
[15] Maillefert JF, Muller G, Falgarone G. Prevalence of hepatitis C virus infection in patients with rheumatoid arthritis. Ann Rheum Dis 2002;61(7):635–7.
[16] Zerrak A, Bour JB, Tavernier C, et al. Usefulness of routine hepatitis C virus, hepatitis B virus, and parvovirus B19 serology in the diagnosis of recent-onset inflammatory arthritides. Arthritis Rheum 2005;53(3):477–8.
[17] Saraux A, Fautrel B, Maillefert JF, et al. Laboratory and imaging studies by French rheumatologists to evaluate patients with early arthritis. J Rheumatol 2006;33(5): 897–902.

[18] Barbosa VS, da Silva NA, Marins RM. Hepatitis C virus seroprevalence and genotypes in patients with diffuse connective tissue diseases and spondyloarthropathies. Braz J Med Biol Res 2005;38(5):801–5.

[19] Martins RM, Vanderborght BO, Rouzere CD, et al. Anti-HCV related to HCV PCR and risk factors analysis in a blood donor population of central Brazil. Rev Inst Med Trop Sao Paulo 1994;36(6):501–6.

[20] Ramos-Casals M, Jara LJ, Medina F, et al. Systemic autoimmune diseases coexisting with chronic hepatitis C virus infection (the HISPAMEC Registry): patterns of clinical and immunological expression in 180 cases. J Intern Med 2005;257(6):549–57.

[21] Niewold TB, Gibofsky A. Concomitant interferon-α therapy and tumor necrosis factor α inhibition for rheumatoid arthritis and hepatitis C. Arthritis Rheum 2006;54(7):2335–7.

[22] Akhtar AJ, Funnyé AS. Hepatitis C virus associated arthritis in absence of clinical, biochemical and histological evidence of liver disease–responding to interferon therapy. Med Sci Monit 2005;11(7):CS37–9.

[23] Zuckerman E, Keren D, Rozenbaum M, et al. Hepatitis C virus-related arthritis: characteristics and response to therapy with interferon alpha. Clin Exp Rheumatol 2000;18(5): 579–84.

[24] Nissen MJ, Fontanges E, Allam Y, et al. Rheumatological manifestations of hepatitis C: incidence in a rheumatology and non-rheumatology setting and the effect of methrotrexate and interferon. Rheumatol 2005;44:1016–20.

[25] Trejo O, Ramos-Casals M, Garcia-Carrasco M, et al. Cryoglobulinemia: study of etiologic factors and clinical and immunologic features in 443 patients from a single center. Medicine 2001;80(4):252–62.

[26] Trendelenburg M, Schifferli JA. Cryoglobulins in chronic hepatitis C virus infection. Clin Exp Immunol 2003;133(2):153–5.

[27] Morra E. Cryoglobulinemia. Hematology Am Soc Hematol Educ Program 2005;368–72.

[28] Arnett FC, Edworthy SM, Bloch DA, et al. The American Rheumatism Association 1987 revised criteria for the classification of rheumatoid arthritis. Arthritis Rheum 1988;31(3): 315–24.

[29] van Boekel M, Vossenaar ER, van den Hoogen FH, et al. Autoantibody systems in rheumatoid arthritis: specificity, sensitivity and diagnostic value. Arthritis Res 2002;4(2):87–93.

[30] Bombardieri M, Alessandri C, Labbadia G, et al. Role of anti-cyclic citrullinated peptide antibodies in discriminating patients with rheumatoid arthritis from patients with chronic hepatitis C infection-associated polyarticular involvement. Arthritis Res Ther 2004;6(2): R137–41.

[31] Girelli F, Foschi FG, Bedeschi E, et al. Is anti cyclic citrullinated peptide a useful laboratory test for the diagnosis of rheumatoid arthritis? Allerg Immunol (Paris) 2004;36(4): 127–30.

[32] Cojocaru M, Cojocaru IM, Iacob SA. Clinical relevance of antikeratin antibodies in rheumatoid arthritis and symmetric polyarthritis associated with hepatitis C infection. Rom J Intern Med 2004;42(4):709–14.

[33] Ueno Y, Kinoshita R, Kishimoto I, et al. Polyarthritis associated with hepatitis C virus infection. Br J Rheumatol 1994;33(3):289–91.

[34] Cimmino MA, Picciotto A, Sinelli N, et al. Has hepatitis C virus a specific tropism for the synovial membrane? Br J Rheumatol 1997;36(4):505–6.

[35] D'Amico E, Palazzi C, Cacciatore P, et al. Anti-ENA antibodies in patients with chronic hepatitis C virus infection. Dig Dis Sci 2002;47(4):755–9.

[36] Wu YY, Hsu TC, Chen TY, et al. Proteinase 3 and dihydrolipoamide dehydrogenase (E3) are major autoantigens in hepatitis C virus (HCV) infection. Clin Exp Immunol 2002; 128(2):347–52.

[37] Dalekos GN, Kristis KG, Boumba DS, et al. Increased incidence of anti-cardiolipin antibodies in patients with hepatitis C is not associated with aetiopathogenetic link to antiphospholipid syndrome. Eur J Gastroenterol Hepatol 2000;12(1):67–74.

[38] Lienesch DW, Sherman KE, Metzger A, et al. Anti-Clq antibodies in patients with chronic hepatitis C infection. Clin Exp Rheumatol 2006;24(2):183–5.

[39] Bogdanos DP, Rigipoulou EI. Self-mimicking autoimmune domains of hepatitis C virus core antigen. Vaccine 2006;24:6173–4.

[40] Misiani R, Bellavita P, Fenili D, et al. Hepatitis C virus infection in patients with essential mixed cryoglobulinemia. Ann Intern Med 1992;117(7):573–7.

[41] Mariette X. Hepatitis C virus, arthritides, and arthromyalgia. Joint Bone Spine 2003;70(4): 246–7.

[42] National Institute of Diabetes and Digestive and Kidney Diseases (NIDDK). Chronic hepatitis C: current disease management. Available at: http://digestive.niddk.nih.gov/ddiseases/pubs/chronichepc/index.htm. Accessed August 25, 2006.

[43] Ioannou Y, Isenberg DA. Current evidence for the induction of autoimmune rheumatic manifestations by cytokine therapy. Arthritis Rheum 2000;43:1431–42.

[44] Selmi C, Lleo A, Zuin M, et al. Interferon alpha and its contribution to autoimmunity. Curr Opin Investig Drugs 2006;7(5):451–6.

[45] Wilson LE, Widman D, Dikman SH, et al. Autoimmune disease complicating antiviral therapy for hepatitis C virus infection. Semin Arthritis Rheum 2002;32(3):163–73.

[46] Murata K, Shiraki K, Takase K, et al. Mono-arthritis following intensified interferon beta therapy for chronic hepatitis C. Hepatogastroenterology 2002;49(47):1418–9.

[47] Sood A, Midha V, Sood N. Rheumatoid arthritis probably induced by pegylated interferon in a patient with chronic hepatitis C. Indian J Gastroenterol 2004;23(1):28–9.

[48] Cacoub P, Saadoun D, Limal N, et al. PEGylated interferon alfa-2b and ribavirin treatment in patients with hepatitis C virus-related systemic vasculitis. Arthritis Rheum 2005;52(3): 911–5.

[49] Mazzaro C, Zorat F, Caizzi M, et al. Treatment with peg-interferon alfa-2b and ribavirin of hepatitis C virus-associated mixed cryoglobulinemia: a pilot study. J Hepatology 2005;42(5): 632–8.

[50] Teoh NC, Farrell GC. Hepatotoxicity associated with non-steroidal anti-inflammatory drugs. Clin Liver Dis 2003;7(2):401–13.

[51] De Lédinghen V, Heresbach D, Fourdan O, et al. Anti-inflammatory drugs and variceal bleeding: a case-control study. Gut 1999;44(2):270–3.

[52] Rostom A, Goldkind L, Laine L. Nonsteroidal anti-inflammatory drugs and hepatic toxicity: a systematic review of randomized controlled trials in arthritis patients. Clin Gastroenterol Hepatol 2005;3(5):489–98.

[53] Riley TR, Smith JP. Ibuprofen-induced hepatotoxicity in patients with chronic hepatitis C: a case series. Am J Gastroenterol 1998;93(9):1563–5.

[54] Andrade RJ, Lucena MI, Garcia-Cortes M, et al. Chronic hepatitis C, ibuprofen, and liver damage. Am J Gastroenterol 2002;97(7):1854–5.

[55] Brok J, Mellerup MT, Krogsgaard K, et al. Glucocorticosteroids for viral hepatitis C. Cochrane Database Syst Rev 2004;2:CD002904. Available at:. http://www.cochrane.org/reviews/en/ab002904.html. Accessed August 29, 2006.

[56] Lovy MR, Starkebaum G, Uberoi S. Hepatitis C infection presenting with rheumatic manifestations: a mimic of rheumatoid arthritis. J Rheumatol 1996;23(6):979–83.

[57] Mok MY, Ng WL, Yuen MF, et al. Safety of disease modifying anti-rheumatic agents in rheumatoid arthritis patients with chronic viral hepatitis. Clin Exp Rheumatol 2000;18(3): 363–8.

[58] Khanna M, Shirodkar MA, Gottlieb AB. Etanercept therapy in patients with autoimmunity and hepatitis C. J Dermatol Treatment 2003;14:229–32.

[59] Peterson JR, Hsu FC, Simkin PA, et al. Effect of tumor necrosis factor α antagonists on serum transaminases and viraemia in patients with rheumatoid arthritis and chronic hepatitis C infection. Ann Rheum Dis 2003;62:1078–82.

[60] Parke FA, Reveille JD. Anti-tumor necrosis factor agents for rheumatoid arthritis in the setting of chronic hepatitis C infection. Arthritis Rheum 2004;51(5):800–4.

[61] Marotte H, Fontanges E, Bailly F, et al. Etanercept treatment for three months is safe in patients with rheumatological manifestations associated with hepatitis C virus. Rheumatology (Oxford) 2006 (doi:10.1093/rheumatology/kel191). Available at: http://rheumatology. oxfordjournals.org/cgi/reprintkel191v1. Accessed October 16, 2006. [Epub ahead of print.]

[62] Magliocco MA, Gottlieb AB. Etanercept therapy for patients with psoriatic arthritis and concurrent hepatitis C virus infection: report of 3 cases. J Am Acad Dermatol 2004;51:580–4.

[63] Rokhsar C, Rabhan N, Cohen SR. Etanercept monotherapy for a patient with psoriasis, psoriatic arthritis, and concomitant hepatitis C infection. J Am Acad Dermatol 2006; 54(2):361–2.

[64] Roux CH, Brocq O, Breuil V, et al. Safety of anti-TNF-α therapy in rheumatoid arthritis and spondylarthropathies with concurrent B or C chronic hepatitis. Rheumatology (Oxford) 2006;45:1294–7.

[65] Pritchard C. Etanercept and hepatitis C. J Clin Rheumatol 1999;5:179–80.

[66] Kremer JM, Alarcon GS, Lightfoot RW Jr, et al. Methotrexate for rheumatoid arthritis: suggested guidelines for monitoring liver toxicity. Arthritis Rheum 1994;37(3):316–28.

[67] Kujawska A, Clements M, Wise CM, et al. Hepatitis C and methotrexate. Arthritis Rheum 2003;49(6):843–5.

[68] Palazzi C, Olivieri I, Cacciatore P, et al. Management of hepatitis C virus-related artritis. Expert Opi Pharmacother 2005;6(1):27–34.

[69] Kayali Z, Buckwold VE, Zimmerman B, et al. Hepatitis C, cryoglobulinemia, and cirrhosis: a meta-analysis. Hepatology 2002;36(4 Pt 1):978–85.

ELSEVIER
SAUNDERS

Infect Dis Clin N Am
20 (2006) 891–912

INFECTIOUS
DISEASE CLINICS
OF NORTH AMERICA

Rheumatic Manifestations of Human Immunodeficiency Virus Infection

Francisco Medina, MD[a,b,*],
Leticia Pérez-Saleme, MD[c], José Moreno, MD[b]

[a]*Rheumatology Department, Hospital de Especialidades, Centro Médico Nacional "Siglo XXI", Instituto Mexicano del Seguro Social, 330 Cuauhtemoc Avenue, México City, DF 06720, Mexico*
[b]*Research Unit on Autoimmune Diseases, Hospital de Especialidades, Centro Médico Nacional "Siglo XXI", Instituto Mexicano del Seguro Social, 330 Cuauhtemoc Avenue, México City, DF 06720, Mexico*
[c]*Infectology Department, Hospital de Especialidades, Centro Médico Nacional "Siglo XXI", Instituto Mexicano del Seguro Social, 330 Cuauhtemoc Avenue, Mexico City, DF 06720, Mexico*

AIDS is the result of infection by HIV. This syndrome is characterized by a myriad of clinical manifestations affecting almost every organ system in the body. Untreated HIV infection follows an inexorable course, leading to profound immunosuppression and death from opportunistic infections or the development of lymphoproliferative malignancy and Kaposi's sarcoma. A quarter century into the pandemic, HIV infection is widely distributed; to date over 65 million people have been infected with HIV, and AIDS has killed more than 25 million people since it was first recognized in 1981 [1]. In 2005 AIDS claimed the lives of 2.8 million people and over 4 million people were newly infected with HIV. The number of people living with HIV worldwide has increased by 1.6 million since 2003 according to World Health Organization (WHO-OMS) estimates in 2005 [2]. Although in May 2006 UNAIDS-WHO global estimates (38.6 million) showed a downward revision, the lower estimates are partly caused by genuine declines in HIV prevalence in several countries [3].

Besides its well-known signs and symptoms, HIV infection presents sometimes with rheumatic manifestations, similar to those associated with

* Corresponding author. Rheumatology Department, Hospital de Especialidades, Centro Médico Nacional "Siglo XXI", Instituto Mexicano del Seguro Social, 330 Cuauhtemoc Avenue, México City, DF 06720, Mexico.
   E-mail address: fmedina99@gmail.com (F. Medina).

infection by human T-cell lymphotropic virus type I, the causative agent of adult T-cell leukemia [4]. Almost any rheumatic syndrome has been found associated with HIV infection. Although rheumatic manifestations can develop at any time during the clinical course of HIV infection, they tend to appear preferentially in late stages [5,6]. AIDS is the new great mimic disease.

Its worldwide distribution, and the fact that HIV infection is systemic, contributes to the common finding of rheumatic manifestations in HIV-infected patients. A variety of rheumatic disorders have been recognized in HIV-positive patients. Since the classic first known report of AIDS association with Reiter's syndrome (reactive arthritis [ReA]) in 1987, HIV infection has been linked to HLA-B27–positive seronegative spondyloarthritides and psoriatic arthritis (PsA), infectious arthritis, pyomyositis, inflammatory myopathies, undifferentiated arthralgias and arthritis without other lesions and unrelated to any known genetic marker [7], and fibromyalgia [8]. Moreover, autoimmune syndromes, such as Sjögren's syndrome, necrotizing vasculitis [9], fibromyalgia [8], and scleroderma [10], also have been associated with HIV infection.

Rheumatic clinical syndromes

Rheumatic diseases include many syndromes of different origins and pathogenic mechanisms. These range from autoimmune diseases to nonspecific inflammation, purely pain noninflammatory syndromes, and infectious rheumatic diseases. Initially, most of these syndromes have been described in AIDS patients, which makes it difficult to ascertain whether each of these disease groups are truly associated with AIDS or it is merely a casual co-occurrence and that these rheumatic complaints are detected only because of the increased awareness of any clinical symptoms during the follow-up of HIV-infected individuals. Nevertheless, some syndromes seem to be true associations and HIV infection seems to predispose to them. These are the ReA variants of the seronegative spondyloarthritides; autoimmune syndromes; and, expectedly, infectious rheumatic diseases. Lastly, there are the rheumatic complaints resulting from antiretroviral therapy and other therapeutic measures of HIV infection. It is predictable that the basis of the associations of each group, although all related to HIV infection or its treatment, differ.

Clinical manifestations

Arthritis can occur at any stage of HIV infection, but the true prevalence of arthritic syndromes and the nature of their association with HIV infection remain unclear. The pattern of HIV-associated arthritis is similar to that of other viral disorders: acute onset, short duration, no recurrences, and no erosive changes [11]. Prospective studies have shown a high prevalence of rheumatic complaints in 30% to 40% of HIV-infected patients, with arthralgias the most common rheumatic manifestation in approximately 25% to 40% of cases [12–14]. Knees, shoulders, and elbows are more frequently involved, although any joint can be affected. Transient but sometimes severe arthralgias also occur [12,13,15]. Arthralgias and myalgias are common in advanced stages of HIV infection, suggesting they are reactive in nature [12]. Jaccoud's arthropathy, a nonerosive deforming arthropathy reported to occur in cases of chronic rheumatic fever and systemic lupus erythematosus (SLE), has also been reported in HIV-infected patients [16].

Seronegative spondyloarthritides

Spondyloarthritis are frequently seen in HIV-positive patients, and initial descriptions uniformly reported seronegative spondyloarthritides including ReA, PsA, and undifferentiated spondyloarthritis as the most common rheumatic diseases associated with HIV infection. Early descriptions also reported a very low incidence of osteoarticular septic complications in HIV patients from the Western world in whom homosexual behavior was the most common risk factor [1–4,17–21]. At variance with these findings were the Spanish reports describing osteoarticular infection, including septic arthritis and pyomyositis as the most common osteoarticular manifestations associated with HIV infection [15,16,20]. This difference was attributed to geographic differences and differences in risk factors with a high prevalence of intravenous drug use [22].

The pandemic of HIV infection in Africa has resulted in an increased awareness of the different types of arthritis that can accompany HIV infection and AIDS. HIV-positive patients have an increased prevalence of ReA [17,19–21,23]. These arthritides are similar to those reported in other parts of the world, although risk factors are different in Africa where heterosexual transmission is a more common cause than homosexual transmission or intravenous drug usage. The changing epidemiology of spondyloarthritides in this region of the world has important practical and educational implications. In Zambia, the prevalence of spondyloarthritis is calculated at approximately 180 per 100,000 in HIV-positive versus 15 per 100,000 in HIV-negative individuals in the general population [24]. ReA was the most common inflammatory joint disorder in black Zambians (272 of 595 newly seen patients), and was closely linked to HIV infection but not with HLA-B27, with clinical and radiologic characteristics similar to those reported in HLA-B27–positive whites.

HLA-B27 is less common among blacks with idiopathic spondyloarthritis. In HIV-positive African AIDS patients, clinical, diagnostic, and radiographic features of seronegative spondyloarthropathies are indistinguishable from those of conventional (HLA-B27 related) disease, but with a higher overall frequency of uveitis, keratoderma, and onycholysis [25–28].

Conventional treatment of rheumatic lesions, including intra-articular steroids, seems to be safe and reasonably effective, even in AIDS patients. Anecdotal evidence suggests that treatment with methotrexate and azathioprine leads to exacerbation of HIV disease and should be avoided [29–31]. In a patient with severe HIV-associated ReA, MRI and sonographic imaging of inflamed knees had extensive polyenthesitis and adjacent osteitis. The arthritis deteriorated despite conventional antirheumatic treatment, but improved dramatically after highly active antiretroviral therapy (HAART), which was accompanied by a significant rise in CD4 T-lymphocyte counts [32].

ReA in HIV-positive patients has been widely documented. Some authors consider that CD4-positive lymphocyte subpopulation does not play a determinant role in ReA [33]. The pathogenesis of ReA seems to be linked to HLA-B27, which has been described as the major susceptibility factor for the disease [34]. The association between AIDS and ReA could be explained by the severe immunosuppression, which predisposes to the invasion by arthritogenic microorganisms. Furthermore, AIDS patients have a wide spectrum of gastrointestinal and genitourinary infections (*Shigella* sp, *Chlamydia trachomatis*, *Entamoeba histolytica*, *Giardia lamblia*, *Cryptosporidium* sp, *Isospora belli*, *Candida* sp, and cytomegalovirus). Some of these infections have been related to the pathogenesis of ReA, and are usually asymptomatic even in HIV-positive patients [20], although other studies suggest the direct or reactive role of retrovirus in the genesis of ReA [15,35,36]. Only limited data are available, however, on synovial immunopathology. Nonspecific chronic synovial inflammation and high synovial fluid cell counts are present in some patients. In other patients, the evidence of inflammatory changes is minimal. The course of ReA in HIV infection may be more severe, progressive, and refractory to treatment than in non–HIV-positive patients [37]. The presence of malar rash in these patients has been reported as the clue for early diagnosis of HIV infection [38]. In an HIV-positive patient with active Reiter's syndrome despite HAART and undetectable plasmatic viral load, acitretin without nonsteroidal anti-inflammatory drugs was effective [39].

In sub-Saharan Africa a dramatic upsurge in the prevalence of rheumatic complaints, directly related to increase of HIV infection, has been observed. These manifestations are mostly spondyloarthritides, primarily ReA and undifferentiated forms of the disease, and less often PsA. HLA-B27 is virtually absent in most of the sub-Saharan Africa populations, and ankylosing spondylitis is rare; only a few cases have been reported from central and southern Africa [40]. The prevalence of HLA-B27 in African blacks is 10 times lower than in white populations. There is also a virtual absence of ankylosing spondylitis even in the West African countries of Gambia and Senegal, where 3% to 6% of the general population is HLA-B27 positive. The clinical features of the disease are similar to those in white HLA-B27–positive patients with ankylosing spondylitis. Acute anterior uveitis and familial occurrence are rare. In Togo, spondyloarthritis was diagnosed in 31 of 2030 patients. Of these 31 patients, eight were HIV-positive patients and had no sacroiliitis [41]. The same authors reported 44 patients with spondyloarthritides; 15 had ankylosing spondylitis and 11 of these were HIV-positive [42]. The symptoms of ankylosing spondylitis in these patients were comparable with those of European patients. The results of these studies contradict the reputed scarcity of ankylosing spondylitis in black Africa [43]. The epidemiology of spondyloarthritides in sub-Saharan Africa has changed by the expanding HIV epidemic, despite the low prevalence of HLA-B27 [44]. More studies are needed to evaluate risk and protective factors for seronegative spondyloarthritis in sub-Saharan African populations and better dissect the relative importance of genetic and environmental factors in the pathogenesis of spondyloarthritis [45].

An increased prevalence of PsA has been clearly established with HIV infection, mostly in AIDS patients [13,30,46]. A variety of psoriatic manifestations may accompany HIV infection, with nail involvement present in most HIV-positive patients with inflammatory articular involvement. The articular pattern most frequently observed is polyarticular and symmetric with enthesopathy and dactylitis, but sacroiliac or spinal affection can also occur [46,47]. Of 702 new Zambian patients with inflammatory arthritis, 28 had PsA and 27 of these were HIV positive. At first consult, 16 patients (60%) were in WHO clinical stage I. PsA is almost universally associated with HIV infection in black Zambians. The clinical features are similar to those described for whites with AIDS-associated PsA [48]. The course of psoriatic arthropathy during HIV infection is variable but tends to progress together with the decrease of $CD4^+$ cell count and to be refractory to conventional treatment. In this regard, the presence of psoriasis can be considered a sign of poor prognosis in HIV infection [47,49].

Infectious rheumatic diseases

In contrast, in HIV-infected patients addicted to intravenous drugs and hemophiliacs, there was an absence of ReA, and a low frequency of symptoms of articular swelling, and a marked presence of septic arthritis. Skeletal infections were caused predominantly by *Staphylococcus aureus* (60%) and *Candida albicans* (20%), although uncommon pathogens, such as septic arthritis by *Stenotrophomonas maltophilia*, *Prototheca wickerhamii* [50], and so forth have been reported in HIV-infected patients.

The practices that lead to HIV infection (the route of entry) seem to play a more decisive role in the appearance of rheumatic manifestations in these patients than the presence of the virus itself or the immunologic alterations thereby produced [51–53]. This suggests that the relative prevalence of associated infections for the routes of entry have a major influence in the types of rheumatic manifestations associated with HIV infection and provide clues to the ethiopathogenesis of the particular syndromes even in HIV-negative individuals.

In a study of 43 cases of hemophiliacs with AIDS and septic arthritis, the spectrum of pathogen microorganisms was somewhat different than in other risk groups. The clinical picture mimics that of hemarthrosis, with high erythrocyte sedimentation rate and fever, often causing a delay in diagnosis, exclusively affecting joints with hemophilic arthropathy, with absence of peripheral leukocytosis, varying CD4$^+$ cell counts. Treatment with systemic antibiotics is often sufficient, obviating the need for arthrotomy and open drainage. Prognosis regarding joint function is relatively good, but the prognosis for the medium- to long-term survival of the patient is poor [54–57].

Soft tissue infections are rarely seen in patients with HIV infection. When present, they tend to occur in the presence of low CD4$^+$ cell counts (<200 cells/mm^3) [58]; intravascular indwelling catheters; extra-articular infection; intravenous drug users; hemophiliacs; and trauma. A wide spectrum of clinical manifestations, however, ranging from cellulitis and soft tissue abscesses to pyomyositis are seen in these patients. In general, the clinical picture, causal microorganisms, and response to therapy are similar to that of HIV-negative patients. Tropical pyomyositis is an acute bacterial infection of skeletal muscles characterized by rapid formation of abscesses. Occurrence of tropical pyomyositis is a criterion for classification of HIV-infected patients in WHO disease stage III; tropical pyomyositis in HIV-infected patients may simulate septic arthritis of the hip and knee, respectively [59]. The most common infectious agent is *S aureus* [60], although *Salmonella enteritidis* [61] has been found. Musculoskeletal manifestations caused by congenital and secondary syphilis usually subside completely after diagnosis and antibiotic therapy in HIV-positive and AIDS patients [62].

Autoimmune diseases

Infection with HIV-1 continues to provide important insights into autoimmunity and rheumatic diseases [63]. Sjögren's-like syndrome, inflammatory myopathy, and systemic vasculitis are associated with HIV infection. HIV-positive patients share a number of clinical and serologic features with SLE. Whether this is true SLE or not is controversial and discussed later. Nevertheless, for the unaware, these similarities may lead to diagnostic confusion [64].

There are few reported cases of concomitant HIV and SLE, generally in patients with long-standing HIV infection that presents with fever, arthralgias and arthritis, photosensitive rash, oral ulcers, alopecia, headache, pleuritic chest pain, and lymphadenopathy. Laboratory tests show leukopenia, thrombocytopenia, nephropathy and diverse autoantibodies against antinuclear antibodies, antiribonucleoprotein, anti-Smith, anti–ribosomal-P protein, and anticardiolipin (aCL). Review of the literature revealed less than

40 cases of concomitant SLE and HIV; in these patients, rheumatologic signs and symptoms were common and overlapped significantly with SLE. Nevertheless, regardless of whether there is an increased prevalence of SLE among HIV-positive patients, autoantibodies, such antinuclear antibodies, anti-DNAds, anti-Smith, anti–smooth muscle, anti–parietal cell, antiglomeruli, antithyroid, and anti–neutrophil cytoplasm antibodies seem to be increased in AIDS [65].

Although it has been suggested that these diseases can be mutually exclusive, distinguishing between the two of them can be difficult because of the high degree of rheumatic complaints and autoantibodies in HIV-positive patients. SLE should be considered in HIV-positive patients with rheumatologic complaints [66].

Moreover, false-positive syphilis tests and the lupus anticoagulant have been reported in 40% to 50% of HIV-positive patients in advanced stages. High-titers of aCL have been detected in a significant proportion of HIV-positive patients without any known clinical relationship. In acute infectious episodes with *Pneumocystis carinii* aCL may be present, and may become negative when the infection is cleared. The IgG aCL isotype has been found in 85% to 95% of patients with advanced HIV infection [67]. In one study, aCL were detected in 17 (50%) of 34 HIV-positive patients, and their presence was significantly associated with the detection of cerebral perfusion abnormalities by Tc 99m hexamethylpropyleneamine oxime single-photon emission CT [68]. Identification of the epitopes recognized by antiphospholipid antibodies induced by HIV-1 will offer insight into the mechanism of thrombosis associated with antiphospholipid antibodies found in the rheumatic diseases.

Muscular complications of HIV infection are classified as follows: (1) HIV-associated myopathy and related conditions including polymyositis, inclusion-body myositis, nemaline myopathy, diffuse infiltrative lymphocytosis syndrome, HIV-wasting syndrome, vasculitis, myasthenic syndromes, and chronic fatigue; (2) iatrogenic conditions including mitochondrial myopathy, HIV-associated lipodystrophy syndrome, and immune restoration syndrome; (3) tumor infiltrations of skeletal muscle; and (4) rhabdomyolysis [69].

Pathogenesis of HIV/AIDS-associated autoimmunity

In viral diseases, after an acute infection some viruses undergo a prolonged latency period in the host, whereas other agents directly produce chronic infections following the primary stage. The mechanisms whereby these infections produce arthritis are diverse and still poorly understood, but are influenced by both host and viral factors [70].

HIV-1 specifically infects CD4+ T lymphocytes, especially those expressing the chemokine receptor CCR5, which serves as a co-receptor for HIV-1. In acute HIV infections, there is a massive expansion of HIV that massively depletes CD4+ cells, particularly in extra lymphoid tissues that contain the majority of CCR5+ T cells and the majority of effector and memory T cells. As CD4+ T cells include several functional populations [71], their depletion can result in a variety of immune alterations. Clearly, depletion of the Th1-type of CD4+ cells favors infections by viruses and intracellular pathogens and predisposes to allergy, whereas depletion of Th2-type cells could increase overall T cells responses and susceptibility to parasitic infections. Whereas depletion of these cells can account for the increased susceptibility to infectious complications of AIDS, it is unlikely that it can contribute to the increased autoimmunity and autoimmune syndromes seen in AIDS.

A subset of CD4+ T cells that constitutively express CD25 and the transcription factor FoxP3 has regulatory functions of immune responses [72]. Expression of the x-chromosome-linked FoxP3 gene is actively involved in the acquisition of the immunoregulatory phenotype of these cells, and genetic defects of FoxP3 cause severe autoimmunity leading to death within the first two years of life in males affected. It has recently been shown that CD4+/CD25+ T cells (T_{REG}) express CCR5 and can be infected by HIV-1. Although the levels of T_{REG} in HIV-positive individuals with autoimmune manifestations have not been reported, it seems plausible to propose that preferential depletion of T_{REG} in some individuals could account for the increased autoimmune phenomena in some AIDS patients.

The caprine arthritis encephalitis virus Vif protein is necessary for a productive infection of susceptible goat cells. The vif gene is conserved among all primate and most nonprimate lentiviruses. Nevertheless, one study reported in vitro interactions between different Vif proteins and nucleocapsid domains of heterologous Gag precursors, supporting the notion that species specificity of lentiviral infection is not caused by molecular interactions between Vif and viral components [73]. There is some similarity in the sequences of a portion of the HIV-1 envelope glycoprotein 120 and several types of human collagen and collagen-like molecules. This observation led to the suggestion that the antibodies against the third hypervariable region (V3) of HIV-1 glycoprotein 120 (V3-specific antibodies) could play a role in the autoimmune phenomena occurring in HIV-infected patients. Such V3-reactive antibodies purified by affinity chromatography are highly specific for the V3-peptide. Moreover, there is cross-reactivity with the separate chains of the human Clq and with the chicken collagen type VI [74].

The chemokine receptor-5 mediates chemotaxis by CC chemokines and is expressed by Th1-type lymphocytes and monocyte-macrophages. In these diseases chemokine receptor-5 is expressed by most T cells and monocytes in the inflammatory infiltrates of rheumatoid arthritis (RA) and multiple sclerosis, but not on RA and multiple sclerosis peripheral blood leukocytes. Moreover, chemokine receptor-5 is the major coreceptor for M-tropic HIV-1 strains [75]. A 32-base pair deletion in chemokine receptor-5 (chemokine receptor-5δ 32 allele) abolishes receptor expression in homozygotes, whereas chemokine receptor-5δ 32 carriers express less receptor than wild-type homozygotes. This polymorphism is related to the resistance to HIV-1 infection and progression towards AIDS [76]. Polymorphisms of the chemokine receptor-2 gene (CCR2-64I) and the chemokine receptor-5 promoter (pCCR5-59029G) have also been correlated with slower progression of HIV-1 disease [77].

The mechanisms of host-virus interactions leading to rheumatic disease continue to be studied in HIV-positive patients with a host-response HIV-1 infection characterized by circulating and tissue infiltrative CD8 T-cell lymphocytosis, termed "diffuse infiltrative lymphocytosis syndrome." This syndrome primarily occurs in the salivary glands, lungs, renal interstitium, and gastrointestinal tract [78]. It differs from Sjögren's syndrome in the degree of salivary gland enlargement, high frequency of extraglandular manifestations, paucity of autoantibodies, and distinct immunogenetic associations, although anti–52-kd Ro/SSA positive has been reported [79]. Salivary gland B-cell lymphoma is a complication common to both conditions. The circulating CD8 T cells in diffuse infiltrative lymphocytosis syndrome have a memory phenotype. Dense infiltrates of $CD8^+$, potentially antiviral killer cells, are characteristically found in the salivary glands of patients who express a certain HLA genotype and who are, typically, long-term survivors of the disease [80]. Tissue cell damage seems to be a consequence of the host immune response to viral proteins present within macrophages in the target tissues. Because similar mechanisms seem to be involved in polymyositis associated with human T-cell lymphotropic virus type I infection, studies into a primate model of polymyositis induced by human T-cell lymphotropic virus type I may be particularly informative. Intracisternal A-type particles, antigenically related to HIV, have been reported in H9 cells co-cultured with homogenates of salivary glands obtained from patients with Sjögren's syndrome and with synovial fluid of patients with RA [81]. Human A-type retroviral particles reverse transcriptase activity and anti–human A-type retroviral particle autoantibodies have been detected in patients with Sjögren's syndrome. A second type of a human intracisternal A-type retrovirus, human A-type retroviral particle-II, was detected in a subset of patients with idiopathic CD4 lymphocytopenia, an AIDS-like immunodeficiency disease. Most human A-type retroviral particle-II positive patients were also antinuclear antibodies positive [82]. Anti–human A-type retroviral particles and anti-HIV p24 autoantibodies are seen in SLE, primary biliary cirrhosis, and multiple sclerosis [83].

Combined antiretroviral treatment

From its introduction in 1997, HAART has become the cornerstone of HIV therapy [84]. Lipodystrophy, hyperlipidemia, hypertriglyceridemia, insulin resistance [85], hyperglycemia, cardiovascular symptoms [86], and hypothyroidism have been described as long-term side effects of HAART. From

Table 1
Rheumatic manifestations in HIV-positive patients before (group 1) and after (group 2) the advent of highly active antiretroviral therapy

Rheumatic manifestation	Group 1 N = 173	Group 2 N = 185	P
Arthralgias	46	9	1 vs 2 < .03
Arthritis	21	1	1 vs 2 < .02
Myalgias	31	10	1 vs 2 < .02
Reactive arthritis	12	1	1 vs 2 .001
Fibromyalgia	11	12	NS
Infectious arthritis	7	4	NS
Pyomyositis	4	5	NS
Tuberculosis	1	5	2 vs 1 < .05
Osteoporosis	0/25	17/75	2 vs 1 .000
Osteonecrosis	0/50	7/96	2 vs 1 .000

Data from Medina F, Perez-Saleme L, Fuentes J, et al. Impact of highly active antiretroviral therapy on rheumatic manifestations in human immunodeficiency virus infected patients. Arthritis Rheum 2004;48:S185.

the advent of HAART, the spectrum of rheumatic manifestations in HIV infection changed. ReA, PsA, and myopathies have fallen, maybe as a result of immune restoration, and osteonecrosis, urate abnormalities, and chronic infections (tuberculosis [TB]) started to report, maybe as a result of metabolic shifts (Table 1). HAART itself, however, is associated with rheumatic complications whose pathogenesis is poorly understood. Indinavir has been associated with case reports of monoarthritis [87,88], frozen shoulder, temporomandibular dysfunction, and Dupuytren's disease [89]. New HIV treatments also may ameliorate these rheumatic conditions; the impact of changes in HIV treatment on these disorders requires further assessment [90].

Earlier studies failed to detect a higher presence of osteoporosis or excessive loss in bone mineral density in HIV-positive patients [91]. Subsequently, however, combined antiretroviral therapy, mainly HAART, has been associated with significant osteopenia and osteoporosis associated in HIV infection. Dual-energy radiographic absorptiometry was performed in 112 men. Those receiving protease inhibitor had a higher incidence of osteopenia and osteoporosis according to WHO definitions (relative risk, 2.19; 95% confidence interval, 1.13–4.23; $P = .02$) and the authors concluded that osteopenia and osteoporosis are independent side effects of HAART associated with protease inhibitor–containing regimens that seem to be independent of adipose tissue maldistribution [92]. Nonexclusive risk factors for osteopenia and osteoporosis could be drug interactions, cytokine activation, and liver dysfunction, in addition to decreased physical activity and hypogonadism [93]. Because the use of HAART is increasing, it is important to establish the meaning of these findings. Moreover, calcium and antiresorptive therapy should be considered in HIV-positive patients on this therapeutic regimen.

Osteonecrosis of the femoral head has been observed in HIV-positive patients receiving protease inhibitor–containing HAART, in the absence of classic risk factors for osteonecrosis [94,95]. Recently, it has been reported that 4% of HIV-positive patients may unknowingly have the bone disorder osteonecrosis [96], and the authors suggest that avascular osteonecrosis should be considered as a late complication of HIV infection.

As a possible explanation of these findings, osteoprotegerin ligand (OPGL, TNFS11) and its receptor RANK (TNFRS11A) are essential for the development and activation of osteoclasts and are critical regulators of physiologic bone remodeling and osteoporosis. Production of osteoprotegerin ligand by activated T cells can directly regulate osteoclastogenesis and bone remodeling. This process may explain why autoimmune diseases and chronic viral infections, such as hepatitis and HIV, result in systemic and local bone loss. Inhibition of osteoprotegerin ligand binding to RANK by the natural decoy receptor osteoprotegerin prevents bone loss in postmenopausal osteoporosis and cancer metastases and completely blocks crippling in a rat model of arthritis [97].

Hypouricemia and hyperuricemia may be considered markers of neoplasia. Urate abnormalities have been detected in HIV-positive patients, with hyperuricemia in 41% and hypouricemia in 5% of these patients, compared with none in the HIV-negative group ($P < .001$) [15]. Acute gout attacks in HIV-positive patients also have been described. Another possibility may be related to therapy, because asymptomatic hyperuricemia has been associated with ritonavir, but gout has rarely been reported. In a retrospective cohort of 1825 HIV-positive patients, 18 patients had gout, of whom 15 were on HAART. Seven of the 18 patients had lipodystrophy and dyslipidemia. Gout was seen in patients with known risk factors for gout or who were receiving ritonavir as a boosted protease inhibitor and who also had lipodystrophy [98]. Properly conducted epidemiologic studies are needed to confirm these preliminary reports. African countries are a valuable source of clinical material for comparative studies to help elucidate factors that influence the development of rheumatic diseases.

Antiphospholipid syndrome

Antiphospholipid syndrome is an autoimmune disease characterized by arterial or venous thrombosis and often by multiple fetal losses and thrombocytopenia, in association with the presence of antiphospholipid antibodies (mainly aCL and lupus anticoagulant); antiphospholipid antibodies have also been detected in patients with acute and chronic infections and malignant diseases [99]. Initially, a high prevalence of antiphospholipid antibodies with a low frequency of associated thrombosis has also been noted among patients with HIV infection, but with HAART, more secondary antiphospholipid syndrome cases have been reported [100]. Hepatitis C virus–HIV coinfected patients have a higher frequency of specific antiphospholipid syndrome–related features, such as myocardial infarction, cutaneous necrosis, renal microangiopathy, avascular bone necrosis, and optic neuropathy. Several autoimmune phenomena related to hepatitis C virus–HIV infections [101], such as the presence of antiphospholipid antibodies, thrombocytopenia, digital ischemia, or cutaneous necrosis, may mimic antiphospholipid syndrome in some patients or, because of the frequent detection of antiphospholipid antibodies in hepatitis C virus–HIV coinfected patients, a casual association with thrombotic events might lead to the fulfillment of the antiphospholipid syndrome classification criteria. Hepatitis C virus and HIV, however, might act as etiopathogenic agents for the development of a true antiphospholipid syndrome in a small subset of patients. To differentiate both etiopathogenic associations, determination of β_2-glycoprotein (GPI) antibodies in these patients might play a key role in distinguishing the pathogenic or β_2-GPI–dependent aCL (etiopathogenic association) from the nonpathogenic β_2-GPI–independent aCL (mimicry or casual association) [102].

Tuberculosis

In many countries of the world, there is now a dual epidemic of TB and HIV disease. HIV specifically eliminates the tissue macrophages and CD4 lymphocytes, the very cells that provide immunity against TB [103]. The WHO estimates that worldwide more than 4 million people are infected with TB, 95% of them living in third-world countries. TB is once again the most frequent infectious disease. Extrapulmonary forms frequently appear with HIV-associated TB. In 10% to 25% of the cases, TB manifests itself in extrapulmonary organs. Musculoskeletal manifestations occur in only about 2% of TB cases. These manifestations can vary and present as spondylitis; osteomyelitis; or monoarthritis, oligoarthritis, or polyarthritis [104].

The symptoms of TB spondylitis are unspecific, and the course is creeping, making an early diagnosis difficult [105]. Spinal TB is more common in the eastern countries than in the Western world. Pott's disease is an uncommon extrapulmonary form of TB, even among HIV-infected patients in whom extrapulmonary disease has increased [106–109]. Dissimilar data about location, diagnosis, and treatment from various hospitals and different countries are reported [110]. The classic radiologic picture of two vertebral diseases with the destruction of the intervertebral disk is easily recognized and readily treated, but its atypical forms are often misdiagnosed and mistreated [111]. Typical findings concerning either etiology or characteristic features of the classic spondylodiscitis are observed less often in HIV-positive patients than in HIV-negative patients; an increasingly common atypical form characterized by spondylitis without disk involvement also has been reported [112,113]. Spondylitis with osteolysis or bone sclerosis at single or multiple levels was also seen. Tuberculous lesion of the posterior arch may be present. In most cases CT scans showed a fragmentary vertebral destruction that was characteristic of the disease. MRI revealed the precise extent of the lesions into the spinal canal [113–115]. Intramedullary tuberculoma [116] also has been described. Poncet disease, a ReA-like form of TB infection, or tuberculous dactylitis has been increasingly reported in HIV-positive patients.

Atypical mycobacterial infection also has been increased in HIV-positive patients. Infectious arthritis and tenosynovitis caused by *Mycobacterium kansasii* has been observed, and infectious arthritis by *M kansasii* [117,118] and *Mycobacterium szulgai* [119] in this population. *Mycobacterium xenopi* may cause bone and joint infections, particularly spondylodiscitis in immunocompromised patients and more often in AIDS patients. Most of the cases reported to date have involved the thoracic or lumbar spine. Antibiotic combinations using fluoroquinolones, new macrolides, and etambuthol are usually prescribed [120].

Therapy for TB, like HAART therapy, has been associated with autoimmune and rheumatic complications. Use of rifabutin with clarithromycin may precipitate acute uveitis in patients with AIDS being treated for systemic *Mycobacterium avium* complex infection. Acute tendonitis may develop with the use of quinolones. Clarithromycin and fluconazole elevate levels of rifabutin by inhibiting metabolism through cytochrome P-450 pathway [121]. Regarding surgical treatment, adequate preoperative nutritional support and compliance with antituberculous treatment are essential to get a satisfactory outcome [122,123].

Pyogenic vertebral osteomyelitis were identified in 2 of 29 patients of a retrospective report and *S aureus* was cultured in both [124]. Pneumococcal spondylitis has been reported as the presenting manifestation of HIV infection [125]. It is important to obtain a tissue diagnosis to exclude pyogenic vertebral osteitis. *Candida* sp spondylodiscitis [126] and cryptococcal spondylitis with neurologic deficit also have been described in an HIV-positive patient. Amphotericin-B and 5-flucytosine were used with a complete neurologic recovery [127]. Because these lesions mimic spinal TB, they may be included in the differential diagnosis.

Immune reconstitution inflammatory syndrome

Immune reconstitution inflammatory syndrome has been described as a syndrome attributed to immune reconstitution occasionally observed following initiation of HAART. During the first 8 to 12 weeks following suppression of HIV replication with HAART, there is a rapid influx of memory T cells that have been trapped within inflamed lymphatic tissues and a slow recovery of naive T cells that seem to derive from both redistribution from the periphery and new thymic production [128,129]. Functional studies demonstrate that despite normalization of CD4 cell numbers, HIV-specific immunity and complete immune restoration seldom occurs. Despite this limitation, post-HAART immune reconstitution inflammatory syndrome seems capable of providing protection from opportunistic infections, although the restoration of immunity can also have adverse consequences. An inflammatory reaction following institution of HAART has been described and is believed to result from an augmented immune response to pathogens that are prevalent in the host but have been clinically occult. It has been showed by numerous reports of immune reconstitution inflammatory syndrome in response to intracellular pathogens (*Mycobacterium avium-intracellulare* [MAI] complex, *Mycobacterium tuberculosis*, *Histoplasma capsulatum*, cytomegalovirus, hepatitis B and C) [130–134]. The mean onset to immune reconstitution inflammatory syndrome appearance following HAART was up to 9 months and most resolved with little or no therapy. Although immune reconstitution inflammatory syndrome is best understood when it occurs in response to a microbial pathogen, it should not be surprising that a similar response manifesting as either the de novo appearance or exacerbation of a previously quiescent or occult neoplasia, such as Kaposi's sarcoma [135], or an autoimmune syndrome (RA [136], SLE [137,138], Reiter's syndrome [RS] [139]) may also occur. Additionally in this context, less than 50 cases have been individually described with sarcoidosis and autoimmune thyroid disease being most common with arthritis and various forms of connective tissue disease making up the rest [133].

Neoplasia

AIDS-associated malignancies are a major complication associated with AIDS patients on immunosuppression [140]. Three cancers are considered an AIDS-defining neoplasm: (1) Kaposi's sarcoma, (2) high-grade B-cell non-Hodgkin's lymphoma, and (3) invasive cervical cancer [141]. Before the introduction of HAART, non-Hodgkin's lymphoma represented one of the most prevalent causes of neoplasia in HIV-infected people [142–145]. The incidence of Kaposi's sarcoma and non-Hodgkin's lymphoma, have fallen sharply since the advent of HAART, as a result of immune restoration rather than of a specific effect on the tumoral process [146]. Recent epidemiologic studies have identified higher rates of non–AIDS-defining neoplasia: carcinoma of the anus, lung, breast, skin, conjunctiva, liver, and prostate in HIV-positive patients [147]. The role of HIV-induced immunosuppression in the development of non–AIDS-defining cancers seems less important than lifestyle habits like smoking and sun exposure, and coinfection with human papilloma, hepatitis B virus, hepatitis C virus, and Epstein-Barr virus. In the era of HAART, with HIV-infected patients living longer, there is a clear need to address this increased risk and be aware of atypical muscle, articular, and skeletal manifestations of neoplasia.

Treatment

The clinical management of HIV-associated arthritides remains difficult, likely reflecting the role of HIV-1 gene products in initiating or amplifying inflammatory joint disease. Most HIV-positive patients with mild rheumatic symptoms do well with conventional anti-inflammatory therapy, but some require the use of immunosuppressive-cytotoxic therapy. Indomethacin can directly inhibit HIV-1 replication and may be useful in combination with conventional antiviral agents [148]. Sulfasalazine has shown efficacy in patients with HIV-associated seronegative arthritis [149]. Hydroxychloroquine inhibits the posttranslational modification of glycoprotein 120 in T cells and monocytes, presumably by increasing endosomal pH and altering enzymes required for glycoprotein 120 production. Hydroxychloroquine suppressed HIV-1 replication in a dose-dependent manner. An additive effect of hydroxychloroquine with zidovudine was observed in the newly infected T and monocytic cells but not in the chronically infected cells [150]. Thalidomide was reintroduced for the treatment of a few skin diseases and recent reports of original pharmacologic properties including inhibition of angiogenesis, modulation of cytokine production (mainly reduced tumor necrosis factor production), and effects on leukocyte functions through expression of cell adhesion molecules indicate that thalidomide may be useful in autoimmune disorders, such as RA, and a treatment for complications of HIV-1 infection [151–153]. Aurothioglucose contains monovalent gold ion and inhibits the DNA-binding of nuclear factor kappa B in vitro. These observations indicate that aurothioglucose is a potentially useful drug for the treatment of HIV-positive patients and arthritic complaints [154]. Steroid and cytostatic treatment of rheumatic diseases may worsen the HIV disease [155]. Etanercept has been successfully used for the treatment of HIV-associated PsA, but the clinical course was complicated by frequent polymicrobial infections. The experience with this patient dictates that caution and careful follow-up must be exercised when prescribing anti–tumor necrosis factor therapy in the setting of HIV infection [156].

Summary

Rheumatic complaints are common in patients with HIV, and HIV positivity confers an increased susceptibility in populations with similar risk factors for HIV infection. With the advent of the modern combined antiretroviral treatment, HAART has had a profound beneficial effect on survival in HIV-infected patients, with lifelong control of HIV infection and normalization of life expectancy; but it has also contributed to both an altered frequency and a different nature of rheumatic complications now being observed in this population, with new rheumatic complications, such as osteoporosis, osteonecrosis, gout, mycobacterial, mycotic osteoarticular infections, and neoplasia perhaps more prevalent. Rheumatologists, internists, and general physicians need to be aware of these changes to provide optimal diagnosis and how to disclose the results to their patients. They also need to be familiar with the management of HIV infection and to direct careful attention to the prevention of HIV transmission in health care facilities.

References

[1] Merson MH. The HIV-AIDS pandemic at 25: the global response. N Engl J Med 2006;354: 2414–6.
[2] Epidemic Update December AIDS. 2005. UNAIDS/ WHO ISBN 92 9 173439 X. Available at: http://www.who.int/hiv/epiupdates/en/index.html. Accessed August 18, 2006.
[3] Understanding the latest estimates of the 2006 report on the global AIDS epidemic. Available at: http://www.who.int/hiv/epiupdates/en. Accessed August 18, 2006.
[4] Vassilopoulos D, Calabrese LH. Rheumatologic manifestations of HIV-1 and HTLV-1 infections. Cleve Clin J Med 1998;65:436–41.
[5] Berman A, Cahn P, Perez H, et al. Prevalence and characteristics of rheumatic manifestations in patients infected with human immunodeficiency virus undergoing antiretroviral therapy. J Rheumatol 1997;24:2492.
[6] Cuellar ML, Espinoza LR. Rheumatic manifestations of HIV-AIDS. Baillieres Best Pract Res Clin Rheumatol 2000;14:579–93.
[7] Buskila D, Gladman DD, Langevitz P, et al. Rheumatologic manifestations of infection with the human immunodeficiency virus (HIV). Clin Exp Rheumatol 1990;8:567–73.
[8] Simms RW, Zerbini CA, Ferrante N, et al. Fibromyalgia syndrome in patients infected with human immunodeficiency virus. Am J Med 1992;92:368–74.
[9] Jeandel P, Chouc PY, Laroche R. Rheumatological aspects of infection with human immunodeficiency virus. Med Trop (Mars) 1990;50:231–5.
[10] Sikdar S, Grover C, Kubba S, et al. An uncommon cause of scleroderma. Scand J Rheumatol 2005;34:242–5.
[11] Berman A, Cahn P, Perez H, et al. Human immunodeficiency virus infection associated arthritis: clinical characteristics. J Rheumatol 1999;26:1158–62.
[12] Berman A, Espinoza LR, Díaz JD, et al. Rheumatic manifestations of human immunodeficiency virus infection. Am J Med 1988;85:59–64.
[13] Buskila D, Gladman D. Musculoskeletal manifestations of infection with human immunodeficiency virus. Rev Infect Dis 1990;12:223–35.
[14] Hacbarth ET, Freire CA, Atra E. Rheumatic manifestations of acquired immunodeficiency syndrome (AIDS). Rev Assoc Med Bras 1992;38:90–4.
[15] Medina-Rodriguez F, Guzman C, Jara LJ, et al. Rheumatic manifestations in human immunodeficiency virus positive and negative individuals: a study of 2 populations with similar risk factors. J Rheumatol 1993;20:1880–4.
[16] Weeratunge CN, Roldan J, Anstead GM. Jaccoud arthropathy: a rarity in the spectrum of HIV-associated arthropathy. Am J Med Sci 2004;328:351–3.
[17] Berman A, Reboredo G, Spindler A, et al. Rheumatic manifestations in populations at risk for HIV infection: the added effect of HIV. J Rheumatol 1991;18:1564–7.
[18] Brantus JF, Meunier PJ. Rheumatic manifestations associated with human immunodeficiency virus infection. Rev Rhum Mal Osteoartic 1992;59:428–35.
[19] Calabrese LH. Rheumatic manifestations of HIV infection. Cleve Clin J Med 1993;60: 484–5.
[20] Espinoza LR, Jara LJ, Espinoza CG, et al. There is an association between human immunodeficiency virus infection and spondyloarthropathies. Rheum Dis Clin North Am 1992; 18:257–66.

[21] Rivera J, Garcia-Monforte A. Human immunodeficiency virus infection and arthritis. J Rheumatol 2000;27:1322–3.

[22] Carreño Perez L. Septic arthritis. Baillieres Best Pract Res Clin Rheumatol 1999;13:37–58.

[23] Brantus JF, Meunier PJ. Rheumatic manifestations associated with human immunodeficiency virus infection. Rev Rhum Mal Osteoartic 1992;59:428–35.

[24] Njobvu P, McGill P, Kerr H, et al. Spondyloarthropathy and human immunodeficiency virus infection in Zambia. J Rheumatol 1998;25:1553–9.

[25] Njobvu P, McGill P. Human immunodeficiency virus related reactive arthritis in Zambia. J Rheumatol 2005;32:1299–304.

[26] Adebajo A, Davis P. Rheumatic diseases in African blacks. Semin Arthritis Rheum 1994; 24:139–53.

[27] Cuellar ML, Espinoza LR. Human immunodeficiency virus associated spondyloarthropathy: lessons from the Third World. J Rheumatol 1999;26:2071–3.

[28] Chinniah K, Mody GM, Bhimma R, et al. Arthritis in association with human immunodeficiency virus infection in black African children: causal or coincidental? Rheumatology (Oxford) 2005;44:915–20.

[29] Keat A, Rowe I. Reiter's syndrome and associated arthritides. Rheum Dis Clin North Am 1991;17:25–42.

[30] Saveuse H, Rouveix E, de Bandt M, et al. HLA-B27 inflammatory spondyloarthropathy, psoriasis and HIV infection. Presse Med 1988;17:698–9.

[31] De Bandt M, Saveuse H, Rouveix E, et al. Joint manifestations and HIV infections. Ann Med Interne (Paris) 1988;139:516–22.

[32] McGonagle D, Reade S, Marzo-Ortega H, et al. Human immunodeficiency virus associated spondyloarthropathy: pathogenic insights based on imaging findings and response to highly active antiretroviral treatment. Ann Rheum Dis 2001;60:696–8.

[33] Forster SM, Seifert MH, Keat AC, et al. Inflammatory joint disease and human immunodeficiency virus infection. BMJ 1988;296:1625–7.

[34] Altman EM, Centeno LV, Mahal M, et al. AIDS-associated Reiter's syndrome. Ann Allergy 1994;72:307–16.

[35] Calabrese LH, O'Connell M, Kelley DM, et al. A longitudinal study of patients infected with the human immunodeficiency virus (HIV). The influence of rheumatic symptoms on the natural history of retroviral infections. Arthritis Rheum 1991;34:257–63.

[36] Iwakura Y, Tosu M, Yoshida E, et al. Induction of inflammatory arthropathy resembling rheumatoid arthritis in mice transgenic for HTLV-1. Science 1991;253:1026–8.

[37] Medina F, Jara LJ, Miranda JM, et al. Successful outcome in HIV+ patients with Reiter's syndrome treated with bromocriptine. Arthritis Rheum 1993;36:727–8.

[38] Buskila D, Langevitz P, Tenenbaum J, et al. Malar rash in a patient with Reiter's syndrome: a clue for the diagnosis of human immunodeficiency virus infection. J Rheumatol 1990;17: 843–5.

[39] Blanche P. Acitretin and AIDS-related Reiter's disease. Clin Exp Rheumatol 1999;17: 105–6.

[40] Lassoued S, Lassoued K, Marchou B, et al. Course of ankylosing spondylitis (AS) in patients with human immunodeficiency virus (HIV). J Rheumatol 1991;18:1939–40.

[41] Mijiyawa M. Spondyloarthropathies in patients attending the rheumatology unit of Lome Hospital. J Rheumatol 1993;20:1167–9.

[42] Mijiyawa M, Oniankitan O, Kolani B, et al. Low back pain in hospital outpatients in Lome (Togo). Joint Bone Spine 2000;67:533–8.

[43] Mijiyawa M, Grunitzky K, Agbanouvi EA, et al. Spondyloarthritis in Togolese patients. Ann Med Interne (Paris) 1991;142:582–6.

[44] Sipsas NV, Panayiotakopoulos GD, Zormpala A, et al. HIV infection and ankylosing spondylitis. Which benefits from the coexistence? Clin Rheumatol 2000;19:512.

[45] Mijiyawa M, Oniankitan O, Khan MA. Spondyloarthropathies in sub-Saharan Africa. Curr Opin Rheumatol 2000;12:281–6.

[46] Espinoza LR, Berman A, Vasey FB, et al. Psoriatic arthritis and acquired immunodeficiency syndrome. Arthritis Rheum 1988;31:1034–40.

[47] Arnett FC, Reveille JD, Duvic M. Psoriasis and psoriatic arthritis associated with human immunodeficiency virus infection. Rheum Dis Clin North Am 1991;17:59–78.

[48] Njobvu P, McGill P. Psoriatic arthritis and human immunodeficiency virus infection in Zambia. J Rheumatol 2000;27:1699–702.

[49] Schewe CK, Kellner H. Rapidly progressive seronegative spondylarthropathy with atlantodental subluxation in a patient with moderately advanced HIV infection. Clin Exp Rheumatol 1996;14:83–5.

[50] Pascual JS, Balos LL, Baer AN. Disseminated Prototheca wickerhamii infection with arthritis and tenosynovitis. J Rheumatol 2004;31:1861–5.

[51] Belzunegui J, Rodriguez-Arrondo F, Gonzalez C, et al. Musculoskeletal infections in intravenous drug addicts: report of 34 cases with analysis of microbiological aspects and pathogenic mechanisms. Clin Exp Rheumatol 2000;18:383–6.

[52] Monteagudo I, Rivera J, Lopez-Longo J, et al. AIDS and rheumatic manifestations in patients addicted to drugs: an analysis of 106 cases. J Rheumatol 1991;18:1038–41.

[53] Medina F, Hermida C, Jara LJ, et al. Staphylococcal arthritis in human immunodeficiency virus infection. Br J Rheumatol 1995;34:397–8.

[54] Barzilai A, Varon D, Martinowitz U, et al. Characteristics of septic arthritis in human immunodeficiency virus-infected haemophiliacs versus other risk groups. Rheumatology 1999;38:139–42.

[55] Tanaka S, Hachisuka K, Okazaki T, et al. Health status and satisfaction of asymptomatic HIV-positive haemophiliacs in Kyushu, Japan. Haemophilia 1999;5:56–62.

[56] Muñoz-Fernández S, Cardenal A, Balsa A, et al. Rheumatic manifestations in 556 patients with human immunodeficiency virus infection. Semin Arthritis Rheum 1991;21:30–9.

[57] Medina F, Jara LJ, Miranda JM, et al. Artritis séptica: reporte de 65 casos. Rev Mex Rheumatol 1995;10:175–9.

[58] Casado E, Olive A, Holgado S, et al. Musculoskeletal manifestations in patients positive for human immunodeficiency virus: correlation with CD4 count. J Rheumatol 2001;28:802–4.

[59] Abouzahir A, Bouchama R, Azennag M, et al. Tropical pyomyositis simulating septic arthritis in AIDS patients. Two cases. Med Trop (Mars) 2004;64:372–4.

[60] Espinoza LR, Berman A. Soft tissues and osteo-articular infections in HIV-infected patients and other immunodeficient states. Baillieres Best Pract Res Clin Rheumatol 1999;13:115–28.

[61] Medina F, Fuentes M, Jara LJ, et al. Salmonella pyomyositis in patients with the human immunodeficiency virus. Br J Rheumatol 1995;34:568–71.

[62] Reginato AJ. Syphilitic arthritis and osteitis. Rheum Dis Clin North Am 1993;19:379–98.

[63] Solomon G, Brancato L, Winchester R. An approach to the human immunodeficiency virus-positive patient with a spondyloarthropathic disease. Rheum Dis Clin North Am 1991;17:43–58.

[64] Chowdhry IA, Tan IJ, Mian N, et al. Systemic lupus erythematosus presenting with features suggestive of human immunodeficiency virus infection. J Rheumatol 2005;32:1365–8.

[65] Massabki PS, Accetturi C, Nishie IA, et al. Clinical implications of autoantibodies in HIV infection. AIDS 1997;11:1845–50.

[66] Daikh BE, Holyst MM. Lupus-specific autoantibodies in concomitant human immunodeficiency virus and systemic lupus erythematosus: case report and literature review. Semin Arthritis Rheum 2001;30:418–25.

[67] McNeil HP, Chesterman CN, Krillis SA. Immunology and clinical importance of antiphospholipids antibodies. Adv Immunol 1991;49:193–280.

[68] Rubbert A, Bock E, Schwab J, et al. Anticardiolipin antibodies in HIV infection: association with cerebral perfusion defects as detected by 99mTc-HMPAO SPECT. Clin Exp Immunol 1994;98:361–8.

[69] Authier FJ, Gherardi RK. Muscular complications of human immunodeficiency virus (HIV) infection in the era of effective anti-retroviral therapy. Rev Neurol (Paris) 2006; 162:71–81.

[70] Calabrese LH, Naides SJ. Viral arthritis. Infect Dis Clin North Am 2005;19:963–80.

[71] Reinhardt RL, Kang SJ, Liang HE, et al. T helper cell effector fates - who, how and where? Curr Opin Immunol 2006;18:271–7.

[72] Fontenot JD, Rasmussen JP, Williams LM, et al. Regulatory T cell lineage specification by the forkhead transcription factor foxp3. Immunity 2005;22:329–41.

[73] Seroude V, Audoly G, Gluschankof P, et al. Viral and cellular specificities of caprine arthritis encephalitis virus Vif protein. Virology 2002;292:156–61.

[74] Petkovic M, Metlas R. Cross–reactivity of the V3-specific antibodies with the human C1q. Z Naturforsch [C] 2001;56:1135–43.

[75] Bruhl H, Cihak J, Stangassinger M, et al. Depletion of CCR5-expressing cells with bispecific antibodies and chemokine toxins: a new strategy in the treatment of chronic inflammatory diseases and HIV. J Immunol 2001;166:2420–6.

[76] Zapico I, Coto E, Rodriguez A, et al. CCR5 (chemokine receptor-5) DNA-polymorphism influences the severity of rheumatoid arthritis. Genes Immun 2000;1:288–9.

[77] Shieh B, Liau YE, Hsieh PS, et al. Influence of nucleotide polymorphisms in the CCR2 gene and the CCR5 promoter on the expression of cell surface CCR5 and CXCR4. Int Immunol 2000;12:1311–8.

[78] Itescu S. Diffuse infiltrative lymphocytosis syndrome in children and adults infected with HIV-1: a model of rheumatic illness caused by acquired viral infection. Am J Reprod Immunol 1992;28:247–50.

[79] Hansen A, Feist E, Hiepe F, et al. Diffuse infiltrative lymphocytosis syndrome in a patient with anti-52-kd Ro/SSA and human immunodeficiency virus type 1. Arthritis Rheum 1999; 42:578–80.

[80] Weyand CM, Goronzy JJ. HIV infection and rheumatic diseases: autoimmune mechanisms in immunodeficient hosts. Z Rheumatol 1992;51:55–64.

[81] Fierabracci A, Upton CP, Hajibagheri N, et al. Lack of detection of retroviral particles (HIAP-1) in the H9 T cell line co-cultured with thyrocytes of Graves' disease. J Autoimmun 2001;16:457–62.

[82] Sander DM, Szabo S, Gallaher WR. Involvement of human intracisternal A-type retroviral particles in autoimmunity. Microsc Res Tech 2005;68:222–34.

[83] Obermayer-Straub P, Manns MP. Hepatitis C and D, retroviruses and autoimmune manifestations. J Autoimmun 2001;16:275–85.

[84] Stellbrink HJ, van Lunzen J. Lymph node during antiretroviral treatment. Curr Opin Infect Dis 2001;14:17–22.

[85] Carr A, Samaras K, Burton S, et al. A syndrome of peripheral lipodystrophy, hyperlipidemia and insulin resistance in patients receiving HIV-protease inhibitors. AIDS 1998;12:F51–8.

[86] Behrens G, Schmidt H, Meyer D, et al. Vascular complications associated with use of HIV protease inhibitors. Lancet 1998;351:1958.

[87] Brooks JI, Gallicano K, Garber G, et al. Acute monoarthritis complicating therapy with indinavir. AIDS 2000;14:2064–5.

[88] Allroggen A, Frese A, Rahmann A, et al. HIV associated arthritis: case report and review of the literature. Eur J Med Res 2005;10:305–8.

[89] Florence E, Schrooten W, Verdont K, et al. Rheumatological complication associated with the use of indinavir and other protease inhibitors. Ann Rheum Dis 2002;61:82–4.

[90] Reveille JD. The changing spectrum of rheumatic disease in human immunodeficiency virus infection. Semin Arthritis Rheum 2000;30:147–66.

[91] Paton NIJ, Macallan DC, Griffin GE, et al. Bone mineral density in patients with human immunodeficiency virus infection. Calcif Tissue Int 1997;61:30–2.

[92] Tebas P, Powderly WG, Claxton S, et al. Accelerated bone mineral loss in HIV-infected patients receiving potent antiretroviral therapy. AIDS 2000;10:F63–7.

[93] Medina F, Pérez L, Sartorius C, et al. Osteoporosis in human immunodeficiency virus in-fected patients. Arthritis Rheum 2000;43:S203.

[94] Blangy H, Loeuille D, Chary-Valckenaere I, et al. Osteonecrosis of the femoral head in HIV-1 patients: four additional cases. AIDS 2000;14:2214.

[95] Meyer D, Behrens G, Schmidt RE, et al. Osteonecrosis of the femoral head in patients re-ceiving HIV protease inhibitors. AIDS 1999;13:1147.

[96] Miller KD, Masur H, Jones EC, et al. High prevalence of osteonecrosis of the femoral head in HIV-infected adults. Ann Intern Med 2002;137:17–25.

[97] Kong YY, Penninger JM. Molecular control of bone remodeling and osteoporosis. Exp Gerontol 2000;35:947–56.

[98] Creighton S, Miller R, Edwards S, et al. Is ritonavir boosting associated with gout? Int J STD AIDS 2005;16:362–4.

[99] Khamashta MA, Hughes GRV. Antiphospholipid antibodies and antiphospholipid syn-drome. Curr Opin Rheumatol 1995;7:389–94.

[100] Asherson RA, Shoenfeld Y. Human immunodeficiency virus infection, antiphospholipid antibodies, and the antiphospholipid syndrome. J Rheumatol 2003;30:214–9.

[101] Cervera R, Asherson RA, Acevedo ML, et al. Antiphospholipid syndrome associated with infections: clinical and microbiological characteristics of 100 patients. Ann Rheum Dis 2004;63:1312–7.

[102] Ramos-Casals M, Cervera R, Lagrutta M, et al. Clinical features related to antiphospho-lipid syndrome in patients with chronic viral infections (hepatitis C virus/HIV infection): description of 82 cases. Clin Infect Dis 2004;38:1009–15.

[103] Jellis JE. Bacterial infections: bone and joint tuberculosis. Baillieres Clin Rheumatol 1995; 9:151–9.

[104] Friedmann RJ, Stevanovic L. Chronic spondylogenic pain syndrome: TB-spondylitis? Schweiz Rundsch Med Prax 1994;83:519–24.

[105] Pszolla N, Strecker W, Hartwig E, et al. Tuberculous spondylitis of the cervical spine. Un-fallchirurg 2000;103:322–5.

[106] Mallolas J, Gatell JM, Rovira M, et al. Vertebral arch tuberculosis in two human immuno-deficiency virus-seropositive heroin addicts. Arch Intern Med 1988;148:1125–7.

[107] Schinina V, Rizzi EB, Rovighi L, et al. Infectious spondylodiscitis: magnetic reso-nance imaging in HIV-infected and HIV-uninfected patients. Clin Imaging 2001;25: 362–7.

[108] Trapiella L, Caminal L, Bernaldo De Quiros JI, et al. Poncet's disease in HIV infected pa-tients. Med Clin (Barc) 2001;117:557.

[109] Leibert E, Schluger NW, Bonk S, et al. Spinal tuberculosis in patients with human immu-nodeficiency virus infection: clinical presentation, therapy and outcome. Tuber Lung Dis 1996;77:329–34.

[110] Garcia-Lechuz JM, Julve R, Alcala L, et al. Experience in a general hospital. Enferm Infecc Microbiol Clin 2002;20:5–9.

[111] Narlawar RS, Shah JR, Pimple MK, et al. Isolated tuberculosis of posterior elements of spine: magnetic resonance imaging findings in 33 patients. Spine 2002;27:275–81.

[112] Pertuiset E, Beaudreuil J, Liote F, et al. Spinal tuberculosis in adults: a study of 103 cases in a developed country,1980-1994. Medicine (Baltimore) 1999;78:309–20.

[113] Whiteman ML. Neuroimaging of central nervous system tuberculosis in HIV-infected pa-tients. Neuroimaging Clin N Am 1997;7:199–214.

[114] Cotten A, Flipo RM, Drouot MH, et al. Spinal tuberculosis: study of clinical and radiolog-ical aspects from a series of 82 cases. J Radiol 1996;77:419–26.

[115] Villoria MF, Fortea F, Moreno S, et al. MR imaging and CT of central nervous system tu-berculosis in the patient with AIDS. Radiol Clin North Am 1995;33:805–20.

[116] Borges MA, Carmo MI, Sambo MR, et al. Intramedullary tuberculoma in a patient with human immunodeficiency virus infection and disseminated multidrug-resistant tuberculo-sis: case report. Int J Infect Dis 1998;2:164–7.

[117] Casado-Burgos E, Muga-Bustamante R, Olive-Marques A, et al. Infectious arthritis by *Mycobacterium kansasii* in a patient with human immunodeficiency virus. Med Clin (Barc) 2001;116:237–8.

[118] Pintado V, Antela A, Corres J, et al. Arthritis and tenosynovitis caused by *Mycobacterium kansasii* associated with human immunodeficiency virus infection. Rev Clin Esp 1999;199: 863.

[119] Hakawi AM, Alrajhi AA. Septic arthritis due to *Mycobacterium szulgai* in a patient with human immunodeficiency virus: case report. Scand J Infect Dis 2005;37:235–7.

[120] Ollagnier E, Fresard A, Guglielminotti C, et al. Osteoarticular *Mycobacterium xenopi* infection. Presse Med 1998;27:800–3.

[121] Gioulekas J, Hall A. Uveitis associated with rifabutin therapy. Aust N Z J Ophthalmol 1995;23:319–21.

[122] Govender S, Parbhoo AH, Kumar KP, et al. Anterior spinal decompression in HIV-positive patients with tuberculosis: a prospective study. J Bone Joint Surg Br 2001;83:864–7.

[123] Govender S, Annamalai K, Kumar KP, et al. Spinal tuberculosis in HIV positive and negative patients: immunological response and clinical outcome. Int Orthop 2000;24:163–6.

[124] Leitao J, Govender S, Parbhoo AH. Pyogenic spondylitis. S Afr J Surg 1999;37:79–82.

[125] Touchard P, Chouc PY, Fulpin J, et al. HIV infection manifesting as a pneumococcal spondylodiscitis. Med Trop (Mars) 1996;56:275–8.

[126] Boix V, Tovar J, Martin-Hidalgo A. Candida spondylodiscitis: chronic illness due to heroin analgesia in an HIV positive person. J Rheumatol 1990;17:563–5.

[127] Govender S, Mutasa E, Parbhoo AH. Cryptococcal osteomyelitis of the spine. J Bone Joint Surg Br 1999;81:459–61.

[128] Autran B, Carcelain G, Li TS, et al. Positive effects of combined antiretroviral therapy on CD4+ T cell homeostasis and function in advanced HIV disease. Science 1997;277:112–6.

[129] Lange CG, Lederman MM. Immune reconstitution with antiretroviral therapies in chronic HIV-1 infection. J Antimicrob Chemother 2003;51:1–4.

[130] DeSimone JA, Pomerantz RJ, Babinchak TJ. Inflammatory reactions in HIV-1-infected persons after initiation of highly active antiretroviral therapy. Ann Intern Med 2000;133: 447–54.

[131] Shelburne SA III, Hamill RJ, Rodriguez-Barradas MC, et al. Immune reconstitution inflammatory syndrome: emergence of a unique syndrome during highly active antiretroviral therapy. Medicine 2002;81:213–27.

[132] French MA, Price P, Stone SF. Immune restoration disease after antiretroviral therapy. AIDS 2004;18:1615–27.

[133] Calabrese LH, Kirchner E, Shrestha R. Rheumatic complications of human immunodeficiency virus infection in the era of highly active antiretroviral therapy: emergence of a new syndrome of immune reconstitution and changing patterns of disease. Semin Arthritis Rheum 2005;35:166–74.

[134] Breton G, Adle-Biassette H, Therby A, et al. Immune reconstitution inflammatory syndrome in HIV-infected patients with disseminated histoplasmosis. AIDS 2006;20:119–21.

[135] Leidner RS, Aboulafia DM. Recrudescent Kaposi's sarcoma after initiation of HAART: a manifestation of immune reconstitution syndrome. AIDS Patient Care STDS 2005;19: 635–44.

[136] Wegrzyn J, Livrozet JM, Touraine JL, et al. Rheumatoid arthritis after 9 years of human immunodeficiency virus infection: possible contribution of tritherapy. J Rheumatol 2002; 29:2232–4.

[137] Diri E, Lipsky PE, Berggren RE. Emergence of systemic lupus erythematosus after initiation of highly active antiretroviral therapy for human immunodeficiency virus infection. J Rheumatol 2000;27:2711–4.

[138] Calza L, Manfredi R, Colangeli V, et al. Systemic and discoid lupus erythematosus in HIV-infected patients treated with highly active antiretroviral therapy. Int J STD AIDS 2003;14: 356–9.

[139] Neumann S, Kreth F, Schubert S, et al. Reiter's syndrome as a manifestation of an immune reconstitution syndrome in an HIV-infected patient: successful treatment with doxycycline. Clin Infect Dis 2003;36:1628–9.

[140] Wood C, Harrington W Jr. AIDS and associated malignancies. Cell Res 2005;15:947–52.

[141] Bower M, Palmieri C, Dhillon T. AIDS-related malignancies: changing epidemiology and the impact of highly active antiretroviral therapy. Curr Opin Infect Dis 2006;19:14–9.

[142] Biviji AA, Paiement GD, Steinbach LS. Musculoskeletal manifestations of human immunodeficiency virus infection. J Am Acad Orthop Surg 2002;10:312–20.

[143] Peeva E, Davidson A, Keiser HD. Synovial non-Hodgkin's lymphoma in a human immunodeficiency virus infected patient. J Rheumatol 1999;26:696–8.

[144] Nyagol J, Leucci E, Onnis A, et al. The effects of HIV-1 Tat protein on cell cycle during cervical carcinogenesis. Cancer Biol Ther 2006;5:684–90.

[145] Grulich AE, Vajdic CM. The epidemiology of non-Hodgkin lymphoma. Pathology 2005; 37:409–19.

[146] Grabar S, Abraham B, Mahamat A, et al. Differential impact of combination antiretroviral therapy in preventing Kaposi's sarcoma with and without visceral involvement. J Clin Oncol 2006;24:3408–14.

[147] Pantanowitz L, Schlecht HP, Dezube BJ. The growing problem of non-AIDS-defining malignancies in HIV. Curr Opin Oncol 2006;18:469–78.

[148] Itescu S. Rheumatic aspects of acquired immunodeficiency syndrome. Curr Opin Rheumatol 1996;8:346–53.

[149] Adebajo AO, Mijiyawa M. The role of sulphasalazine in African patients with HIV-associated seronegative arthritis. Clin Exp Rheumatol 1998;16:629.

[150] Chiang G, Sassaroli M, Louie M, et al. Inhibition of HIV-1 replication by hydroxychloroquine: mechanism of action and comparison with zidovudine. Clin Ther 1996;18:1080–92.

[151] Combe B. Thalidomide: new indications? J Bone Spine 2001;68:582–7.

[152] Neiger BL. The re-emergence of thalidomide: results of a scientific conference. Teratology 2000;62:432–5.

[153] Settles B, Stevenson A, Wilson K, et al. Down-regulation of cell adhesion molecules LFA-1 and ICAM-1 after in vitro treatment with the anti-TNF-alpha agent thalidomide. Cell Mol Biol 2001;47:1105–14.

[154] Traber KE, Okamoto H, Kurono C, et al. Anti-rheumatic compound aurothioglucose inhibits tumor necrosis factor-alpha-induced HIV-1 replication in latently infected OM10.1 and Ach2 cells. Int Immunol 1999;11:143–50.

[155] Melaku Z, Haga HJ. Rheumatological manifestations in HIV infections. Tidsskr Nor Laegeforen 2000;120:1326–8.

[156] Aboulafia DM, Bundow D, Wilske K, et al. Etanercept for the treatment of human immunodeficiency virus-associated psoriatic arthritis. Mayo Clin Proc 2000;75:1093–8.

INFECTIOUS
DISEASE CLINICS
OF NORTH AMERICA

ELSEVIER
SAUNDERS

Infect Dis Clin N Am
20 (2006) 913–929

Role of Endogenous Retroviruses in Autoimmune Diseases

Ines Colmegna, MD[a], Robert F. Garry, PhD[b],*

[a]Section of Rheumatology, Department of Medicine, Louisiana State University Health
Sciences Center, 2020 Gravier Street, New Orleans, LA 70112, USA
[b]Department of Microbiology and Immunology, Tulane University Health Sciences Center,
1430 Tulane Avenue, New Orleans, LA 70112, USA

Definition and characteristics of human endogenous retroviruses

The human genome sequencing project and similar initiatives for other species have revealed that a large portion of vertebrate genomic DNA consists of genetic elements that are present in multiple copies. These repetitive elements can be subdivided into those that are interspersed (transposons and other mobile elements, processed pseudogenes) or tandemly arrayed (satellites and telomeres) in the genome. Human endogenous retroviruses (HERVs) represent a class of interspersed mobile repetitive elements known as retrotransposons. HERVs are closely related to certain members of the Retroviridae, an important family of human and animal viruses that includes HIV and human T-lymphotropic virus (HTLV), causes of the AIDS and adult T-cell leukemia, respectively. Before the pandemic emergence of HIV, the study of this virus family lead to the discovery of oncogenes, a quantum advance in the field of cancer genetics. In contrast to exogenous retroviruses, which are transmitted horizontally as infectious particles in a manner similar to other viruses, HERVs typically do not form infectious particles, but rather are transmitted vertically by Mendelian mechanisms (Table 1). Recent studies have implicated HERVs in a wide variety of processes, both pathologic (ie, autoimmune diseases and cancer) and physiologic (ie, placental function and morphogenesis [1], and protection from exogenous retroviral infection [2,3]). This article discusses studies that implicate HERVs in many human autoimmune diseases.

* Corresponding author.
E-mail address: rfgarry@tulane.edu (R.F. Garry).

Table 1
Differential characteristics of exogenous and endogenous retroviruses

Type	Transmission	Examples	Disease associations	Physiologic functions
Exogenous	Infectious particles	HIV-I	Immunodeficiency	—
		HTLV-I	T-cell leukemia/ lymphoma	—
		HTLV-II	Myelopathy/tropical spastic paraparesis	—
Endogenous	Generally noninfectious germline inheritance (Mendelian)	HERV-W	Multiple sclerosis, schizophrenia	Syncytiotrophoblast formation
		HERV-K10 (HML-2)	Testicular cancer, seminomas	—
		HERV-K18	JRA, type I diabetes	Immune tolerance
		HERV-K113	SS, MS	—

Abbreviations: JRA, juvenile rheumatoid arthritis; MS, multiple sclerosis; SS, Sjögren syndrome.

Evolution of human endogenous retroviruses

The biology of HERVs is best examined in the context of their origins as remnants of past retroviral infections. The defining feature of retroviruses is the requirement for a reverse transcriptase (RT) step in the replication cycle. Retroviral RT creates a double-stranded DNA intermediate (provirus) from the virion-associated single-stranded RNA, thereby reversing the typical flow of genetic information (ie, from DNA to mRNA). During the RT step repeated sequences at the ends of the retroviral RNA are combined with unique 3' and 5' sequences to create the proviral long terminal repeats (LTR). Integration of the proviral DNA into host chromosomal DNA, catalyzed by the retroviral integrase (IN), is a required step in the replication cycle of most infectious retroviruses. After integration, binding of cellular transcription factors to the LTR can drive transcription of proviral and cellular genes. The rare infection of germline cells by a retrovirus would be expected to establish proviruses in stable chromosomal locations thereby creating an HERV. Further copying by way of RT, then integrating in different locations within the genome, produces a "family" of related HERVs.

HERVs can serve as models for other retrotransposons that replicate in the genome by making a DNA copy from an mRNA by way of RT, then pasting copies back into the genome in multiple places using IN (in word processing: command c, then command v). Other retroelements include the human long and short interspersed nuclear elements (LINEs, SINEs). HERVs are distinguished from LINEs and SINEs by the presence of their LTRs (Fig. 1). Replication of HERVs and other retrotransposons increases

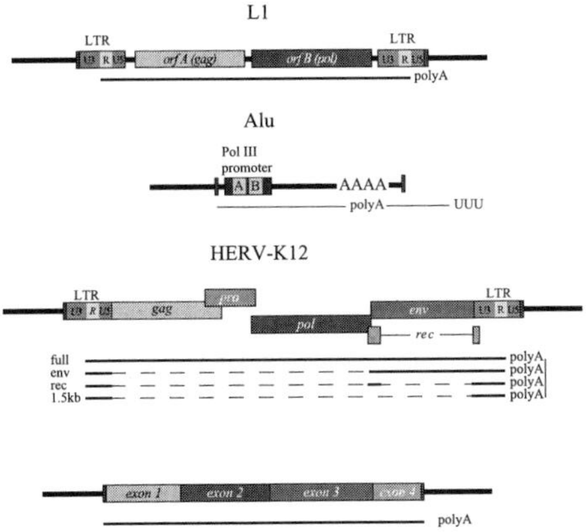

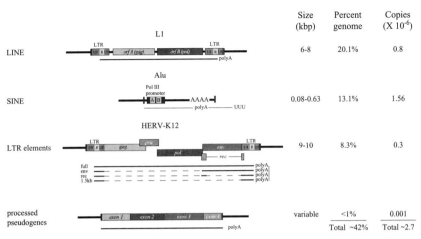

	Size (kbp)	Percent genome	Copies (X 10^{-6})
LINE	6-8	20.1%	0.8
SINE	0.08-0.63	13.1%	1.56
LTR elements	9-10	8.3%	0.3
processed pseudogenes	variable	<1%	0.001
		Total ~42%	Total ~2.7

Fig. 1. Diagrams of the major classes of retrotransposable elements and their transcripts. L1, a LINE, is a non-LTR retrotransposon that uses an RNA polymerase II promoter. Transcription of L1 produces a full-length RNA encoding two proteins. ORF1 encodes an RNA-binding protein. ORF2 encodes endonuclease and RT. Alu elements are SINEs that use an RNA polymerase III promoter (A and B boxes) and generally use LINE enzymes for transposition. Some members of the HERV-K family have intact *gag*, *pol*, and *env* genes (see text). In addition, HERV-K may encode Rec, which is functionally homologous to the Rev protein encoded by HIV. LINEs also may insert copies of cell mRNA (lacking introns) at low efficiency to form pseudogenes.

genome size, and by inserting near or within genes they can either disrupt or increase transcription of genes. In contrast to retroelements, another abundant class of repetitive sequences DNA transposons cut and paste (command x, then command v) using a transposase.

Human endogenous retrovirus structure

HERVs contain all or a subset of the three genes universally present in the genomes of replication-competent retroviruses. The *gag* (group antigen) gene encodes proteins that in exogenous retroviruses comprise the nucleocapsid of the virus (major capsid protein, CA) and a matrix layer (matrix, MA). The *gag* gene is named because antibodies produced against the Gag proteins cross-react with Gag proteins of retroviruses of the same group (species), but not others. The *pol* gene encodes several enzymes associated with the retrovirus core, including protease (PR), RT, and IN. Exogenous retroviruses are enveloped; virions contain lipid and products of the *env* gene designated surface (SU) and transmembrane (TM) glycoproteins. Most HERVs contain partial deletions or mutations that disrupt the reading frames of the genes for each structural protein. HERVs also may have deletions in one or both LTRs. The human genome does contain HERVs, however, such as members of the HERV K family, with long open reading frames encoding functional proteins (see Fig. 1). Notably, the W family of HERVs expresses a functional Env, called syncytin, which functions as a fusogen during syncytiotrophoblast formation of the placenta [4]. Newly discovered HERV 113 also seems capable of synthesizing *gag*, *pol*, and *env* protein products [5]. Certain HERVs (for example: HERV-K family members) contain accessory genes analogous to those of complex retroviruses, such as HTLV or HIV, that regulate genome expression or replication (see Fig. 1).

Human endogenous retrovirus classification, distribution, and diversity

The human genome contains abundant numbers of incomplete and complete HERV copies that collectively make up approximately 8.3% of the human genome (see Fig. 1). Currently recognized HERVs have been classified into more than 40 different families or lineages, according to sequence similarities. Classification of HERVS follows that of exogenous retrovirus classification, a scheme based on comparisons of the size of the genome and morphologic characteristics (Table 2). Class I contains HERVs related to gamma retroviruses, class II HERVs are related to beta retroviruses, and class III HERVs are related to spumaviruses. HERV families have been tentatively named according to the tRNA that is used to prime RT (Table 3).

Table 2
Viruses of the family *Retroviridae*

Subfamily	Distinguishing feature	Example	Related HERV
Alpharetroviridae	Genome <8 kb; assembly at cell membrane; C-type	Avian leukosis virus	None
Betaretroviridae	Intracytoplasmic assembly (B- or D-type)	Mouse mammary tumor virus	Class II
Deltaretroviridae	Genome <9 kb; C-type	Bovine leukemia virus	None
Gammaretroviridae	Genome >8 kb; assembly at cell membrane; C-type	Murine leukemia virus	Class I
Epsilonretrovidae	Assembly at cell membrane;	Walleye dermal sarcoma virus	None
Lentiviridae	Genome >9 kb; bar-shaped and concentric core	Human immunodeficiency virus	None
Spumaviridae	Assembly as intracytoplasmic particles	Chimpanzee foamy spumavirus	Class III

Table 3
Classification of human endogenous retroviruses

Class	Examples	Disease associations
I (gamma; C-type)	HERV-H[a]	
	HERV-F[a]	
	HERV-W[a]	MS, schizophrenia psoriasis
	HERV-R/erv9 (ERV9)	
	HERV-P (HuERS-P, HuRRS-P)	
	HERV-E (4-1, ERVA, NP-2)	SLE
	HERV-R/erv 3 (HERV3)[a]	
	RRHERV-I (HERV 15)	
	HERV T (S71, CRTK1, CRTK6)[a]	
	HERV-I (RTVL-I)	
	HERV-IP-T47D (ERV-FTD)	
	HERV-FRD[a]	
II (beta; A, B, and D)	HERV-K (HML-1.1)	
	HERV-K10 (HML-2)[a]	Testicular cancer
	HERV-K18[a]	JRA, type I diabetes
	HERV-K-T47D (HML-4)	
	HERV-K-NMWV2 (HML-5)	
	HERV K (HML-6p)	
	HERV-K-NMWV7 (HML-7)	
	HERV-K-NMWV3 (HML-8)	
	HERV-K-NMWV9 (HML-9)	
	HERV-KC4 (HML-10)	
	HERV-K113[a]	SS, MS
	HERV K115[a]	
III (spuma)	HERV-L	
	HERV-S (HERV18)	
	HERV-U	
	HERV-U3	

Abbreviations: JRA, juvenile rheumatoid arthritis; MS, multiple sclerosis; SLE, systemic lupus erythematosus; SS, Sjögren syndrome.
[a] coding env genes.

Human endogenous retroviruses and autoimmunity

Both exogenous and endogenous retroviruses display a marked variety of interactions with their host and, in a susceptible individual, may be inciting, contributory, or perpetuating factors in the pathogenesis of autoimmune conditions [6]. Studies looking at the role of HERVs have been conducted in most organ-specific and systemic autoimmune conditions, including rheumatoid arthritis (RA), juvenile rheumatoid arthritis (JRA), psoriasis, systemic lupus erythematosus (SLE), systemic sclerosis, Sjögren syndrome (SS), multiple sclerosis (MS), alopecia areata, type I diabetes, primary biliary cirrhosis, essential thrombocythemia (ET), and Graves disease. Although disease associations have been established, there is as yet no proven definite causative association between HERVs and disease [7]. Evidence for a relationship between HERVs and autoimmune diseases is suggested by the finding of circulating antibodies reactive with endogenous retroviral proteins and endogenous retroviral gene expression (mRNA transcripts and proteins) in autoimmune diseases, and the evidence that human endogenous retroviruses can encode superantigenic activity [8].

The proposed mechanisms by which expression of defective retroviruses might lead to the dysregulation of the immune response include:

- *Transcriptional activation.* HERVs may act as insertional mutagens or *cis*-regulatory elements causing activation, inhibition, or alternative splicing of cellular genes involved in immune function. A-type retroviruses, for example, can function as transpositional elements, and sequences in their transcriptional control region (LTR) can activate cellular genes, including those of cytokines or oncogenes. HERVs also may encode elements like *tat* in HIV-1 or *tax* in HTLV-1, both of which are capable of transactivating cellular genes. Alternatively, an HERV-encoded protein also may act in *trans* to regulate gene expression.
- *Superantigen (SAg) motifs that bypass the normal MHC restrictive process of T-cell stimulation.* SAg are microbial proteins that sequentially bind to MHC class II proteins and the Vβ chain of the T-cell receptor and thereby strongly stimulate and expand T cells. EBV and perhaps other DNA viruses can induce endogenous SAg genes encoded by HERV [9]. EBV SAg expression is regulated by type I interferons [10,11]. Recently it has been shown that negative thymic selection to HERV-K18 SAg constitutes a first checkpoint controlling peripheral tolerance compared with SAg reactivity [12].
- *Production of neo-antigens by modification of cellular components.* Virally encoded components may associate physically with or otherwise modify cellular proteins or structures, thereby rendering them autoantigenic.
- *Molecular mimicry.* Expression of retroviral antigens that cross-react with major histocompatibility complex (MHC) components could disrupt the idiotypic network that regulates the immune system resulting in autoimmunity. Several retroviral proteins share amino acid sequence similarities with cellular proteins, which could explain the humoral immunity reported in autoimmune disease elicited by cross-reactivity with HERV proteins. The 70K protein of U1snRNP was the first lupus autoantigen shown to contain a region of homology and immunologic cross-reactivity with a conserved p30 Gag protein of most mammalian-type C retroviruses. Query and Keene [13] showed that: (1) anti-p30Gag antibodies recognize a recombinant 70K-LacZ fusion protein and U1 snRNPs, and (2) autoantibodies against U1 snRNPs were elicited by immunization with p30Gag. They proposed, therefore, that autoimmunity to U1RNP may be triggered by expression of an endogenous retroviral Gag protein. Anti-Gag antibodies elicited by the HERVs could cross-react with the 70K protein and, subsequently, recognition could expand to additional 70K epitopes [13].

- *Epitope spreading.* T-cell recognition of a self epitope is followed by activation of autoreactive T cells recognizing other epitopes of the same antigen, and, with time, epitopes of other proteins [14].
- *Activation of innate immunity through pattern recognition receptors.* HERV-W Env is able to specifically activate cells of the innate immune system through CD14 and TLR4. This activation is associated with the production of major proinflammatory cytokines [15].

Human endogenous retroviruses and systemic lupus erythematosus

A role of retroviruses in SLE pathogenesis is supported by an increasing body of evidence. A possible retroviral link with SLE was suspected initially because of the similarity of autoimmune manifestations and immune dysregulation between patients who have SLE and those infected with known human retroviruses, such as HIV-1. It has been shown that one third of patients who have SLE produce high-titer antibodies to various retroviral proteins, including Gag, Env, and Nef, and the p24 capsid antigen of HIV-1 and HTLV, in the absence of overt retroviral infection [16–18]. This phenomenon was attributed to molecular mimicry between retroviral antigens and host proteins. Actually, patients who have SLE also produce antibodies to HERV proteins and the striking amino acid similarities between certain Gag proteins and human autoantigens, such as a component of U1 sn-ribonucleoprotein (70K protein), topoisomerase I, and SS-B/La, have suggested that the natural targets of some antibodies in SLE may be HERV proteins. Detection of antibodies reactive with peptides present in the envelope genes of HERV-H [19], HTLV-related endogenous sequence (HRES) [20], ERV-1, human intracisternal A-type retroviral particles (HIAP) [21], ERV3, and HERV-K also have been described in patients who have SLE. Particularly in the case of HRES, there is amino acid sequence homology between HRES-1 and the *gag*-related region of the 70 kDa U1sn-RNP protein [22], and this has been proposed as one of the critical events in the etiopathogenesis of SLE [23]. Interestingly, the presence of anti-HRES-1 antibodies, which was documented in 50% of patients who had SLE by Western blot analysis, has been linked to clinically active disease [20]. A strong linkage between HIAP and SLE has been established. In various reports, 60% to 95% of patients who have SLE react with HIAP preparations. Interestingly, patients who have discoid or cutaneous forms of lupus display reduced seroreactivity with HIAP proteins [21].

Animal models also support a role of HERV in SLE pathogenesis. The expression of 8.4-kb MCF endogenous retroviral transcripts is a primary feature of murine lupus [24]. In the MRL/lpr mouse model for SLE, the integration of HRES-1 into the murine *fas* apoptosis-promoting gene results in a lowered expression of Fas protein and a consequent failure of apoptosis in autoreactive lymphocytes [25]. It seems that defective activation-induced cell death in peripheral autoreactive lymphocytes is the primary mechanism by which these mice develop systemic autoimmunity. Furthermore, the insertion of a retrotransposon into the second intron of the *fas* gene of MRL-lpr/lpr mice, leads to reduced apoptosis, survival of autoreactive lymphocytes, and earlier mortality [26].

HERV clone 4-1, a member of the HERV-E family, is distributed widely in the DNA of Japanese individuals. Studies from Juntendo University reported that HERV clone 4-1 sequences show increased transcription and translation in patients who have SLE compared with normal controls and that the increased transcription of HERV clone 4-1 in patients who have SLE is partially regulated by epigenetic mechanisms. The presence of the *gag* region antigen and messenger RNA for the clone 4-1 *gag* region also was described in peripheral blood mononuclear cells (PBMCs) from patients who had SLE, but not in normal controls [27]. Finally, serum antibodies to recombinant clone 4-1 *gag* products were detected in approximately 50% of patients who had SLE [28]. Synthetic peptides derived from HERV clone 4-1 can induce immune abnormalities observed in patients who have SLE: T-cell activation, cytokine production (increase IL-16 and IL-6 production and inhibit mitogen-mediated IL-2 production), and polyclonal B cell activation [29,30].

Although no correlation with disease activity has been proved yet, treatment with steroids reduced the amount of clone 4-1–like mRNA in patients who had SLE [31]. Furthermore, a possible correlation between plasma concentrations of anti-U1 RNP and anti-Sm antibodies and the presence of HERV-E clone 4-1 gGag mRNA in PBMC of patients who have SLE and a correlation between the level of PBMC HERV-E clone 4-1 Gag transcript and blood plasma content of antiSm antibody have been suggested. Because the U1 70-kDa protein and Sm polypeptide antigens are located on the same molecule of the spliceosome complex, the correlations described may suggest a cross-reactivity between an unknown viral antigen and anti-Sm antibody [32].

The use of a demethylating agent (5-aza-deoxycytidine) causes a quantitative increase of the clone 4-1 mRNA [33] and decreases the mRNA for DNA methyltransferase-1 (DNMT-1; methylation-regulating enzyme) in PBMCs from normal individuals. Transcription of DNMT-1 mRNA in PBMC from patients who have SLE is lower than in cells from normal controls [34]. The transcription of endogenous autoantigens, such as HERV, seems to be promoted by DNA hypomethylation, which is implied by low DNMT activity. Interestingly, estrogens may increase the expression of HERVs by reducing DNA methylation through the inhibition of DNMT activity [29].

Finally, in primary epidermal keratinocytes and in the skin of patients who have SLE, UBV radiation has been shown to activate the transcription of various endogenous retroviral *pol* sequences closely related to *pol* sequences of human endogenous retroviruses [35].

Human endogenous retroviruses and multiple sclerosis

Several HERVs (-W, -K, -H) and multiple pathogenic mechanisms have been described in association with MS [14]. Studies on RNA associated with viral particles in leptomeningeal, choroids plexus or B-lymphocyte cultures from patients who have multiple sclerosis have found sequences corresponding to overlapping regions of a retroviral genome that was named MSRV (multiple sclerosis–associated retrovirus virions) [36]. MSRV has genetically high homologous counterparts in normal human DNA, the HERV-W family [37]. Independent studies have confirmed an association of MSRV virion RNA with the temporal and clinical progression of MS [38], and differential MSRV/HERV-W RNA levels between MS and controls were reported in lymphoid cells [39].

Subsequent studies showed that the Env protein of HERV-K18 has superantigen activity in vitro strongly activating T cells and that this SAg activity could be reproduced with the use of a recombinant MSRV Env protein [40].

HERV-W Gag and Env proteins are induced by human herpes simplex (HSV)-1 [41,42] in neuronal and endothelial cells in vitro. The transactivation of HERV-W proteins by HSV-1 could enhance their potential oligodendrotoxic and immunopathogenic effects [42]. Epstein-Barr virus (EBV) infection of B cells also leads to transactivation of HERV-K18 *env* alleles that express a TCRVβ13-specific SAg activity previously identified as an EBV-associated superantigen [9].

To test the pathogenicity of MSRV retroviral particles in vivo, severe combined immunodeficiency (SCID) mice grafted with human lymphocytes were injected intraperitoneally with MSRV virion. These mice developed acute neurologic symptoms and died within 5 to 10 days post injection. By RT-PCR circulating MSRV RNA was detected in serum and overexpression of proinflammatory cytokines in spleen. Necropsy revealed disseminated and major brain hemorrhages that occurred before death in multifocal areas of brain parenchyma and meninges. Interestingly, when MSRV virion was inoculated to SCID mice grafted with T lymphocyte–depleted cells a dramatic reduction in the number of affected mice was observed [43]. A different group confirmed that HERV-W Env (syncytin) is upregulated in glial cells within acute demyelinating lesions of patients who had multiple sclerosis and that conditioned medium of human fetal astrocytes in which an HERV-W Env construct was expressed is cytotoxic to human and rat oligodendrocytes. Even more, syncytin-mediated neuroinflammation and death of oligodendrocytes were prevented by the antioxidant ferulic acid in a mouse model of multiple sclerosis [44].

Another recent study showed that there is a physiologic expression of an HERV-W Env in human brain that mainly is associated with infiltrating lymphoid cells or brain macrophages, whereas expression of HERV-W Gag antigens is observed in neurons (cell body, axons, dendrites). In contrast to this, an MS-specific Gag and Env pattern was described in which these antigens were detected essentially at the level of endothelial and microglial cells. Within demyelinated lesions Gag antigen accumulated in dystrophic axons [45]. Moreover, HERV-W Env can activate the innate immune system through a TLR4/CD14-dependent pathway; therefore it can induce human monocytes to produce major proinflammatory cytokines in a CD14- and TLR4-dependent fashion, induce DC maturation, and confer the capacity to support a Th1-type of T-cell differentiation [15].

In vitro, proinflammatory cytokines that are detrimental in MS, TNF-α, and IFN-γ have been shown to stimulate the release of MSRV by PBMCs, whereas IFN-β blocked virus release [46]. Conversely, the surface unit of MSRV envelope protein also was shown to mediate an increase of IL-6 and IL-12p40 production by the PBMC from patients who have MS and to promote the development of naïve CD4$^+$ CD45RA T cells into IFN-γ– secreting Th1-like cells. The cytokine release correlates with disease severity [47], and it has been proposed that IL-6, which in particular is produced in a TLR4-dependent manner [15], renders naïve CD4$^+$ T cells insensitive to the suppressive activity of CD4$^+$ CD25 T reg, and therefore facilitates the priming of autoreactive T cells [48]. Taken together these data suggest a loop involving inflammation that increases MSRV, which in turn and because of their gliotoxic and superantigenic properties expands the original mechanism. The demonstration of HERV-H virions in the blood of patients who have MS and increased levels of HERV-H and HERV-K RNA levels in brain tissue and a humoral response with elevated levels of antibodies toward HERV-W in serum and HERV-H in CSF is further evidence of a role for HERV in MS [49]. Antibodies with reactivity to HERV are produced locally in MS CSF and reactivity is mainly toward gammaretroviral HERV or similar epitopes [14].

Studies comparing the proliferation of PBMCs after stimulation with MS virions or HERV-H peptides alone or in combination with HERV antigens revealed a synergistic effect on the proliferative response when both antigens were combined [14,50].

Human endogenous retroviruses and diabetes

Several lines of evidence suggest the involvement of HERV-K in the cause of type I DM. HERV-K18 locus seems to be unique among the endogenous retrovirus HERV-K family because of its transcriptional induction by proinflammatory stimuli and its constitutive expression in the thymus [51]. HERV-K18 encodes T-cell SAg, and T cells with HERV-K18 Sag-reactive T-cell receptor Vβ7 chains were found to be enriched in the pancreas, in the spleen, and in circulation at DM onset [51,52]. HERV-K18 mRNA expression also was enhanced in inflammatory lesions of patients who had recent-onset type 1 DM. HERV-K18 transcription and SAg function in cells capable of efficient presentation are induced by proinflammatory stimuli, namely viruses [9] and interferon-α [10].

Human endogenous retroviruses and other autoimmune conditions

Alopecia areata

In this autoimmune condition characterized by an aberrant T-cell response against hair follicle self-antigens, serum antibodies reacting with human intracisternal A-type retrovirus proteins have been found [53].

Rheumatoid arthritis

Evidence implicating retroviruses in rheumatoid arthritis can be drawn from the parallels between human and animal retroviral infections. Animal retroviral pathogens, such as caprine arthritis encephalitis virus and maedi visna virus, cause chronic arthritis in sheep and goats with similarities to human RA. An association of HRV-5 and RA has been claimed based on the detection by nested PCR of proviral DNA in approximately 50% of synovial samples from patients who have RA (12/25) [54]. A recent study evaluated by real time PCR synovial tissue from 75 patients who had RA, the same number of patients who had osteoarthritis (OA), and 50 controls. All tissue specimens tested negative for HRV-5 proviral DNA. The authors emphasize the importance of using strict and reproducible methods for the study of HERV [55]. An elevated multi-epitope–specific antibody response toward HERV-K proteins also has been documented in patients who have RA [56].

Increased levels of HERV-K10 expression were shown in PBMCs from patients who had RA compared with those from OA and healthy controls [57]. Another study evaluated the synovial expression of HERV-K (HML-2) by reverse transcription PCR and immunofluorescence in RA, OA, and healthy controls. HERV-K *env* gene-derived mRNA and the Rec protein were found to be expressed in normal and rheumatoid synovial cells with differences in the transcription levels of certain transcripts (apparent lower expression levels in arthritic synovia) [58].

Juvenile rheumatoid arthritis

The expression levels of HERV-K18 by semiquantitative reverse transcription PCR were evaluated in JRA. HERV-18 superantigen transcripts were found to be elevated in the peripheral blood and in the synovial fluid mononuclear cells in JRA, and its expression was strongly induced by IFN-α. The levels of HERV-K18 in peripheral blood were independent of serum IFN-α levels, seropositivity for EBV, or the percentage of circulating B cells [59]. A concern about this report is the small sample size and the use of semi-quantitative reverse transcription PCR.

Sjögren syndrome

The fact that Sjögren-like syndromes occur in a proportion of HIV and HTLV-1 infections lead to the search for other retroviruses in idiopathic disease. In fact, 33% of the sera from patients who have SS react against the p24 group specific antigen of HIV-1, whereas 47% of the salivary gland biopsies contain an epithelial cytoplasmic protein reactive with a monoclonal antibody to p24 of HIV [60]. The discovery of a human intracisternal A-type retroviral particle that was antigenically related to HIV but distinguishable from this virus by ultrastructural, physical, and enzymatic criteria in lymphoblastoid cells exposed to homogenates of salivary tissue from patients who had SS was the first evidence of an HERV in SS [61].

Subsequently it was shown that 88% of patients who have SS have seroreactivity to HIAP, and that there is a strong correlation between HIAP-1 reactivity and the presence of anti–SS-A and SS-B antibodies [21].

Other viruses have been linked to SS. An increased prevalence of HTLV-reactive antibodies in 36% of Japanese patients who had SS was shown by ELISA, particle agglutination assay, and Western blot [62]. A different study, from an HTLV-1 endemic area, showed that 23% of SS versus 3% of the general population was seropositive for HTLV. In this study, salivary IgA antibodies to HTLV-1 were common among seropositive patients who had SS (5/7), which was interpreted as suggestive of increased viral activity in the salivary glands [63]. In contrast, in the United States and Europe there is no increased reactivity among similar patients to HTLV proteins [16].

Only higher frequency of provirus of HERV-K113 in patients who had SS was found in a study that evaluated the geographic distribution of HERV-K113 and HERV-K115 and their prevalence in different autoimmune diseases. In this study the geographic distribution for both HERVs was similar [64].

Essential thrombocytopenia

By electron microscopy immunostaining, HERV-K10 gag protein was detected in two patients who had ET. In these patients, HERV-K10 formed clusters in the cytoplasm and it was also found in intracellular vacuoles from megakaryocytes [65].

Psoriasis

Recent progress in the genetics of psoriasis showed that within the major locus of susceptibility (6p21.3, PSORS1) an endogenous retroviral sequence was mutated and that this mutation segregated with the disease [66]. By immunofluorescence confocal microscopy, a differential expression and a characteristic dust-like cytoplasmic staining of HERV-E Env protein was reported in psoriatic lesions in contrast to normal skin or atopic dermatitis samples. The intensity of HERV-E Env expression in psoriatic skin was decreased in nonlesional samples compared with lesional or perilesional samples. Furthermore, HERV-E Env expression also could be downregulated by UVB [67]. More recently the expression of three HERV families, namely

HERV-W, -K, and -E, was confirmed in normal and psoriatic skin, the level of expression being higher in psoriatic skin samples. Two types of sequences were mainly represented, which shared homology with the HERV-K and the ERV-9/HERV-W families. Only resident cutaneous cells expressed these sequences in contrast to blood and sera samples that were negative. *Trans*-complementation or *trans*-activation (ie, human papillomavirus, HIV-1) are the postulated mechanisms to explain the endogenous retroviral reactivation [68]. Another study found a high frequency of IgG antibodies against *gag* and *env* genes of the murine leukemia virus–like group of HERVs. Moreover, these antibodies reacted with an epidermal epitope in protein extracts from normal and psoriatic skin cultures [69].

Summary

Molecular epidemiologic proof that HERVs and other retroelements are involved in autoimmunity or other disorders is complicated by their large numbers in the human genome. As discussed, most HERVs are no longer functional or active because of the accumulation of mutations, frameshifts, and deletions. Detection or quantification of HERV transcripts that may be pathologically involved in a particular autoimmune disease thus is often compromised by the presence in great excess of related, but nonfunctional, RNA. This phenomenon should not deter active work in the field, although it will require development of improved methods to discriminate accurately between closely related RNA transcripts. Development of improved immunologic methods to precisely identify epitopes on autoantigens or rare self-reactive T-cell clones may further implicate HERVs and the other repetitive elements in regulation of the immune system in health and disease.

Acknowledgments

The authors acknowledge the previous contribution of Dr. Andras Perl [70]. Many early studies on the possible role of HERVs in autoimmunity, not referenced in the current paper, can be found in this important review.

References

[1] Muir A, Lever A, Moffett A. Expression and functions of human endogenous retroviruses in the placenta: an update. Placenta 2004;18:S16–25.
[2] Nelson PN, Carnegie PR, Martin J, et al. Demystified. Human endogenous retroviruses. Mol Pathol 2003;56:11–8.
[3] Lower R, Lower J, Kurth R. The viruses in all of us: characteristics and biological significance of human endogenous retrovirus sequences. Proc Natl Acad Sci USA 1996;93: 5177–84.

[4] Mi S, Lee X, Li X, et al. Syncytin is a captive retroviral envelope protein involved in human placental morphogenesis. Nature 2000;403:785–9.

[5] Turner G, Barbulescu M, Su M, et al. Insertional polymorphisms of full-length endogenous retroviruses in humans. Curr Biol 2001;11:1531–5.

[6] Nakagawa K, Harrison LC. The potential roles of endogenous retroviruses in autoimmunity. Immunol Rev 1996;152:193–236.

[7] Ryan FP. Human endogenous retroviruses in health and disease: a symbiotic perspective. J R Soc Med 2004;97:560–5.

[8] Portis JL. Perspectives on the role of endogenous human retroviruses in autoimmune diseases. Virology 2002;296:1–5.

[9] Sutkowski N, Conrad B, Thorley-Lawson DA, et al. Epstein-Barr virus transactivates the human endogenous retrovirus HERV-K18 that encodes a superantigen. Immunity 2001;15:579–89.

[10] Stauffer Y, Marguerat S, Meylan F, et al. Interferon-alpha-induced endogenous superantigen: a model linking environment and autoimmunity. Immunity 2001;15:591–601.

[11] Posnett DN, Yarilina AA. Sleeping with the enemy—endogenous superantigens in humans. Immunity 2001;15:503–6.

[12] Meylan F, De Smedt M, Leclercq G, et al. Negative thymocyte selection to HERV-K18 superantigens in humans. Blood 2005;105:4377–82.

[13] Query CC, Keene JD. A human autoimmune protein associated with U1 RNA contains a region of homology that is cross-reactive with retroviral p30gag antigen. Cell 1987;51:211–20.

[14] Christensen T. Association of human endogenous retroviruses with multiple sclerosis and possible interactions with herpes viruses. Rev Med Virol 2005;15:179–211.

[15] Rolland A, Jouvin-Marche E, Saresella M, et al. Correlation between disease severity and in vitro cytokine production mediated by MSRV (multiple sclerosis associated retroviral element) envelope protein in patients with multiple sclerosis. J Neuroimmunol 2005;160:195–203.

[16] Talal N, Dauphinee MJ, Dang H, et al. Detection of serum antibodies to retroviral proteins in patients with primary Sjögren's syndrome (autoimmune exocrinopathy). Arthritis Rheum 1990;33:774–81.

[17] Deas JE, Liu LG, Thompson JJ, et al. Reactivity of sera from systemic lupus erythematosus and Sjögren's syndrome patients with peptides derived from human immunodeficiency virus p24 capsid antigen. Clin Diagn Lab Immunol 1998;5:181–5.

[18] Blomberg J, Nived O, Pipkorn R, et al. Increased antiretroviral antibody reactivity in sera from a defined population of patients with systemic lupus erythematosus. Correlation with autoantibodies and clinical manifestations. Arthritis Rheum 1994;37:57–66.

[19] Bengtsson A, Blomberg J, Nived O, et al. Selective antibody reactivity with peptides from human endogenous retroviruses and nonviral poly(amino acids) in patients with systemic lupus erythematosus. Arthritis Rheum 1996;39:1654–63.

[20] Perl A, Colombo E, Dai H, et al. Antibody reactivity to the HRES-1 endogenous retroviral element identifies a subset of patients with systemic lupus erythematosus and overlap syndromes. Correlation with antinuclear antibodies and HLA class II alleles. Arthritis Rheum 1995;38:1660–71.

[21] Sander DM, Szabo S, Gallaher WR, et al. Involvement of human intracisternal A-type retroviral particles in autoimmunity. Microsc Res Tech 2005;68:222–34.

[22] Gergely P Jr, Pullmann R, Stancato C, et al. Increased prevalence of transfusion-transmitted virus and cross-reactivity with immunodominant epitopes of the HRES-1/p28 endogenous retroviral autoantigen in patients with systemic lupus erythematosus. Clin Immunol 2005;116:124–34.

[23] Adelman MK, Marchalonis JJ. Endogenous retroviruses in systemic lupus erythematosus: candidate lupus viruses. Clin Immunol 2002;102:107–16.

[24] Krieg AM, Khan AS, Steinberg AD. Expression of an endogenous retroviral transcript is associated with murine lupus. Arthritis Rheum 1989;32:322–9.

[25] Wu J, Zhou T, He J, et al. Autoimmune disease in mice due to integration of an endogenous retrovirus in an apoptosis gene. J Exp Med 1993;178:461–8.

[26] Chu JL, Drappa J, Parnassa A, et al. The defect in Fas mRNA expression in MRL/lpr mice is associated with insertion of the retrotransposon, ETn. J Exp Med 1993;178: 723–30.

[27] Ogasawara H, Hishikawa T, Sekigawa I, et al. Sequence analysis of human endogenous retrovirus clone 4–1 in systemic lupus erythematosus. Autoimmunity 2000;33:15–21.

[28] Hishikawa T, Ogasawara H, Kaneko H, et al. Detection of antibodies to a recombinant gag protein derived from human endogenous retrovirus like sequence, clone 4–1, in autoimmune diseases. Viral Immunol 1997;10:137–47.

[29] Sekigawa I, Naito T, Hira K, et al. Possible mechanisms of gender bias in SLE: a new hypothesis involving a comparison of SLE with atopy. Lupus 2004;13:217–22.

[30] Naito T, Ogasawara H, Kaneko H, et al. Immune abnormalities induced by human endogenous retroviral peptides: with reference to the pathogenesis of systemic lupus erythematosus. J Clin Immunol 2003;23:371–6.

[31] Sekigawa I, Ogasawara H, Kaneko H, et al. Retroviruses and autoimmunity. Intern Med 2001;40:80–6.

[32] Piotrowski PC, Duriagin S, Jagodzinski PP. Expression of human endogenous retrovirus clone 4–1 may correlate with blood plasma concentration of anti-U1 RNP and anti-Sm nuclear antibodies. Clin Rheumatol 2005;24:620–4.

[33] Okada M, Ogasawara H, Kaneko H, et al. Role of DNA methylation in transcription of human endogenous retrovirus in the pathogenesis of systemic lupus erythematosus. J Rheum 2002;29:1678–82.

[34] Ogasawara H, Okada M, Kaneko H, et al. Possible role of DNA hypomethylation in the induction of SLE: relationship to the transcription of human endogenous retroviruses. Clin Exp Rheumatol 2003;21:733–8.

[35] Hohenadl C, Germaier H, Walchner M, et al. Transcriptional activation of endogenous retroviral sequences in human epidermal keratinocytes by UVB irradiation. J Invest Dermatol 1999;113:587–94.

[36] Perron H, Garson JA, Bedin F, et al. Molecular identification of a novel retrovirus repeatedly isolated from patients with multiple sclerosis. The Collaborative Research Group on Multiple Sclerosis. Proc Natl Acad Sci USA 1997;94:7583–8.

[37] Grason JA, Tuke PW, Giraud P, et al. Detection of virion-associated MSRV-RNA in serum of patients with multiple sclerosis. Lancet 1998;351:33.

[38] Sotgiu S, Serra C, Mameli G, et al. Multiple sclerosis-associated retrovirus and MS prognosis: an observational study. Neurology 2002;59:1071–3.

[39] Nowak J, Januszkiewicz D, Pernak M, et al. Multiple sclerosis-associated virus-related pol sequences found both in multiple sclerosis and healthy donors are more frequently expressed in multiple sclerosis patients. J Neurovirol 2003;9:112–7.

[40] Perron H, Jouvin-Marche E, Michel M, et al. Multiple sclerosis retrovirus particles and recombinant envelope trigger an abnormal immune response in vitro, by inducing polyclonal Vbeta16 T-lymphocyte activation. Virology 2001;287:321–32.

[41] Lafon M, Jouvin-Marche E, Marche PN, et al. Human viral superantigens: to be or not to be transactivated? Trends Immunol 2002;23:238–9.

[42] Ruprecht K, Obojes K, Wengel V, et al. Regulation of human endogenous retrovirus W protein expression by herpes simplex virus type 1: implications for multiple sclerosis. J Neurovirol 2006;12:65–71.

[43] Firouzi R, Rolland A, Michel M, et al. Multiple sclerosis-associated retrovirus particles cause T lymphocyte-dependent death with brain hemorrhage in humanized SCID mice model. J Neurovirol 2003;9:79–93.

[44] Antony JM, van Marle G, Opii W, et al. Human endogenous retrovirus glycoprotein-mediated induction of redox reactants causes oligodendrocyte death and demyelination. Nat Neurosci 2004;7:1088–95.

[45] Perron H, Lazarini F, Ruprecht K, et al. Human endogenous retrovirus (HERV)-W ENV and GAG proteins: physiological expression in human brain and pathophysiological modulation in multiple sclerosis lesions. J Neurovirol 2005;11:23–33.

[46] Serra C, Mameli G, Arru G, et al. In vitro modulation of the multiple sclerosis (MS)-associated retrovirus by cytokines: implications for MS pathogenesis. J Neurovirol 2003;9: 637–43.

[47] Rolland A, Jouvin-Marche E, Viret C, et al. The envelope protein of a human endogenous retrovirus-W family activates innate immunity through CD14/TLR4 and promotes Th1-like responses. J Immunol 2006;176:7636–44.

[48] Pasare C, Medzhitov R. Toll pathway-dependent blockade of CD4+ CD25+ T cell-mediated suppression by dendritic cells. Science 2003;299:1033–6.

[49] Christensen T, Dissing Sorensen P, Riemann H, et al. Molecular characterization of HERV-H variants associated with multiple sclerosis. Acta Neurol Scand 2000;101:229–38.

[50] Brudek T, Christensen T, Hansen HJ, et al. Simultaneous presence of endogenous retrovirus and herpes virus antigens has profound effect on cell-mediated immune responses: implications for multiple sclerosis. AIDS Res Hum Retroviruses 2004;20:415–23.

[51] Marguerat S, Wang WY, Todd JA, et al. Association of human endogenous retrovirus K-18 polymorphisms with type 1 diabetes. Diabetes 2004;53:852–4.

[52] Conrad B, Weidmann E, Trucco G, et al. Evidence for superantigen involvement in insulin-dependent diabetes mellitus aetiology. Nature 1994;371:351–5.

[53] La Placa M, Vitone F, Bianchi T, et al. Serum antibodies against human intracisternal A-type particle (HIAP) endogenous retrovirus in Alopecia areata patients: a hallmark of autoimmune disease? J Invest Dermatol 2004;123:407–9.

[54] Griffiths DJ, Cooke SP, Herve C, et al. Detection of human retrovirus 5 in patients with arthritis and systemic lupus erythematosus. Arthritis Rheum 1999;42:448–54.

[55] Piper KE, Hanssen AD, Lewallen DG, et al. Lack of detection of human retrovirus-5 pro-viral DNA in synovial tissue and blood specimens from individuals with rheumatoid arthritis or osteoarthritis. Arthritis Rheum 2006;55:123–5.

[56] Herve CA, Lugli EB, Brand A, et al. Autoantibodies to human endogenous retrovirus-K are frequently detected in health and disease and react with multiple epitopes. Clin Exp Immunol 2002;128:75–82.

[57] Ejtehadi HD, Freimanis GL, Ali HA, et al. The potential role of human endogenous retrovirus K10 in the pathogenesis of rheumatoid arthritis: a preliminary study. Ann Rheum Dis 2006;65:612–6.

[58] Ehlhardt S, Seifert M, Schneider J, et al. Human endogenous retrovirus HERV-K(HML-2) Rec expression and transcriptional activities in normal and rheumatoid arthritis synovia. J Rheumatol 2006;33:16–23.

[59] Sicat J, Sutkowski N, Huber BT. Expression of human endogenous retrovirus HERV-K18 superantigen is elevated in juvenile rheumatoid arthritis. J Rheumatol 2005;32: 1821–31.

[60] Yamano S, Renard JN, Mizuno F, et al. Retrovirus in salivary glands from patients with Sjogren's syndrome. J Clin Pathol 1997;50:223–30.

[61] Garry RF, Fermin CD, Hart DJ, et al. Detection of a human intracisternal A-type retroviral particle antigenically related to HIV. Science 1990;250:1127–9.

[62] Eguchi K, Matsuoka N, Ida H, et al. Primary Sjögren's syndrome with antibodies to HTLV-I: clinical and laboratory features. Ann Rheum Dis 1992;51:769–76.

[63] Terada K, Katamine S, Eguchi K, et al. Prevalence of serum and salivary antibodies to HTLV-1 in Sjögren 's syndrome. Lancet 1994;344:1116–9.

[64] Moyes DL, Martin A, Sawcer S, et al. The distribution of the endogenous retroviruses HERV-K113 and HERV-K115 in health and disease. Genomics 2005;86:337–41.

[65] Morgan D, Brodsky I. Human endogenous retrovirus (HERV-K) particles in megakaryocytes cultured from essential thrombocythemia peripheral blood stem cells. Exp Hematol 2004;32:520–5.

[66] Foerster J, Nolte I, Junge J, et al. Haplotype sharing analysis identifies a retroviral dUTPase as candidate susceptibility gene for psoriasis. J Invest Dermatol 2005;124:99–102.

[67] Bessis D, Moles JP, Basset-Seguin N, et al. Differential expression of a human endogenous retrovirus E transmembrane envelope glycoprotein in normal, psoriatic and atopic dermatitis human skin. Br J Dematol 2004;151:737–45.

[68] Moles JP, Tesniere A, Guilhou JJ. A new endogenous retroviral sequence is expressed in skin of patients with psoriasis. Br J Dermatol 2005;153:83–9.

[69] Moles JP, Hadi JC, Guilhou JJ. High prevalence of an IgG response against murine leukemia virus (MLV) in patients with psoriasis. Virus Res 2003;94:97–101.

[70] Perl A. Role of endogenous retroviruses in autoimmune diseases. Rheum Dis Clin N Am 2003;29:123–43.

ELSEVIER
SAUNDERS

Infect Dis Clin N Am
20 (2006) 931–961

INFECTIOUS
DISEASE CLINICS
OF NORTH AMERICA

Impact of Biologic Agents on Infectious Diseases

Lesley Ann Saketkoo, MD, MPH[a,b,c,*],
Luis R. Espinoza, MD[b,c]

[a]Division of Rheumatology, Ochsner Clinic Foundation, New Orleans, LA, USA
[b]Section of Rheumatology, Louisiana State University Health Sciences Center,
New Orleans, LA, USA
[c]Department of Medicine, Louisiana State University Health Sciences Center,
New Orleans, LA, USA

Chronic inflammatory diseases lead to disabling destruction of joints, end-stage organ damage, hematologic derangements, and neurologic compromise. The introduction of biologic agents has produced an astounding transformation by halting or slowing the progression of diseases, such as rheumatoid arthritis (RA), psoriatic arthritis, spondyloarthropathy, collagen vascular disease, inflammatory bowel disease, and multiple sclerosis resulting in marked decrease of disability and improvement in quality of life and health outcomes.

Along with great relief and hope, biologics have brought the need for expert vigilance requiring judicious selection of candidates, close observation, and careful attention to patient education. Biologics are associated with the development of serious life-threatening infections in addition to other well-documented hematologic, immunologic, cardiovascular, and malignant adverse effects. Further complications include the concomitant use of other immunosuppressive therapies, such as prednisone and methotrexate; coexistent morbidities [1]; and underlying immune dysfunction associated with autoimmune diseases [2]. This article focuses on biologics in current and imminent use, predominantly tumor necrosis factor (TNF)-α inhibitors, to provide a reference and gateway to prevention, recognition, and management of potential pathogens of serious infections defined as fatal,

This article is dedicated in sadness and hope to the history, excellence of care, and remarkable medical training provided by West-900–Infectious Disease Unit of Charity Hospital, New Orleans, Louisiana.

* Corresponding author. 618 Robert Street, New Orleans, LA 70115.
E-mail address: saketkoo.md@gmail.com (L.A. Saketkoo).

life-threatening, or causing prolonged hospitalization (Appendix 1). The efficacy and safety of these agents in the management of infectious diseases, such as HIV and hepatitis C virus (HCV), are also touched on briefly.

An extensive literature search of more than 350 publications was conducted using the PubMed database. To be exhaustive and complete, each agent was used as a keyword and cross referenced to a list of pathogens and clinical syndromes. Reference lists were also examined for additional sources. Information not gathered from studies and case reports of patients being treated for inflammatory disease are clearly stated as such. Sources were omitted when a clear effect could not reasonably be attributed to the specific agent (ie, patients treated with cyclophosphamide-hydroxydauno-mycin-Oncovin-prednisone [CHOP] plus rituximab without a nonrituximab group or single case reports clouded by concomitant use of other known highly toxic agents) unless plausible arguments based on supporting reference were included.

Much of this article is built on systematic reviews reliant on data through adverse event reporting systems (AERS) in the United States and abroad. It is imperative to understand the shortcomings of passive reporting systems [3,4]. Underreporting may be caused by an unrecognized association resulting from transfer of care, length of time interval from treatment to event, lack of familiarity with these agents, and because commonly acquired pathogens are less likely to be reported [5]. Clinicians may not be aware of reporting systems, of how to access them, not perceive reporting as a responsibility, or find the reporting system too cumbersome. Difficulties retrieving information from these systems exist [6]. It is presumed that data presented here are incomplete in numbers and that serious infections are of more relevance and far-reaching than this article suggests [7]. Growing frequency and indications of use, the imminent flux of newer agents, and severity of adverse events warrant patient advocacy in the form of stringent registries obligating prescribing practitioners to report major adverse events. Such an information system would allow for deeper understanding, potentially establishing guidelines in prevention and management of serious complications [7].

Tumor necrosis factor-α inhibitors

TNF-α is a multifunctional cytokine that is a chief mediator of inflammation and integral component to a healthy immune response against infection and malignancy. TNF-α is a protein secreted by T cells, natural killer cells, and mast cells but mainly from activated mononuclear phagocytes in response to antigen presentation. Most cells possess TNF receptors. Receptors are either membrane bound or freely circulating. The soluble form acts to neutralize excess circulating TNF. TNF-α has profound pathologic complexity mediating both systemic effects and local damage present in serious systemic complications of infection like sepsis and the destruction seen in many autoinflammatory diseases. TNF-α effects are as follows [8–11]:

- Hypothalamus causing fever
- Muscle to produce catabolism with resultant weight loss and malaise
- Liver to synthesize acute phase reactants
- Macrophage recruitment to site of infection
- Stimulation of granulocyte colony-stimulating factor
- Production of nitric oxide in macrophages needed for killing organisms
- Induction of interleukin-1, another key component in the inflammatory cascade
- Activation of inflammatory and coagulation processes of endothelial cells
- Apoptosis of various tumor cells

Etanercept (Enbrel)

Etanercept is a soluble humanized receptor that decreases circulating TNF-α thereby competing with host receptors normally stimulated by TNF-α. Etanercept does not bind universally or avidly to membrane-bound TNF-α rendering a partial blockade of TNF-α. Etanercept is approved for treatment of RA, juvenile rheumatoid arthritis, psoriatic arthritis, plaque psoriasis, and ankylosing spondylitis. Having a half-life of only 4 days, it is injected subcutaneously twice or once weekly to maintain effective blockade.

Infliximab (Remicade)

Infliximab is a chimeric monoclonal antibody comprised of human and mouse proteins. Antibody development to the murine protein is noted and avoided with use of other immunosuppressants, such as methotrexate or azathioprine. It has high binding affinity for soluble and membrane-bound TNF-α receptors resulting in a more complete blockade. Infliximab is approved for RA, psoriatic arthritis, ankylosing spondylitis, ulcerative colitis and active Crohn's disease. Infliximab is intravenously administered at weeks 0, 2, and 6 and then every 8 weeks and has a half-life of 9 days but may have biologic activity for up to 2 months.

Adalimumab (Humira)

Adalimumab is a fully human monoclonal antibody to TNF-α with high affinity for both soluble and membrane-bound TNF-α receptors. It is approved for use in RA, psoriatic arthritis, and ankylosing spondylitis. Adalimumab has a half-life of approximately 2 weeks and is administered subcutaneously every 2 weeks.

Summary

TNF-α neutralizers (Table 1) are being used with increasing frequency and being approved for a growing number of diseases. Most serious

Table 1
Biologic agents

Biologic	Action	Half-life	Administration	Indications
Infliximab (Remicade)	Chimeric antibody to membrane and soluble TNF-α	9 d	Infusion at wk 0, 2, 6, and then every 8 wks	RA, ankylosing spondylitis, psoriatic arthritis, Crohn's disease, ulcerative colitis
Adalimumab (Humira)	Humanized antibody to membrane and soluble TNF-α	2 wk	Subcutaneous injection every 2 wk	RA, psoriatic arthritis, ankylosing spondylitis
Etanercept (Embrel)	Humanized TNF-α receptor, decreases circulating TNF-α, partial blockade	4 d	Subcutaneous injection twice per week	RA, JRA, psoriatic arthritis, plaque psoriasis, ankylosing spondylitis
Anakinra (Kineret)	Recombinant human IL-1Ra, which blocks IL-1 receptor; signal blockade	4–6 h	Daily subcutaneous injection	RA, JRA
Rituximab (Rituxin)	Chimeric antibody targeting CD20 mediates B-cell lysis	80–400 h	For RA: two infusions 2 wk apart	RA and non-Hodgkin's lymphoma
Abatacept (Orencia)	Humanized protein preventing costimulation between T-cell and APC	8–25 d	Infusion at wk 0, 2, and 4 then every 4 wk	RA
Natalizumab (Tysabri)	Chimeric antibody to leukocyte integrins; prevents migration to tissue	7–15 d	Undetermined for RA and Crohn's	MS, approval pending for Crohn's disease and RA

Abbreviations: APC, antigen presenting cell; IL, interleukin; JRA, juvenile rheumatoid arthritis; MS, multiple sclerosis; RA, rheumatoid arthritis; TNF, tumor necrosis factor.

infections have been associated with this group of biologic agents with infliximab having ($P < .0001$) more frequent serious infections when compared with Etanercept [6]. Infliximab has a more lasting neutralizing effect [12]. Etanercept offers a partial blockade allowing protective mechanisms of TNF-α to be present during infection [13]. Although controversy exists in increased rates of overall infection when compared with disease-modifying antirheumatic drugs [14], there is little question regarding increased rates of extrapulmonary tuberculosis (TB) and serious infections of intracellular bacteria or endemic mycoses.

Other immunomodulating agents

Anakinra (Kineret)

Anakinra is a recombinant human variant of the naturally occurring interleukin (IL)-1 receptor antagonist (IL-1Ra), which blocks the IL-1 signal and inhibits IL-1, which mediates synovial damage and inhibits repair in RA. Half-life is 4 to 6 hours and it is administered as daily subcutaneous injections. Anakinra has a favorable safety profile but poor long-term efficacy in adults and may be of limited use [15]. Infections occur at a similar rate as that of the placebo groups [16,17].

Rituximab (Rituxin)

Rituximab is a chimeric human-mouse monoclonal antibody against CD20 on pre–B lymphocytes and mature B lymphocytes. Binding induces B-lymphocyte lysis, depleting B-cell lineages. B lymphocytes mediate pathogenesis of RA at multiple points in the inflammatory response and are associated with chronic synovitis. Administration for RA is two infusions 2 weeks apart. Half-life is 3.5 to 17 days with B-cell depletion enduring for several months, being detectable in serum 3 to 6 months after treatment. Rituximab is approved for non-Hodgkin's lymphoma and RA. Infectious concern surrounds hepatitis B virus (HBV) and HCV reactivation, and susceptibility to such viruses as cytomegalovirus, herpes simplex virus, varicella-zoster virus, parvovirus B19, and JC virus. Severe fatal infections have occurred up to 1 year after treatment. Live vaccine administration is not recommended [18].

Abatacept (Orencia)

Abatacept is a fully humanized soluble fusion protein that mimics the naturally occurring CTLA-4. CTLA-4 circulates and down-regulates T-cell activity by binding to CD28 on T lymphocytes. This action blocks the costimulatory signal between CD28 and antigen-presenting cell proteins CD80 or CD86, thereby decreasing T-cell activation and proliferation and subsequent B-cell effects with inhibition of TNF-α, IL-2, IL-6, and possibly interferon-γ [19]. Administration is as an infusion at weeks 0, 2, and 4 and then every 4 weeks. Half-life is 8 to 25 days with biologic effects lasting up to 3 months. Live vaccines should not be given until 3 months after treatment. Abatacept is in early postmarketing stages, and establishing trends of associated infectious disease requires time. An increased risk for TB and bacterial pneumonia, however, may exist. One case each of sepsis, aspergillosis, and septic arthritis was reported [20].

Natalizumab (Tysabri)

Natalizumab is a chimeric monoclonal antibody directed at α_4-integrin, a membrane protein on all leukocytes except neutrophils. Leukocytes migrate from the vascular space and into parenchyma by α_4-integrin–recognizing receptors on various cell adhesion molecules. Natalizumab competitively binds α_4-integrin preventing transmigration of inflammatory cells across endothelial cells and into tissue. Half-life is 7 to 15 days administered at four weekly infusions for multiple sclerosis. It is approved for treatment of relapsing-remitting multiple sclerosis and may soon be approved for RA and Crohn's disease. In addition to progressive multifocal leukoencephalopathy (see later), for which there is now black box and bold warnings, premarketing trials identified cases of *Aspergillus, Pneumocystis jiroveci* (formerly *carinii*) pneumonia, pulmonary *Mycobacterium avium* complex, and a fatal case of herpes encephalitis [21].

Tuberculosis

Approval of infliximab in August of 1998 was preceded by only one TB case identified. The immediate months to follow saw a wave of TB cases reported to the Food and Drug Administration (FDA) in striking temporal association with anti–TNF-α use. Keane and colleagues [22], by systematic review, established a temporal and disease pattern that implicated infliximab in causal relation to development of TB. Time to diagnosis was made ≤ 12 weeks from initiation of treatment with greater than 50% of patients presenting with disseminated and extrapulmonary disease involving lymph tissue, bone, bladder, bowel, and meanings.

Since the study by Keane and colleagues [22], studies have examined the use of anti–TNF-α agents in relation to TB. TB is consistently reported with the highest frequency over other severe infections with manifestations of extrapulmonary TB predominating [6,22,23]. The FDA now requires labeling of infliximab and adalimumab to display black box warnings advising of the high risk of TB and a bold warning for etanercept. Reports of other biologics supporting an association with an increased risk of TB with the possible exception of abatacept [20] were not found.

Wolfe and colleagues [24] determined the baseline rate of TB in RA patients before infliximab use was not higher than that of the general population. The study has self-reported ethnic, socioeconomic, and literacy limitations rendering inability to generalize data. This contrasts Askling and colleagues [2], who identified RA patients in Sweden as having a four-fold increased risk of developing TB than did an age- and sex-matched population, as did Carmona and colleagues in Spain [25]. TNF-α blockade increases this risk eight times with infliximab and 4.5 times with etanercept [6,24,26]. It cannot be overemphasized that TNF-α mediates production of fever, weight loss, and night sweats, whereas a deficiency of TNF-α can mask constitutional and other symptoms usually seen in TB infection leading to atypical presentations. [22,27,28].

TNF-α has a role in defense against mycobacteria and in the pathology of the infection. TNF-α is expressed by activated macrophages, T cells, and natural killer cells in response to TB infection and facilitates macrophage ingestion and intracellular destruction of TB. TNF-α recruits proinflammatory cells and fibroblasts required in granuloma formation [29]. The inflammatory machinery descends on the infectious focus working to contain the pathogen preventing dissemination and interfering with the delivery of nutritive material. In the TNF-α–deficient person, the occurrence of these events is unreliable because TNF-α is necessary for the initial immune challenge and the maintenance of latency. Impairment of granuloma formation is the likely mechanism of extrapulmonary disease and the severe clinical course seen with TNF-α inhibition [30].

Saliu and colleagues [31] reported TNF inhibitory effects on antimycobacterial immune functions in whole blood cultures finding that both infliximab and adalimumab reduced $CD69^+$ CD4 cells by 70% and 49% ($P < .05$) and suppressed interferon-γ production by 70% and 64% ($P < .05$). Etanercept did not produce a significant effect. IL-10, however, was equally suppressed by all three agents. These findings may account for differences in occurrence rates. Infliximab is consistently implicated as the anti–TNF-α agent most often associated with TB reactivation and portends a higher risk of developing active TB than etanercept. TB typically presents at 11 to 12 weeks of treatment [6,28] and adalimumab at 30 weeks [32].

Patterns suggest a reactivation of latent disease. Less is known regarding the contribution of de novo infection. Wallis [33] recently examined AERS data by mathematical modeling to distinguish de novo from reactivation. Infliximab reactivated 22% of latent infections during each month of treatment precipitating 75% of latent TB infection (LTBI) in the first year of therapy, whereas the rate for etanercept was only 1.6%. During the first 2 years of anti–TNF-α therapy, new infections accounted for 25% and 52% of TB cases, respectively, even in low-prevalence areas. Both drugs caused at least half of new infections to progress to active disease. Areas with higher TB transmission rates may be more prone to new infection.

Screening with purified protein derivative (PPD) before anti–TNF-α therapy is current practice; however, false-negative results in RA patients are concerning. A prospective study in Peru found PPD placement in RA patients an inadequate determination of TB status because of a preponderance of negative results [34]. In 1997, the Centers for Disease Control and Prevention changed its position on anergy skin testing in HIV-infected patients, stating that anergy testing did not make a useful contribution to decision making in the diagnosis of LTBI or initiating isoniazid treatment [35]. Many experts agree that patients with negative PPD results but a history or clinical finding indicating higher risk be treated as LTBI before TNF-α inhibition [36]. Anti-TNF therapy influence on PPD response [37] requires further examination. T-cell–based interferon-γ assays are a promising and imminently available screening for LTBI. They use antigens highly specific for TB and seem to have superior efficacy to the PPD [38].

Disclosure of LTBI or active TB requires treatment according to established guidelines for immunocompromised patients. The remaining dilemma is deciding to initiate, continue, or postpone anti-TNF therapy and when to restart therapy in relation to antitubercular therapy. No formal guidelines have been established but the Centers for Disease Control and Prevention suggests consideration of halting therapy until TB treatment for latent or active disease is completed. Expert arguments exist for TNF-α use during antitubercular treatment in patients with severe inflammatory disease in whom treatment should not be delayed recommending anti–TNF-α after 1 month of tolerance to isoniazid [39]. A phase I study with 16 HIV-positive patients found that anti-TB therapy with concomitant use of etanercept did not affect response to treatment [40].

Regarding isoniazid-associated hepatotoxicity in patients with autoimmune disease, current best practice applies: screen for pre-existing liver disease, alcohol overuse, and coincidence of another potentially hepatotoxic drug that can possibly be substituted. Serial aminotransferase levels are indicated with a level greater than three times upper limit of normal being cause for concern. If given alone, isoniazid should be given for the 9-month daily course; deviation could result in relapse of active disease [41,42].

Non-TB mycobacteria, such as *M avium* complex and *Mycobacterium leprae* [6], in association with anti–TNF-α therapy are described infrequently [43]. *M avium* complex presenting with a psoas muscle abscess with etanercept use has been described [44]. Despite paucity of reports, systematic review of all reported cases by September 2002 reveals two-times greater frequency of non-TB mycobacteria ($P = .023$) with infliximab over etanercept. In addition, a number of murine studies support the essential mediation of TNF-α in preventing necrotizing progression of *M avium* complex [45–47].

Recommendations for tuberculosis prevention

The following recommendations apply:

- PPD should be obtained before biologic therapy and then every 12 months [48]. Given the high prevalence of anergy, repeat PPD at 2 weeks may disclose cases of LTBI [39]. An induration ≥5 mm is a positive reading for LTBI in patients with possible underlying immunocompromise including autoimmune disorders, HIV, and posttransplant. This value is regardless of *Candida* or other control. An induration of ≤5 mm is a lesser likelihood of LTBI and does not exclude LTBI.
- A positive reading should interrupt therapy at least until treatment for LTBI is initiated with clinical improvement if the patient is symptomatic. An investigation for active TB should ensue. LTBI is treated per

Centers for Disease Control and Prevention guidelines for immunosuppressed patients with 9 months of daily isoniazid unless local resistance patterns dictate otherwise.

- Centers for Disease Control and Prevention recommends consideration in treating patients with negative PPD readings but whose screening history or clinical picture put them at risk.
- Some experts obtain chest radiographs before [39,49] or within 3 months of initiation of treatment [50] and should always follow a positive PPD reading or suggestive history.
- Obtain a thorough TB screening history including travel, country of origin, exposure to known TB case, history of having been incarcerated, in a homeless shelter or nursing home or contact with a person with such residence, a history of substance abuse, employment in health industry, or history of a positive PPD or radiograph suggestive of TB.
- Educate patients on the potential risk of developing TB, symptoms associated with TB infection, instructions to stop medication and contact physician with development of symptoms. Symptoms include persistent fever, weight loss, night sweats, or respiratory symptoms and extrapulmonary disease symptoms, such as malaise, mass, or lymphadenopathy, but TB may present atypically.
- Persistent fever or respiratory symptoms should be taken seriously in all patients receiving biologic agents maintaining a high index of suspicion for TB.
- Cases should be reported to local public health officials to facilitate treatment and identification of additional contacts exposed.
- Cases should be reported to the FDA's adverse event reporting system.

Fungal and parasitic infections

Wallis and colleagues [6] conducted a large systematic review to identify granulomatous disease in coincidence with TNF-α inhibition. In addition to TB, several endemic and opportunistic fungal infections were identified: systemic candidiasis, histoplasmosis, coccidioidomycosis, *Cryptococcus*, and aspergillosis and other bacterial and mycobacterial pathogens. The incidence of these granulomatous infections was found to be greater than two times higher ($P < .0001$) with infliximab than with etanercept and reported in the first 3 months after initiation of treatment. As with TB, in mycotic infection, TNF inhibition interferes with granuloma formation and apoptosis of infected macrophages occurs, which undermines the host's ability to protect against disseminated infection. Beaman [51] demonstrated that TNF-α potentiates antifungicidal capability of human monocytes. Active discovery and dialog are needed to establish screening and empiric treatment guidelines.

Coccidioidomycosis is caused by a dimorphic fungus existing as a mold in soil and dust and is endemic to the southwestern United States and Mexico.

Its spores are aerosolized by occupational and recreational disruption of soil with transmission occurring by inhalation. It causes potentially fatal illness presenting as a flulike illness or pneumonia with fever, cough, headaches, rash, and myalgia. Immunocompromised patients may fail to recover developing chronic pulmonary infection or widespread disseminated infection with central nervous system involvement potentially leading to permanent neurologic damage.

Through a retrospective comparative study of five rheumatology practices and one medical center in areas endemic for coccidioidomycosis, Bergstrom and colleagues [52] demonstrated statistically significant increased risk of patients with inflammatory arthritis being treated with anti–TNF-α agents ($P \leq .01$). From 1998 to 2003 (57 months), 13 symptomatic cases were identified. Twelve cases involved infliximab with onset 2 to 48 weeks from initiation of treatment and one etanercept case with onset at 96 weeks. None of these patients had comorbid conditions that might put them at higher risk, such as HIV, diabetes, or pregnancy. All patients were on methotrexate and one patient was on prednisone and cyclosporine. Before TNF inhibition, two patients had a previous history of coccidioidomycosis, 12 patients had normal pretreatment chest radiographs, no patient had documentation of skin manifestations, and six patients had documentation of negative serology, which confounds arguments that the initial presentation to rheumatology was for an acute primary infection of coccidioidomycosis causing "desert arthritis" mistaken for RA. Two deaths were identified, one of which was caused by posthumous recognition of the pathogen in which antifungal treatment was never initiated. This particular case illustrates the imperative nature in maintaining a high index of suspicion and obtaining thorough birth and travel histories. The findings of Bergstrom and colleagues [52] are corroborated by a greater than six times increased risk established by Wallis and colleagues [6] ($P = .013$) using completely different methods of investigation.

Suggested preventive measures are screening history for residence in endemic areas, central nervous system infections, and chest radiograph and consideration of serology testing of IgM and IgG and then again every 3 months. Patient education regarding transmission and symptoms should be conducted [48]. History of meningitis in an endemic area or a suggestive history demands vigilance. Screening serology by some transplant centers is performed in endemic areas. A positive screening results in fluconazole prophylaxis [53]. Active disease warrants discontinuation of TNF inhibition keeping in mind that relapse rate of disease is high on discontinuation of antifungals [54].

Histoplasmosis, another life-threatening infection to which patients under TNF inhibition are potentially predisposed, is one of the most prevalent mycoses in the United States with the most highly endemic areas being in the Ohio and Mississippi River valleys. Transmission is by inhalation of spores with disruption of soil containing contaminated bird or bat droppings.

Histoplasmosis infection is often asymptomatic in presentation and self-limited. Immunocompromised people are at higher risk of becoming symptomatic, however, and may succumb to substantial morbidity with disseminated disease [5,55–57]. TNF-α is important in both primary and secondary histoplasmosis infection. Inhibition of TNF-α in mouse models conferred 100% mortality with coincident histoplasmosis infection [58].

By May 2002, 22 acute life-threatening cases were identified in the United States by the FDA AERS [55] and by September 2002, 40 cases were further identified [6]. Four remarkable cases were additionally described in the literature [5,56]. These cases illustrate the vast potential for underestimation of postmarketing surveillance because correspondence with the authors suggests these cases were unlikely to have been reported to AERS. Initial presentation was predominantly fever, malaise, weight loss, and cough, with pulmonary nodules or diffuse interstitial pneumonitis, thrombocytopenia, neutropenia, and pancytopenia. Presentation was exceptional in one patient who presented with granulomatous hepatitis. Five patients of the 22 cases reported by May died. Wallis and colleagues [6] established a greater than seven times increased risk ($P < .001$) with infliximab over etanercept.

Suggested screening in patients with history of residence in endemic areas is a chest radiograph with urine histoplasmin antigen at baseline and every 3 months [48,56]. If active histoplasmosis is identified, anti–TNF-α treatment should cease. Pre-emptive or reinitiated treatment during TNF inhibition should be considered with suggestive history [56]. Patients should be counseled on activities associated with transmission of disease (exploring caves, cleaning chicken coops, shifting soil). Further investigation is needed in this area to formulate guidelines.

Aspergillosis presents on a spectrum of allergic in the immunocompetent to invasive in the immunocompromised, which is often fatal. *Aspergillus* sp. is ubiquitous and is transmitted to human hosts by inhalation of spores found on dead or decaying leaves and vegetation, compost, or grain. Development of serious disease is extremely uncommon in immunocompetent people. In mouse models, TNF-α prevents dissemination from lungs to vital organs and mortality, which otherwise was shown to be >40% and 0% in noninhibited mice [59]. TNF-α seems to enhance an early event in host defense system against invasion by *Aspergillus* and a late event via superoxide anion production resulting in hyphal damage and destruction [60].

In 2001, three cases of invasive aspergillosis associated with TNF-α inhibition were reported. The first case was a young man with fistulizing Crohn's disease who developed symptoms of high fever, productive cough, and dyspnea 5 days following initial intravenous infusion of infliximab without other immunesuppressants. Massive bilateral infiltrates were found on chest radiograph, he died 1 month later of multiorgan failure and septic shock. Despite antifungal treatment, serial cultures and autopsy revealed invasive growth of *Aspergillus fumigatus* [61]. The second case was a 73-year-old woman with chronic obstructive pulmonary disease and 10-year history of RA with recent initiation of infliximab, fluctuating doses of prednisone (5–10 mg), and leflunomide. Two months after initiation she was treated for right upper lobe pneumonia discovered on chest radiograph. Another 2 months later she presented afebrile with cough productive of white clumps and recent 20-lb weight loss. Obstructive right upper and middle lobe infiltrates were found on CT of chest and bronchoscopy revealed *A fumigatus* [62]. The third case reported involved a 55-year-old woman with a 10-year history of RA being treated with etanercept and 5-mg prednisone daily for 10 months when she presented with high fever, dyspnea, and productive cough and ultimately respiratory failure and pneumopyothorax. Bronchoscopy revealed *A fumigatus* [63]. By September 2002, there were 30 cases of aspergillosis (20 infliximab, 10 etanercept) reported without clinical description. Although more cases of infliximab were reported, this was not statistically significant [6]. Subsequently, a case has been reported with aspergillosis, disseminated TB, and cutaneous herpes simplex infection during treatment of RA with infliximab and methotrexate [42].

Marty and colleagues [64] discovered a significantly increased risk of invasive fungal infection (adjusted $P = .004$) in patients treated with infliximab for severe graft-versus-host disease after bone marrow transplantation. Prophylaxis against filamentous fungi is strongly suggested in this scenario. De Rosa and colleagues [62] suggest adherence to use of masks in high-risk patients when in close proximity to construction.

Cryptococcal infection is transmitted by inhalation of yeast or spores from soil or dust with contaminated bird droppings. The most common presentation is with pneumonia or disseminated disease with central nervous system involvement. *Cryptococcus* sp. is encapsulated yeast with worldwide distribution. Infection carries an overall mortality rate of 12% and permanent neurologic damage can ensue after resolution of infection [65]. Mouse models reveal inhibition of TNF-α preventing pulmonary clearance of *Cryptococcus neoformans* [66].

Wallis and colleagues [6] found 19 cases of *Cryptococcus* infection in association with TNF-α blockade. Subsequently, there have been five additional [48,67–70] case reports published, one of which describes possible zoonotic transmission from a pet bird [70]. All cases were associated with infliximab with onset from time of treatment being 3 to 5 weeks. Wallis and colleagues [6] found no significant increase of cryptococcal infection between infliximab and etanercept. It is important to recognize that invasive cryptococcal disease can occur with negative cerebrospinal fluid or serum cryptococcal antigen and culture as supported by two case reports [67,68] and a high index of suspicion is critical for prevention of devastating sequelae [68]. There is no discussion of preventive guidelines found on review of literature. It seems a reasonable approach to treat patients with a history of cryptococcal infection with suppressive antifungal therapy during TNF blockade as done in AIDS treatment protocol.

Pneumocystis pneumonia is caused by a ubiquitous fungus *Pneumocystis jiroveci* (formerly *carinii*). This pathogen is of no consequence in healthy individuals. In patients who are immunocompromised, however, illness begins insidiously with dry cough and flulike symptoms leading to dyspnea at rest, rapidly leading to respiratory failure and death. Only 12 cases of *P jiroveci* pneumonia have been described with methotrexate alone since the advent of its use [71]. By June 2001, there were at least 15 cases associated with anti–TNF-α therapy. Ten of these cases were with infliximab onset being between one and three doses with three deaths (one United States). Eight cases were with etanercept time to onset being 1 to 4 months with three deaths (all United States) [72]. HIV status was either reported as negative or not commented on. There were six apparently additional cases published worldwide associating *P jiroveci* pneumonia with infliximab use [73–78]. In vitro and mouse studies suggest TNF blockade prevents both clearance and control of the pneumocystis organism by the host defense system and results in more severe infection [79–81].

Some experts encourage evaluation for prophylaxis on an individual basis considering lymphocyte count and dose and duration of immunosuppressant treatment [32,77]. Prophylaxis is with TMP-SMX or dapsone, atovaquone, or inhaled pentamidine if allergic to sulfa. There is a paucity of data at this time for formal recommendations.

Although there is a paucity of description in the literature of biologic associated candidiasis [82], Wallis and colleagues [6] quantify almost a fivefold increase in systemic *Candida* with infliximab over etanercept ($P = .046$) and 2.3 increase with any candidial presentation ($P = .006$) in the United States. TNF knockout mice had increased susceptibility to both oral and systemic candidiasis [83]. This is an area requiring further investigation.

Other fungal and protozoal pathogens have been associated with TNF-α inhibition in case reports, such as disseminated sporotrichosis [84], toxoplasmosis [85], and a fatal case of myositis involving *Brachiola algerae* via mosquito vector [86].

Bacterial infection

The importance of maintaining high suspicion for the unusual suspects cannot be stressed enough. The Spanish Registry revealed that in serious infections, especially pneumonia, a continuous problem remains to be lack of identification of the implicated bacterial organisms reported as a prevalence of 14.2% [87].

Listeriosis is the result of a gram-positive intracellular organism well known to cause meningitis, encephalitis, and septicemia in newborns, pregnant women, the elderly, and people with compromised immune system. Listeria carries a mortality rate of 15% to 30% [65]. Patients often present with vague to severe flulike, gastrointestinal, or neurologic symptoms; index of suspicion must be high. TNF-α seems to be important in macrophage bactericidal activity in listeriosis [8,9,88,89].

By December 2001, there were 15 cases of listeriosis associated with TNF antagonists and 11 cases were identified 9 months later. Two cases involved etanercept with one death, and 24 cases involved infliximab with 7 deaths. [90] Median onset from initiation of infliximab was two to three doses. There were two additional case reports with infliximab presenting with brain abscess after cholecystectomy and fatal cholecystitis progressing to meningoencephalitis with posthumous culture growth of *Listeria* [91]. The latter patient received empiric treatment with ceftriaxone, metronidazole, and fluconazole lacking *Listeria* coverage. Several case reports of *Listeria* meningoencephalitis with empiric treatment including ampicillin on presentation resulted in rapid resolution of symptoms [92–96].

Preventive efforts in patients receiving anti-TNF therapy include education on food preparation and safety with thorough cooking of meats; washing raw vegetables; and avoidance of unpasteurized dairy products, soft cheeses (eg, as camembert), and precooked meats (hot dogs, deli meats) unless thoroughly reheated [65]. Maintaining a high suspicion for *Listeria* with a low threshold for including ampicillin in patients presenting with neurologic symptoms is advised. TMP-SMX prophylaxis also covers for *Listeria* and might be considered in the elderly or patients with lymphocytopenia.

Pneumococcal infection in elderly and immunocompromised people may lead to sudden severe pneumonia and sepsis. Isolated case reports of pneumococcal pneumonia with one case progressing to fatal acute respiratory distress syndrome, bacteremia, and meningitis related to anti-TNF therapy has been described [48,97–99]. A case of pneumococcal necrotizing fasciitis with fatal sepsis being treated with etanercept and low-dose prednisone was reported whereby etanercept may not have been stopped in timely manner [100]. That necrotizing fasciitis is uncommon in immunocompetent hosts suggests the addition of anti–TNF-α therapy may have led to a predisposing state. TNF-α prevents bacteremia and death in mouse models. TNF-α levels increase proportionally to bacterial burden [101] with TNF-α inhibition conferring impaired clearance of bacteria and early mortality [102] because of pneumococcal pneumonia and fatal peritonitis [103]. Pneumococcal vaccine is preferably administered 2 weeks before anti–TNF-α therapy; however, it may be given during therapy. Patients should be counseled on signs and symptoms, such as shaking chills, fever, and rigor. Ellerin and colleagues [32] support a home dose of fluoroquinolone at hand to be taken with symptoms while patient is on route to medical attention.

Legionellosis is caused by gram-negative bacteria that thrive in aqueous environments, such as air conditioner ducts and shower heads. It manifests as pneumonia in patients who are elderly, immunosuppressed, or who have pulmonary disease with transmission being by inhalation. Case reports with anti–TNF-α therapy have been described [104,105]. Depletion of TNF-α impairs pulmonary host immune response to *Legionella* with persistent pneumonitis in rats [106].

Three cases of salmonella septic arthritis have been reported with etanercept use [107] and one case with infliximab use [108]. One case was of salmonella septicemia associated with adalimumab and the other was a fatal case associated with infliximab. *Salmonella* is transmitted by eggs, meat, and unpasteurized dairy products. It may also be transmitted by pet turtles, iguanas, and other reptiles. Patient education of food safety is similar to that of *Listeria*: undercooked eggs, chicken, and instructions for handwashing after contact with pet reptiles.

Other bacteria reported to the AERS by 2002 included *Bartonella* and *Brucella* [6]. *Nocardia* was found to be 4.85 times higher with infliximab versus etanercept ($P = .046$) [6].

There are limited data regarding the use of biologics perioperatively, most of which are what can be gleaned from surgery in patients with Crohn's disease [109]. Although a fourfold increased risk of skin and soft tissue infection has been reported with anti-TNF agents compared with disease-modifying antirheumatic drug [14], it is uncertain how this relates to perioperative infection. A controlled cohort study reported infliximab before intestinal resection did not result in increased hospital stay or increased rate of postoperative complications ($P < .05$) [110]. Another limited study found that patients with RA receiving unspecified anti–TNF-α therapy who underwent elective foot surgery had similar complication rates and healing times compared with those without anti-TNF therapy [111].

Viruses

TNF-α has variable effects on viral pathogens. In some instances, the presence of TNF-α interferes with viral pathology; in others it may be causative in pathogenesis [112]. Influenza is the most common serious infection likely to be contracted in patients receiving TNF-α inhibition. Administration of influenza vaccine seems to be safe [113].

At least six cases of varicella-zoster virus [114–116] have been described after first infusion of infliximab. Varicella-zoster virus usually occurs as a primary infection in childhood and has a lifetime reactivation of 10% to 15% as shingles, a painful neurocutaneous disorder during times of physiologic stress or immunosuppression that can lead to serious morbidity. The Spanish Registry found that herpes zoster was the second most common infection identified after TB, although these data did not reach statistical significance [87]. Screening for varicella-zoster virus should be done by confirming a history of childhood chickenpox; if uncertain, varicella-zoster virus serology should be considered with subsequent administration of varicella vaccine with negative history or serology. Varicella vaccine was newly approved by the FDA for adults after the vaccine was shown to decrease the incidence and severity of herpes zoster and postherpetic neuralgia [117]. Development of herpetic disease with TNF inhibition and possibly with abatacept warrants dosing of acyclovir as for immunosuppressed patients.

TNF-α has been shown to protect mice from infection with herpes simplex virus-1 and human monocytes infected with herpes simplex virus-1 secrete higher amounts of TNF and are less susceptible to herpes simplex virus-1 infection [112]. TNF-α is critical in both the primary and reactivating phases; inhibition allows free replication of herpes simplex virus-1 [118]. Patients receiving anti-TNF therapy and probably abatacept should be followed closely for recurrent lesions and offered pre-emptive treatment for herpes simplex virus infection.

Cytomegalovirus, also known as HHV-5, is ubiquitous approaching 100% seropositivity in early adulthood. Cytomegalovirus is usually latent without manifestation in the immunocompetent host. It can reactivate with severe immunosuppression as seen in HIV, marrow toxic chemotherapy, or organ transplantation. Its manifestations can be treacherous and fatal presenting as blindness-causing retinitis, pneumonitis, and painful destruction of the gastrointestinal tract. Cytomegalovirus having a predilection for the immunosuppressed state has caused concern about the risk of reactivation with the use of biologic agents.

Torre-Cisneros and colleagues [119] in a prospective study of 15 patients receiving infliximab who were cytomegalovirus positive or had latent infection were found to have no reactivation of cytomegalovirus during or 6 months after treatment of RA with infliximab. A case is described of disseminated cytomegalovirus in a woman treated with infliximab for Crohn's disease. She had initial improvement but subsequently developed fever, worsening diarrhea, and skin lesions and was found to have cytomegalovirus on biopsies. Cessation of infliximab resulted in improvement with authors recommending that cytomegalovirus infection be ruled out with apparent worsening of symptoms before fortification of biologic therapy [120].

A pilot trial for evaluating safety and efficacy of rituximab and alemtuzumab (CD 52 targeted humanized antibody) in 12 patients with lymphoid malignancy who had failed prior chemotherapy found no evidence of cytomegalovirus reactivation during or 6 months after administration [121]. Faderl and colleagues [122] had a different outcome in the treatment of 48 patients, finding that 52% of patients developed infections of which cytomegalovirus was prominent with viremia in 27% and 15% of patients with symptomatic viremia requiring treatment.

Epstein-Barr virus is an ubiquitous herpes virus to which most people have been exposed and retain a low level of circulating Epstein-Barr virus–positive B-cell population in healthy people. In the immunosuppressed, Epstein-Barr virus–positive cells can increase in titers with the most serious complications being development of lymphomas. It is too early to ascertain firm assertions regarding biologics' effects on Epstein-Barr virus activation. Reijasse and colleagues [123] conducted a pilot study that did not reveal an overall difference in Epstein-Barr virus serial viral loads between Epstein-Barr virus–positive Crohn's patients receiving infliximab and Epstein-Barr virus–positive healthy controls over an 18-month period. It was noted, however, that some of the Crohn's disease patients had transiently high viral loads compatible with increased risk of lymphoma advising that long-term outcome need be determined. Cezard and colleagues [124] describe adverse effects in a prospective study of severe pediatric Crohn's disease treated with infliximab. In all eight EBV positive patients, there was reactivation of Epstein-Barr virus with increase of viral load by 100- to 1000-fold as determined by polymerase chain reaction. All patients were EBV PCR negative prior to infliximab administration and became EBV PCR negative again 6 months after discontinuation of treatment, leading the authors to be concerned about development of lymphoma with retreatment. Rituximab has been shown to control Epstein-Barr virus viral load [125,126] and successfully treat Epstein-Barr virus–related lymphoma [127]. Further investigation is required to establish guidelines for monitoring reactivation with anti-TNF therapy and possibly abatacept.

TNF-α has been shown to have antiproliferative effects on strains of human papillomavirus known to mediate cervical cancer. Cervical carcinoma in HIV-positive women is AIDS defining regardless of CD4 counts or viral load because it is an expression of extreme immune suppression. In theory, anti-TNF agents and abatacept potentially allow proliferation of culprit human papillomavirus strains by interference of multiple TNF-α activities. TNF-α induces strong inhibition of transcription of oncogenes E6-E7 required for proliferation in human papillomavirus-16 cervical carcinoma [128,129]. Lysis of tumor cells that express E6 is dependent on TNF-α to stimulate macrophage activity and nitric oxide–mediated apoptosis [130]. Although case reports seem nonexistent, in these early days of new biologics and until time yields more information, a pap smear before biologic therapy and routine surveillance should be considered.

Parvovirus B19 is a single-stranded DNA virus, known as the viral exanthem in childhood called "fifth disease" or "slapped cheek syndrome." It is well known to cause a transient reactive arthritis in adulthood. Its most impressive manifestation is an association with a spectrum of hematologic aplasias. Two case reports suggest immunosuppression with rituximab in causal relation in the development of pure red cell aplasia associated with parvovirus B19 infection [131,132]. Both patients were being treated for lymphoid malignancies with CHOP in addition to rituximab and were without evidence of malignant invasion of bone marrow. The authors assert that aplasia with parvovirus B19 infection is not a known association of CHOP therapy; however, three cases were found possibly to contest this [133–135]. There was also a report of red cell aplasia during a large phase II trial with rituximab alone for treatment of relapsed indolent lymphoma for which cause was not disclosed [132,136]. Polymerase chain reaction for virus may be required for detection, because serology could be negative with first exposures [132].

JC virus is a double-stranded DNA virus and is ubiquitous in that sero-positivity tends to occur before 20 years old worldwide with a prevalence of 80% to 90% [137]. There has been no syndrome associated with primary infection nor has the mode of transmission been identified. Once contracted it seems that it lies dormant in the bone marrow and lymphoid tissues of individuals. Any manifestation of the JC virus is exceedingly rare unless the subject develops immunosuppression or granulomatous disease at which time there is potential for development of progressive multifocal leukoencephalopathy. Progressive multifocal leukoencephalopathy is a rare, invariably fatal demyelinating disorder with increased prevalence since the introduction HIV. Progressive multifocal leukoencephalopathy may present with symptoms similar to those of stroke, seizure, or dementia. Berger and Houff [137] report "best evidence to date suggests that JC virus is not latent in the brain—to establish infection in the brain, it must traffic there," suggesting facility of transit by a predisposing circumstance.

Concern arose when natalizumab had been taken off the market in February 2005. Three patients had developed progressive multifocal leukoencephalopathy during drug trials with data suggesting that patients receiving natalizumab may be at particular risk [138]. Later, Yousry and colleagues [139] quantified this associated risk to be 1 per 1000 with mean treatment time of 17.9 months (95% confidence interval).

These events prompted Roos and Oster [140] to argue for a high index of suspicion and evaluation for the JC virus with polymerase chain reaction of cerebrospinal fluid in all patients receiving immunomodulating therapy whose presentation suggests encephalopathy or demyelination, ring-enhancing lesions, or mass effect on imaging [141]. Their arguments were based on a review of literature that included the following salient points: Mohan and colleagues [142] reported in 2001 the development of demyelination in 18 cases of patients receiving etanercept and two receiving infliximab for RA as reported to the FDA AERS. The diagnosis of progressive multifocal leukoencephalopathy is easily missed and likely to be underreported and underdiagnosed in patients receiving anti–TNF-α therapy [143].

Goldberg and colleagues [144] describe two patients who underwent autologous blood stem cell transplant and rescue and, after established immune reconstitution, received rituximab, who developed progressive multifocal leukoencephalopathy while in remission at 9 and 20 months after transplantation. Although these patients also underwent high-dose chemotherapy in addition to receiving rituximab, it is worth noting that only 10 cases of bone marrow transplant–associated progressive multifocal leukoencephalopathy had been documented before these two cases documented by Goldberg and colleagues [144], which suggests possible significance.

Effects of biologic agents on chronic viral diseases: hepatitis B virus, hepatitis C virus, and HIV

Hepatitis B virus

Case reports differ in regard to HBV reactivation in patients with chronic HBV being treated with TNF-α. There are abbreviated case reports that have been published describing observed safety with anti–TNF-α in patients with chronic hepatitis B [145,146]. Anelli and colleagues [147] describe a patient with RA and chronic hepatitis B in which HBV DNA was undetectable after treatment with infliximab. Others, however, describe a growing number of cases of HBV reactivation in patients with rheumatic disease on TNF-α inhibitors leading to serious complications [148–150]. Case reports describe coadministration of lamivudine with an anti-TNF agent is not associated with HBV reactivation [145,148,151]. In regard to rituximab, there have also been several case reports of fulminant hepatitis and subclinical reactivation [152–155]. Case reports suggest tandem use of lamivudine is preventive [156,157].

Calabrese and colleagues [148] offer guidelines for assessment, prevention, and treatment of HBV-positive patients undergoing anti–TNF-α therapy. These might be well considered for initiation of all immunomodulant therapy. Best practice strongly suggests HBV screening before initiation of any immunosuppressant agent, especially anti–TNF-α agents and rituximab, with serial transaminases and viral load along with consideration of pre-emptive lamivudine if results so indicate [148–150].

Hepatitis C virus

Hepatitis C is associated with the development of a wide spectrum of rheumatic diseases. These include various manifestations of vasculitis, arthritis, and connective tissue disorders that are ordinarily treated with immunosuppressive therapy in nonhepatitis patients. Preliminary studies reveal anti–TNF-α to be a safe and effective treatment of co-existing rheumatic disease in patients with chronic HCV without significant side effects, worsening of disease, or increase of HCV markers. [146,151,158,159]. Studies demonstrate significance between etanercept and placebo ($P = .04$) in achieving negative HCV RNA and normal alanine transaminase in patients being treated for chronic HCV disease with interferon and ribavirin. The etanercept arm experienced fewer side effects [151]. High levels of circulating TNF in HCV are known to be present in patients with HCV who are refractory to standard HCV treatment. This is likely caused by TNF suppressive effects on peripheral T cells resulting in decreases of interferon-γ with resultant lack of viral suppression [151].

Multiple case reports describe successful and safe use of rituximab in patients with HCV cryoglobulinemic vasculitis [160–162]. A prospective study of 20 patients in Italy reported 75% complete response and 75% lasting remission at 1 year in patients treated with adjuvant rituximab in patients who were intolerant or refractory to interferon-α. In patients who had responsive disease, however, the HCV viral load was found progressively to increase and be doubled 1 year later, a potentially harmful outcome suggesting strong consideration of tandem antiviral use in patients with HCV receiving rituximab [163]. Aksoy and colleagues [164] report a case with a pejorative outcome in a patient with dramatic acceleration of viral load replication after being treated with rituximab for HCV-related non-Hodgkin's lymphoma who died 6 months later because of infiltrative neurologic disease.

Again, best practice with use of immunosuppressant therapy is ascertainment of HCV status, if positive results follow transaminases and viral load closely and strong consideration of a concomitant antiviral, such as ribavirin.

HIV

Rheumatic and autoimmune disease is a well known association of HIV disease. Entities include vasculitis, arthropathy, arthritis, myopathy, psoriatic disease, and diseases resembling sarcoidosis and Sjögren's disease. This is likely caused by both manifestation of primary disease and resultant dysregulation and hyperactivity of immune response and a consequence of subsequent effective immune reconstitution with highly active antiretroviral therapy [165,166].

Rheumatic disease in HIV prompts consideration of treatment with immunosuppressive therapy in patients who are at risk for life-threatening deterioration of immune defense. TNF-α is required for host response to intracellular pathogens, suggesting use of anti-TNF agents in HIV disease is a worrisome prospect. Anti-TNF therapy has been used successfully in HIV-positive patients with progressive psoriatic arthritis [167,168] and Reiter syndrome [169]. Etanercept given as pretreatment against immune activation of IL-2 revealed no effect on HIV viral load [170]. As in other chronic viruses, circulating TNF levels are found to be elevated in HIV disease proportionately to degree of compromise and presence of opportunistic infections. TNF-α may facilitate lymphocyte depletion and dysfunction and viral replication [166,171]. Etanercept given adjuvantly to TB therapy in HIV-positive patients not on highly active antiretroviral therapy was without adverse events and increased $CD4^+$ T-cells by 25%; however, there was no reduction of viral load [40]. Oral anti-TNF-alpha agents with a half-life of mere hours requiring twice daily dosing may be imminently available and confer a safer treatment profile for HIV rheumatic disease. Further studies regarding the use of anti-TNF therapy in HIV rheumatic disease are warranted.

Acknowledgments

The authors thank Dr. Robert Quinet for support and generosity; Dr. Raquel Cuchacovich for expertise in immunology; Ms. Carol Kelly for patience and kind assistance; Ms. Amanda Riley, librarian; Drs. Portia Harris and Joythi Mallepalli; Dr. Robert Wallis for thoughtfulness, prepublication transmission of JID article, and sharing unpublished data on de novo TB infection; Dr. Leonard Calabrese for prepublication transmission; Drs. Karen Wood, Joan Bathon, Shunsuke Mori, and Raymond Chung for assistance in queries of their articles; Dr. Goodarz Saketkoo for insight; and the clinicians and researchers cited here for excellent efforts in reporting and education of the medical community.

Appendix 1. Recommendations for prevention and avoidance of serious complications

General precautions:

Evaluate patient for risk or presence of infection and obtain recent travel history with each encounter.

Respiratory or neurologic symptoms, fever, and constitutional symptoms should prompt thorough investigation.

Stop biologic agents with signs of serious illness.

Maintain a high suspicion for and consider coverage for unusual pathogens during serious illness.

Empiric treatment for meningitis should include coverage for Listeria.

Recall that TNF-α mediates fever, weight loss, and night sweats and serious infection may present atypically.

Viral Hepatitis and HIV

Obtain hepatitis panel before use of biologic agents.

If positive, obtain transaminase, coagulation, and viral load studies.

Consider baseline liver biopsy before initiation.

Consider co-administration of antiviral, such as lamivudine for HBV or ribavirin for HCV.

Enlist concurrent care with an HIV specialist when considering use of these agents in patients with HIV.

Tuberculosis

Conduct a thorough assessment for LTBI: PPD, chest radiograph, birth, social, lifetime travel, and contact histories.

A negative PPD does not exclude LTBI. Consider two-step testing. Repeat PPD every 12 months while on therapy.

An induration of ≥5 mm is positive and requires treatment for LTBI including those with history of bacille Calmette-Guérin vaccine.

Strongly consider prophylaxis for suspected LTBI or patients at very high risk.

Consider postponing TNF inhibition until completion of treatment for LTBI.

Educate patients on signs, symptoms, and risk factors for TB.

Endemic mycoses

Consider serum and urine screening studies for endemic mycoses or suggestive history before biologic therapy.

Educate patients on risk factors, signs, and symptoms of endemic mycotic disease.

Instruct patients to stop medication and contact physician with development of high fever and respiratory symptoms.

Counsel on recreational and occupational activities leading to transmission.

Preventive measures include mask-wearing when gardening, in proximity to construction, and tending bird roosts.

Food safety

Educate patients on food preparation and safety.

Thoroughly wash vegetables to be eaten raw.

Thoroughly cook meat and eggs; avoid precooked meats, such as hot dogs and deli-meats, unless thoroughly recooked.

Avoid unpasteurized dairy products and soft cheeses, such as camembert and feta.

Vaccines

Influenza vaccine seems to be safe during TNF-α blockade.

Provide pneumococcal vaccine at least 2 weeks before biologic use.

Administer pneumococcal vaccine if patient on anti-TNF therapy and has not received vaccine.

Consider meningococcal vaccine

Consider HBV immunization series.

Consider hepatitis A vaccine for patients in communities with high incidence and for men who have sex with men.

Varicella vaccine should be considered in patients being considered for immunosuppressive therapy.

Avoid live vaccines during use of infliximab, adalimumab, etanercept, rituximab, and abatacept.

Avoid live vaccines for 2 months and 3 months after treatment with infliximab and abatacept, respectively.

Additional preventive measures against serious infection

Consider oral home dose of fluoroquinolone to take with onset of fever, chills, and rigors on route to medical facility.

TMP-SMX prophylaxes against *P carinii* pneumonia; *Listeria;* toxoplasmosis; and possibly *Aspergillus, nocardiasis,* and *Pneumococcus.*

Sexually transmitted diseases:

Obtain routine pap smears for women before biologic therapy and in accordance with current guidelines.
Counsel patients on impact of safer sex.

Finally:

Consider above guidelines for all biologic agents until specifics about infectious pathology can be delineated.
REPORT ALL ADVERSE EVENTS to: www.fda.gov/medwatch.

References

[1] Hyrich K, Symmons D, Watson K, et al. British Society for Rheumatology Biologics Register. Baseline comorbidity levels in biologic and standard DMARD treated patients with rheumatoid arthritis: results from a national patient register. Ann Rheum Dis 2006;65: 895–8.

[2] Askling J, Fored CM, Brandt L, et al. Risk and case characteristics of tuberculosis in rheumatoid arthritis associated with tumor necrosis factor antagonists in Sweden. Arthritis Rheum 2005;52:1986–92.

[3] Wood AJ. Thrombotic thrombocytopenic purpura and clopidogrel: a need for new approaches to drug safety. N Engl J Med 2000;342:1824–6.

[4] Kane-Gill SL, Devlin JW. Adverse drug event reporting in intensive care units: a survey of current practices. Ann Pharmacother 2006;40(7–8):1267–73.

[5] Giles JT, Bathon JM. Serious infections associated with anticytokine therapies in the rheumatic diseases. J Intensive Care Med 2004;19:320–34.

[6] Wallis RS, Broder MS, Wong JY, et al. Granulomatous infectious diseases associated with tumor necrosis factor antagonists. Clin Infect Dis 2004;38:261–5 [correction: 2004;39: 1254–5].

[7] Kremer JM. The CORRONA database. Autoimmun Rev 2006;5:46–54.

[8] Beretich GR Jr, Carter PB, Havell EA. Roles for tumor necrosis factor and gamma interferon in resistance to enteric listeriosis. Infect Immun 1998;66:2368–73.

[9] Havell EA. Evidence that tumor necrosis factor has an important role in antibacterial resistance. J Immunol 1989;143:2894–9.

[10] Sullivan KE. Regulation of inflammation. Immunol Res 2003;27:529–38.

[11] Strieter RM, Belperio JA, Keane MP. Host innate defenses in the lung: the role of cytokines. Curr Opin Infect Dis 2003;16:193–8.

[12] Scallon B, Cai A, Solowski N, et al. Binding and functional comparisons of two types of tumor necrosis factor antagonists. J Pharmacol Exp Ther 2002;301:418–26.

[13] Zganiacz A, Santosuosso M, Wang J, et al. TNF-alpha is a critical negative regulator of type 1 immune activation during intracellular bacterial infection. J Clin Invest 2004;113: 401–13.

[14] Dixon WG, Watson K, Lunt M, et al. Rates of serious infection, including site-specific and bacterial intracellular infection, in rheumatoid arthritis patients receiving anti-tumor necrosis factor therapy. Arthritis Rheum 2006;54:2368–76.

[15] den Broeder AA, de Jong E, Franssen MJ, et al. Observational study on efficacy, safety, and drug survival of anakinra in rheumatoid arthritis patients in clinical practice. Ann Rheum Dis 2006;65:760–2.

[16] Fleishmann RM. Safety of anakinra, a recombinant interleukin-1 receptor antagonist (r-metHuIL-1ra), in patients with rheumatoid arthritis and comparison to anti-TNF-α agents. Clin Exp Rheumatol 2002;20(Suppl 27):S35–41.

[17] Schiff MH, DiVittorio G, Tesser J, et al. The safety of anakinra in high-risk patients with active rheumatoid arthritis. Arthritis Rheum 2004;50:1752–60.

[18] Rituximab package insert. Biogen Idec Inc. and Genetech, Inc; California; 2003.

[19] Kremer JM. Selective costimulation modulators: a novel approach for the treatment of rheumatoid arthritis. J Clin Rheumatol 2005;11(3 Suppl):S55–62.

[20] Kremer JM, Genant HK, Moreland LW, et al. Effects of abtacept in patients with methotrexate-resistant active rheumatoid arthritis: a randomized trial. Ann Intern Med 2006;144: 865–76.

[21] Natalizumab package insert. Biogen Idec; California; 2006.

[22] Keane J, Gershon S, Wise RP, et al. Tuberculosis associated with infliximab, a tumor necrosis factor alpha-neutralizing agent. N Engl J Med 2001;345:1098–104.

[23] Gomez-Reino JJ, Carmona L, Valverde VR, et al. Treatment of rheumatoid arthritis with tumor necrosis factor inhibitors may predispose to significant increase in tuberculosis risk: a multicenter active-surveillance report. Arthritis Rheum 2003;48:2122–7.

[24] Wolfe F, Michaud K, Anderson J, et al. Tuberculosis infection in patients with rheumatoid arthritis and the effect of infliximab therapy. Arthritis Rheum 2004;50:372–9.

[25] Carmona L, Hernandez-Garcia C, Vadillo C, et al. Increased risk of tuberculosis in patients with rheumatoid arthritis. J Rheumatol 2003;30:1436–9.

[26] Keane J. TNF-blocking agents and tuberculosis: new drugs illuminate an old topic. Rheumatology (Oxford) 2005;44:714–20.

[27] Magro F, Pereira P, Veloso Tavarela F, et al. Unusual presentation of tuberculosis after infliximab therapy. Inflamm Bowel Dis 2005;11:82–4.

[28] Mohan AK, Cote TR, Block JA, et al. Tuberculosis following the use of etanercept, a tumor necrosis factor inhibitor. Clin Infect Dis 2004;39:295–9.

[29] Gardam MA, Keystone EC, Menzies R, et al. Anti-tumour necrosis factor agents and tuberculosis risk: mechanisms of action and clinical management. Lancet Infect Dis 2003;3:148–55.

[30] Stenger S. Immunological control of tuberculosis: role of tumour necrosis factor and more. Ann Rheum Dis 2005;64(Suppl 4):iv24–8.

[31] Saliu OY, Sofer C, Stein DS, et al. Tumor-necrosis-factor blockers: differential effects on mycobacterial immunity. J Infect Dis 2006;194:486–92.

[32] Ellerin T, Rubin RH, Weinblatt ME. Infections and anti-tumor necrosis factor alpha therapy. Arthritis Rheum 2003;48:3013–22.

[33] Wallis RS. Infectious complications of TNF antagonists. Presented at the IDSA 44th Annual Meeting. Toronto, Canada, November 2006.

[34] Ponce de Leon D, Acevedo-Vasquez E, Sanchez-Torres A, et al. Attenuated response to purified protein derivative in patients with rheumatoid arthritis: study in a population with a high prevalence of tuberculosis. Ann Rheum Dis 2005;64:1360–1.

[35] Centers for Disease Control and Prevention. Anergy skin testing and tuberculosis [corrected] preventive therapy for HIV-infected persons: revised recommendations. MMWR Recomm Rep 1997;46:1–10.

[36] Centers for Disease Control and Prevention (CDC). Tuberculosis associated with blocking agents against tumor necrosis factor-alpha–California, 2002–2003. MMWR Morb Mortal Wkly Rep 2004;53:683–6.

[37] Joven BE, Almodovar R, Galindo M, et al. Does anti-tumour necrosis factor alpha treatment modify the tuberculin PPD response? Ann Rheum Dis 2006;65:699.

[38] Pai M, Kalantri S, Dheda K. New tools and emerging technologies for the diagnosis of tuberculosis: part I. Latent tuberculosis. Expert Rev Mol Diagn 2006;6:413–22.

[39] Long R, Gardam M. Tumour necrosis factor-alpha inhibitors and the reactivation of latent tuberculosis infection. CMAJ 2003;168:1153–6.

[40] Wallis RS, Kyambadde P, Johnson JL, et al. A study of the safety, immunology, virology, and microbiology of adjunctive etanercept in HIV-1-associated tuberculosis. AIDS 2004; 18:257–64.

[41] Parra Ruiz J, Ortego Centeno N, Raya Alvarez E. Development of tuberculosis in a patient treated with infliximab who had received prophylactic therapy with isoniazid [letter]. J Rheumatol 2003;30:1657–8.

[42] van der Klooster JM, Bosman RJ, Oudemans-van Straaten HM, et al. Disseminated tuberculosis, pulmonary aspergillosis and cutaneous herpes simplex infection in a patient with infliximab and methotrexate. Intensive Care Med 2003;29:2327–9.

[43] Peno-Green L, Lluberas G, Kingsley T, et al. Lung injury linked to etanercept therapy. Chest 2002;124:1174–5.

[44] Phillips K, Husni ME, Karlson EW, et al. Experience with etanercept in an academic medical center: are infection rates increased? Arthritis Rheum 2002;47:17–21.

[45] Ehlers S, Benini J, Kutsch S, et al. Fatal granuloma necrosis without exacerbated mycobacterial growth in tumor necrosis factor receptor p55 gene-deficient mice intravenously infected with Mycobacterium avium. Infect Immun 1999;76:3571–9.

[46] Appelberg R, Castro AG, Pedrosa J, et al. Role of gamma interferon and tumor necrosis factor alpha during T-cell-independent and –dependent phases of Mycobacterium avium infection. Infect Immun 1994;62:3962–71.

[47] Bermudez LE, Young LS. Tumor necrosis factor, alone or in combination with IL-2, but not IFN-γ, is associated with macrophage killing of Mycobacterium avium complex. J Immunol 1988;140:3006–13.

[48] Crum NF, Lederman ER, Wallace MR. Infections associated with tumor necrosis factor-alpha antagonists. Medicine (Baltimore) 2005;84:291–302.

[49] Cunnane G, Doran M, Bresnihan B. Infections and biological therapy in rheumatoid arthritis. Best Pract Res Clin Rheumatol 2003;17:345–63.

[50] British Thoracic Society Standards of Care Committee. BTS recommendations for assessing risk and for managing Mycobacterium tuberculosis infection and disease in patients due to start anti-TNF-alpha treatment. Thorax 2005;60:800–5.

[51] Beaman L. Effects of recombinant gamma interferon and TNF on in vitro interactions of human mononuclear phagocytes with Coccidioides immitis. Infect Immun 1995;63: 4178–80.

[52] Bergstrom L, Yocum DE, Ampel NM, et al. Increased risk of coccidioidomycosis in patients treated with tumor necrosis factor alpha antagonists. Arthritis Rheum 2004;50:1959–66.

[53] Blair JE, Douglas DD, Mulligan DC. Early results of targeted prophylaxis for coccidioidomycosis in patients undergoing orthotopic liver transplantation within an endemic area. Transpl Infect Dis 2003;5:3–8.

[54] Dewsnup DH, Galgiani JN, Graybill JR, et al. Is it ever safe to stop azole therapy for Coccidioides immitis meningitis? Ann Intern Med 1996;124:305–10.

[55] Lee JH, Slifman NR, Gershon SK, et al. Life-threatening histoplasmosis complicating immunotherapy with tumor necrosis factor alpha antagonists infliximab and etanercept. Arthritis Rheum 2002;46:2565–70.

[56] Wood KL, Hage CA, Knox KS, et al. Histoplasmosis after treatment with anti-tumor necrosis factor-alpha therapy. Am J Respir Crit Care Med 2003;167:1279–82.

[57] Wallis RS, Broder M, Wong J, et al. Reactivation of latent granulomatous infections by infliximab. Clin Infect Dis 2005;41(Suppl 3):S194–8.

[58] Allendoerfer R, Deepe GS Jr. Regulation of infection with Histoplasma capsulatum by TNFR1 and -2. J Immunol 2000;165:2657–64.

[59] Nagai H, Guo J, Choi H, et al. Interferon-gamma and tumor necrosis factor-alpha protect mice from invasive aspergillosis [abstract]. J Infect Dis 1995;172:1554–60.

[60] Roilides E, Dimitriadou-Georgiadou A, Sein T, et al. Tumor necrosis factor alpha enhances antifungal activities of polymorphonuclear and mononuclear phagocytes against Aspergillus fumigatus. Infect Immun 1998;66:5999–6003.

[61] Warris A, Bjorneklett A, Gaustad P. Invasive pulmonary aspergillosis associated with infliximab therapy. N Engl J Med 2001;344:1099–100.

[62] De Rosa FG, Shaz D, Campagna AC, et al. Invasive pulmonary aspergillosis soon after therapy with infliximab, a tumor necrosis factor-alpha-neutralizing antibody: a possible healthcare-associated case? Infect Control Hosp Epidemiol 2003;24:477–82.

[63] Lassoued S, Sire S, Farny M, et al. Pulmonary aspergillosis in a patient with rheumatoid arthritis treated by etanercept. Clin Exp Rheumatol 2004;22:267–8.

[64] Marty FM, Lee SJ, Fahey MM, et al. Infliximab use in patients with severe graft-versus-host disease and other emerging risk factors of non-*Candida* invasive fungal infections in aller-genic hematopoietic stem cell transplant recipients: a cohort study. Blood 2003;102:2768–76.

[65] Centers for Disease Control. Disease listings. Available at: http://www.cdc.gov. Accessed August 10, 2006.

[66] Herring AC, Lee J, McDonald RA, et al. Induction of interleukin-12 and gamma interferon requires tumor necrosis factor alpha for protective T1-cell-mediated immunity to pulmo-nary *Cryptococcus neoformans* infection. Infect Immun 2002;70:2959–64.

[67] Shrestha RK, Stoller JK, Honari G, et al. Pneumonia due to *Cryptococcus neoformans* in a patient receiving infliximab: possible zoonotic transmission from a pet cockatiel. Respir Care 2004;49:606–8.

[68] Hage CA, Wood KL, Winer-Muram HT, et al. Pulmonary cryptococcosis after initiation of anti-tumor necrosis factor-α therapy [letter]. Chest 2003;124:2395–7.

[69] Arend SM, Kuijper EJ, Allaart CF, et al. Cavitating pneumonia after treatment with inflix-imab and prednisone. Eur J Clin Microbiol Infect Dis 2004;23:638–41.

[70] True DG, Penmetcha M, Peckham SJ. Disseminated cryptococcal infection in rheumatoid arthritis treated with methotrexate and infliximab. J Rheumatol 2002;29:1561–3.

[71] Stenger AA, Houtman PM, Bruyn GA, et al. *Pneumocystis carinii* pneumonia associated with low dose methotrexate treatment for rheumatoid arthritis. Scand J Rheumatol 1994;23:51–3.

[72] Arthritis Drugs Advisory Committee. Safety update on TNF-α antagonists: infliximab and etanercept. Available at: http://www.fda.gov. Accessed August 7, 2006.

[73] Seddik M, Melliez H, Seguy D, et al. *Pneumocystis jiroveci (carinii)* pneumonia after initi-ation of infliximab and azathioprine therapy in a patient with Crohn's disease. Inflamm Bowel Dis 2005;11:618–20.

[74] Mori S, Imamura F, Kiyofuji C, et al. *Pneumocystis jiroveci* pneumonia in a patient with rheumatoid arthritis as a complication of treatment with infliximab, anti-tumor necrosis factor alpha neutralizing antibody [abstract]. Mod Rheumatol 2006;16:58–62.

[75] Kaur N, Mahl TC. *Pneumocystis carinii* pneumonia with oral candidiasis after infliximab therapy for Crohn's disease. Dig Dis Sci 2004;49:1458–60.

[76] Velayos FS, Sandborn WJ. *Pneumocystis carinii* pneumonia during maintenance anti-tumor necrosis factor-alpha therapy with infliximab for Crohn's disease. Inflamm Bowel Dis 2004;10:657–60.

[77] Minnee RC, Stokkers P, Riemens SC, et al. Pneumocystis pneumonia during infliximab treatment for active Crohn's colitis [abstract]. Ned Tijdschr Geneeskd 2005;149:2290–5.

[78] Tai TL, O'Rourke KP, McWeeney M, et al. *Pneumocystis carinii* pneumonia following a second infusion of infliximab. Rheumatology (Oxford) 2002;41:951–2.

[79] Chen W, Havell EA, Harmsen AG. Importance of endogenous tumor necrosis factor alpha and gamma interferon in host resistance against *Pneumocystis carinii* infection. Infect Immunol 1992;60:1979–84.

[80] Tamburrini E, De Luca A, Ventura G, et al. *Pneumocystis carinii* stimulates in vitro produc-tion of tumor necrosis factor-alpha by human macrophages [abstract]. Med Microbiol Immunol (Berl) 1991;180:15–20.

[81] Kolls JK, Lei D, Vasquez C, et al. Exacerbation of murine *Pneumocystis carinii* infection by adenoviral-mediated gene transfer of a TNF inhibitor [abstract]. Am J Respir Cell Mol Biol 1997;16:112–8.

[82] Belda A, Hinojosa J, Serra B, et al. Systemic candidiasis and infliximab therapy [abstract]. Gastroenterol Hepatol 2004;27:365–7.

[83] Farah CS, Hu Y, Riminton S, et al. Distinct roles for interleukin-12p40 and tumour necrosis factor in resistance to oral candidiasis defined by gene-targeting. Oral Microbiol Immunol 2006;21:252–5.

[84] Gottlieb GS, Lesser CF, Holmes KK, et al. Disseminated sporotrichosis associated with treatment with immunosuppressants and tumor necrosis factor-alpha antagonists. Clin Infect Dis 2003;37:838–40.

[85] Gonzalez-Vicent M, Diaz MA, Sevilla J, et al. Cerebral toxoplasmosis following etanercept treatment for idiopathic pneumonia syndrome after autologous peripheral blood progenitor cell transplantation. Ann Hematol 2003;82:649–53.

[86] Coyle CM, Weiss LM, Rhodes LV III, et al. Fatal myositis due to the microsporidian Brachiola algerae, a mosquito pathogen. N Engl J Med 2004;351:42–7.

[87] Carmona L, Gomez-Reino J, Gonzalez-Gonzalez R. Spanish Registry of Adverse Events of Biological Therapies in Rheumatic Diseases (BIOBADASER) [spanish]. Reumatología Clínica 2005;1(2):95–104.

[88] Kato K, Nakane A, Minagawa T, et al. Human tumor necrosis factor increases the resistance against Listeria infection in mice [abstract]. Med Microbiol Immunol (Berl) 1989; 178:337–46.

[89] Nishikawa S, Miura T, Sasaki S, et al. The protective role of endogenous cytokines in host resistance against an intragastric infection with Listeria monocytogenes in mice [abstract]. FEMS Immunol Med Microbiol 1996;16:291–8.

[90] Slifman NR, Gershon SK, Lee JH, et al. Listeria monocytogenes infection as a complication of treatment with tumor necrosis factor alpha-neutralizing agents. Arthritis Rheum 2003; 48:319–24.

[91] Gluck T, Linde HJ, Scholmerich J, et al. Anti-tumor necrosis factor therapy and Listeria monocytogenes infection: report of two cases. Arthritis Rheum 2002;46:2255–7.

[92] Aparicio AG, Munoz-Fernandez S, Bonilla G, et al. Report of an additional case of anti-tumor necrosis factor therapy and Listeria monocytogenes infection. Arthritis Rheum 2003; 48:1764–5.

[93] Joosten AA, van Olffen GH, Hageman G. Meningitis due to Listeria monocytogenes as a complication of infliximab therapy [abstract]. Ned Tijdschr Geneeskd 2003;147: 1470–2.

[94] Morelli J, Wilson FA. Does administration of infliximab increase susceptibility to listeriosis? Am J Gastroenterol 2000;95:841–2.

[95] Bowie VL, Snella KA, Gopalachar AS, et al. Listeria meningitis associated with infliximab. Ann Pharmacother 2004;38:58–61.

[96] Pagliano P, Attanasio V, Fusco U, et al. Does etanercept monotherapy enhance the risk of Listeria monocytogenes meningitis? Ann Rheum Dis 2004;63:462–3.

[97] Ritz MA, Jost R. Severe pneumococcal pneumonia following treatment with infliximab for Crohn's disease. Inflamm Bowel Dis 2001;7:327.

[98] Zimmer C, Beiderlinden M, Peters J. Lethal acute respiratory distress syndrome during anti-TNF-alpha therapy for rheumatoid arthritis. Clin Rheumatol 2006;25: 430–2.

[99] Killingley B, Carpenter V, Falnagan K, et al. Pneumococcal meningitis and etanercept: chance or association? J Infect 2005;51:49–51.

[100] Baghai M, Osmon DR, Wolk DM, et al. Fatal sepsis in a patient with rheumatoid arthritis treated with etanercept. Mayo Clin Proc 2001;76:573–5.

[101] Takashima K, Tateda K, Matsumoto T, et al. Role of tumor necrosis factor alpha in pathogenesis of pneumococcal pneumonia in mice. Infect Immun 1997;65:257–60.

[102] Van der Poll T, Keogh CV, Buurman WA, et al. Passive immunization against tumor necrosis factor-alpha impairs host defense during pneumococcal pneumonia in mice. Am J Respir Crit Care Med 1997;155:603–8.

[103] Wellmer A, Gerber J, Ragheb J, et al. Effect of deficiency of tumor necrosis factor alpha or both of its receptors on *Streptococcus pneumoniae* central nervous system infection and peritonitis. Infect Immun 2001;69:6881–6.

[104] Gobbi FL, Benucci M, Del Rosso A. Pneumonitis caused by *Legionella pneumoniae* in a patient with rheumatoid arthritis treated with anti-TNF-[alpha] therapy (infliximab). J Clin Rheumatol 2005;11:119–20.

[105] Wondergem MJ, Voskuyl AE, van Agtmael MA. A case of legionellosis during treatment with a TNF-alpha antagonist. Scand J Infect Dis 2004;36:310–1.

[106] Skerret SJ, Bagby GJ, Schmidt RA, et al. Antibody-mediated depletion of tumor necrosis factor-alpha impairs pulmonary host defenses to *Legionella pneumophila*. J Infect Dis 1997; 176:1019–28.

[107] Makkuni D, Kent R, Watts R, et al. Two cases of serious food-borne infection in patients treated with anti-TNF-alpha. Are we doing enough to reduce the risk? Rheumatology (Oxford) 2006;45:237–8.

[108] Katsarolis I, Tsiodras S, Panagopoulous P. Septic arthritis due to *Salmonella enteritidis* associated with infliximab sue. Scand J Infect Dis 2005;37:304–6.

[109] Rosandich PA, Kelley JT III, Conn DL. Perioperative management of patients with rheumatoid arthritis in the era of biologic response modifiers. Curr Opin Rheumatol 2004;16: 192–8.

[110] Marchal L, D'Haens G, Van Assche G, et al. The risk of post-operative complications associated with infliximab therapy for Crohn's disease: a controlled cohort study. Aliment Pharmacol Ther 2004;19:749–54.

[111] Bibbo C, Goldberg JW. Infectious and healing complications after elective orthopaedic foot and ankle surgery during tumor necrosis factor–alpha inhibition therapy [abstract]. Foot Ankle Int 2004;25:331–5.

[112] Herbein G, O'Brien WA. Tumor necrosis factor (TNF)-alpha and TNF receptors in viral pathogenesis. Proc Soc Exp Biol Med 2000;223:241–57.

[113] Fomin I, Caspi D, Levy V, et al. Vaccination against influenza in rheumatoid arthritis: the effect of disease modifying drugs, including TNFα blockers. Ann Rheum Dis 2006;65: 191–4.

[114] Baumgart DC, Dignass AU. Shingles following infliximab infusion. Ann Rheum Dis 2002; 61:661.

[115] Gottenberg JE, Merle-Vincent F, Bentaberry F, et al. Anti-tumor necrosis factor alpha therapy in fifteen patients with AA amyloidosis secondary to inflammatory arthritides: a followup report of tolerability and efficacy. Arthritis Rheum 2003;48: 2019–24.

[116] Stephens MC, Shepanski MA, Mamula P, et al. Safety and steroid-sparing experience using infliximab for Crohn's disease at a pediatric inflammatory bowel disease center [abstract]. Am J Gastroenterol 2003;98:104–11.

[117] Oxman MN, Levin MJ, Johnson GR, et al. A vaccine to prevent herpes zoster and postherpetic neuralgia in older adults. N Engl J Med 2005;352:2271–84.

[118] Minagawa H, Hashimoto K, Yanagi Y. Absence of tumour necrosis factor facilitates primary and recurrent herpes simplex virus-1 infections. J Gen Virol 2004;85(Pt 2): 343–7.

[119] Torre-Cisneros J, Del Castillo M, Caston JJ, et al. Infliximab does not activate replication of lymphotropic herpesviruses in patients with refractory rheumatoid arthritis. Rheumatology (Oxford) 2005;44:1132–5.

[120] Helbling D, Breitbach TH, Krause M. Disseminated cytomegalovirus infection in Crohn's disease following infliximab therapy. Eur J Gastroenterol Hepatol 2002;14:1393–5.

[121] Nabhan C, Patton D, Gordon LI, et al. A pilot trial of rituximab and alemtuzumab combination therapy in patients with relapsed and/or refractory chronic lymphocytic leukemia. Leuk Lymphoma 2004;45:2269–73.

[122] Faderl S, Thomas DA, O'Brien S, et al. Experience with alemtuzumab plus rituximab in patients with relapsed and refractory lymphoid malignancies. Blood 2003;101:3413–5.

[123] Reijasse D, Le Pendeven C, Cosnes J, et al. Epstein-Barr virus viral load in Crohn's disease: effect of immunosuppressive therapy. Inflamm Bowel Dis 2004;10:85–90.

[124] Cezard JP, Nouaili N, Talbotec C, et al. A prospective study of the efficacy and tolerance of a chimeric antibody to tumor necrosis factors (remicade) in severe pediatric Crohn disease. J Pediatr Gastroenterol Nutr 2003;36:632–6.

[125] Daibata M, Bandobashi K, Kuroda M, et al. Induction of lytic Epstein-Barr virus (EBV) infection by synergistic action of rituximab and dexamethasone renders EBV-positive lymphoma cells more susceptible to gancyclovir cytotoxicity in vitro and in vivo. J Virol 2005; 79:5875–9.

[126] Clave E, Agbalika F, Bajzik V, et al. Epstein-Barr virus (EBV) reactivation in allogeneic stem-cell transplantation: relationship between viral load, EBV-specific T-cell reconstitution and rituximab therapy. Transplantation 2004;77:76–84.

[127] Kelaidi C, Tulliez M, Lecoq-Lafon C, et al. Long-term remission of an EBV-positive B cell lymphoproliferative disorder associated with rheumatoid arthritis under methotrexate with anti-CD20 monoclonal antibody (rituximab) monotherapy. Leukemia 2002;16: 2173–4.

[128] Yuan H, Fu F, Zhuo J, et al. Human papillomavirus type 16 E6 and E7 oncoproteins upregulate c-IAP2 gene expression and confer resistance to apoptosis. Oncogene 2005;24: 5069–78.

[129] Lembo D, Donalisio M, De Andrea M, et al. A cell-based high-throughput assay for screening inhibitors of human papillomavirus-16 long control region activity. FASEB J 2006;20: 148–50.

[130] Routes JM, Morris K, Ellison MC, et al. Macrophages kill human papillomavirus type 16 E6-expressing tumor cells by tumor necrosis factor alpha- nitric oxide- dependent mechanisms. J Virol 2005;79:116–23.

[131] Sharma VR, Fleming DR, Slone SP. Pure red cell aplasia due to parvovirus B19 in a patient treated with rituximab. Blood 2000;96:1184–6.

[132] Song KW, Mollee P, Patterson B, et al. Pure red cell aplasia due to parvovirus following treatment with CHOP and rituximab for B-cell lymphoma. Br J Haematol 2002;119:125–7.

[133] Toyota S, Nakamura N, Dan K. Coexistence of pure red cell aplasia and autoimmune hemolytic anemia occurring during remission of malignant lymphoma [abstract]. Rinsho Ketsueki 2002;43:493–5.

[134] McNall RY, Head DR, Pui CH, et al. Parvovirus B19 infection in a child with acute lymphoblastic leukemia during induction therapy. J Pediatr Hematol Oncol 2001;23:309–11.

[135] Azzi A, Macchia PA, Favre C, et al. Aplastic crisis caused by B19 virus in a child during induction therapy for acute lymphoblastic leukemia. Haematologica 1989;74:191–4.

[136] McLaughlin P, Grill-Lopez AJ, Link BK, et al. Rituximab chimeric anti- CD 20 monoclonal antibody therapy for relapsed indolent lymphoma [abstract]. J Clin Oncol 1998;16: 2825–33.

[137] Berger JR, Houff S. Progressive multifocal leukoencephalopathy: lessons from AIDS and natalizumab. Neurol Res 2006;28:299–305.

[138] Food and Drug Administration. Natalizumab (marketed as Tysabri) information. June 2006. Available at: http://www.fda.gov. Accessed July 17, 2006.

[139] Yousry TA, Major EO, Ryschkewitsch C, et al. Evaluation of patients treated with natalizumab for progressive multifocal leukoencephalopathy. N Engl J Med 2006;354:924–33.

[140] Roos JCP, Oster AJK. Anti-tumour necrosis factor α therapy and the risk of JC virus infection [letter]. Arthritis Rheum 2006;54:381–2.

[141] Kleinschmidt-DeMasters BK, Tyler KL. Progressive multifocal leukoencephalopathy complicating treatment with natalizumab and interferon β-1a for multiple sclerosis. N Engl J Med 2005;353:369–74.

[142] Mohan N, Edwards ET, Cupps TR, et al. Demyelination occurring during anti–tumor necrosis factor α therapy for inflammatory arthritides. Arthritis Rheum 2001;44:2862–9.

[143] Van Assche G, van Ranst M, Sciot R, et al. Progressive multifocal leukoencephalopathy after natalizumab therapy for Crohn's disease. N Engl J Med 2005;353:362–8.

[144] Goldberg SL, Pecora AL, Alter RS, et al. Unusual viral infections (progressive multifocal leukencephalopathy and cytomegalovirus disease) after high-dose chemotherapy with autologous blood stem cell rescue and peri-transplantation rituximab. Blood 2002;99:1486–8.

[145] Roux CH, Brocq O, Breuil V, et al. Safety of anti-TNF-{alpha} therapy in rheumatoid arthritis and spondylarthropathies with concurrent B or C chronic hepatitis. Rheumatology (Oxford) 2006;45(10):1294–7.

[146] Oniankitan O, Duvoux C, Challine D, et al. Infliximab therapy for rheumatic diseases in patients with chronic hepatitis B or C. J Rheumatol 2004;31:107–9.

[147] Anelli MG, Diletta DT, Manno C, et al. Improvement of renal function and disappearance of hepatitis B virus DNA in a patient with rheumatoid arthritis and renal amyloidosis following treatment with infliximab. Arthritis Rheum 2005;52:2519–20.

[148] Calabrese LH, Zein N, Vassilopoulos D. Hepatitis B virus (HBV) reactivation with immunosuppressive therapy in rheumatic diseases: assessment and preventive strategies. Ann Rheum Dis 2006;65:983–9.

[149] Ostuni P, Botsios C, Punzi L, et al. Hepatitis B reactivation in a chronic hepatitis B surface antigen carrier with rheumatoid arthritis treated with infliximab and low dose methotrexate [letter]. Ann Rheum Dis 2003;62:686–7.

[150] Millonig G, Kern M, Ludwiczek O, et al. Subfulminant hepatitis B after infliximab in Crohn's disease: need for HBV-screening? World J Gastroenterol 2006;12:974–6.

[151] Calabrese LH, Zein N, Vassilopoulos D. Safety of antitumour necrosis factor (anti-TNF) therapy in patients with chronic viral infections: hepatitis C, hepatitis B, and HIV infection. Ann Rheum Dis 2004;63(Suppl II):ii18–24.

[152] Sera T, Hiasa Y, Michitaka K, et al. Anti-HBs-positive liver failure due to hepatitis B virus reactivation induced by rituximab. Intern Med 2006;45:721–4.

[153] Sarrecchia C, Cappelli A, Aiello P. HBV reactivation with fatal fulminating hepatitis during rituximab treatment in a subject negative for HBsAg and positive for HBsAb and HBcAb. J Infect Chemother 2005;11(4):189–91.

[154] Tsutsumi Y, Kanamori H, Mori A, et al. Reactivation of hepatitis B virus with rituximab. Expert Opin Drug Saf 2005;4:599–608.

[155] Dai MS, Chao TY, Kao WY, et al. Delayed hepatitis B virus reactivation after cessation of preemptive lamivudine in lymphoma patients treated with rituximab plus CHOP. Ann Hematol 2004;83:769–74.

[156] Tsutsumi Y, Tanaka J, Kawamura T, et al. Possible efficacy of lamivudine treatment to prevent hepatitis B virus reactivation due to rituximab therapy in a patient with non-Hodgkin's lymphoma. Ann Hematol 2004;83:58–60.

[157] Hamaki T, Kami M, Kusumi E, et al. Prophylaxis of hepatitis B reactivation using lamivudine in a patient receiving rituximab. Am J Hematol 2001;68:292–4.

[158] Peterson JR, Hsu FC, Simkin PA, et al. Effect of tumour necrosis factor alpha antagonists on serum transaminases and viraemia in patient with rheumatoid arthritis and chronic hepatitis C infection. Ann Rheum Dis 2003;62:1078–82.

[159] Parke FA, Reveille JD. Anti-tumor necrosis factor agents for rheumatoid arthritis in the setting of chronic hepatitis C infection. Arthritis Rheum 2004;51:800–4.

[160] Pekow J, Chung RT. Treatment of type II cryoglobulinemia associated with hepatitis C with rituximab [letter]. J Clin Gastroenterol 2006;40:450.

[161] Lamprecht P, Lerin-Lozano C, Merz H, et al. Rituximab induces remission in refractory HCV associated cryoglobulinaemic vasculitis. Ann Rheum Dis 2003;62:1230–3.

[162] Cai FZ, Ahern M, Smith M. Treatment of cryoglobulinemia associated peripheral neuropathy with rituximab. J Rheumatol 2006;33:1197–8.

[163] Sansonno D, De Re V, Lauletta G, et al. Monoclonal antibody treatment of mixed cryoglobulinemia resistant to interferon alpha with an anti-CD20. Blood 2003;101:3818–26.

[164] Aksoy S, Abali H, Kilickap S, et al. Accelerated hepatitis C virus replication with rituximab treatment in a non-Hodgkin's lymphoma patient. Clin Lab Haematol 2006;28:211–4.

[165] Marquez J, Restrepo CS, Candia L, et al. Human immunodeficiency virus-associated rheumatic disorders in the HAART era. J Rheumatol 2004;31:741–6.

[166] Calabrese LH, Kirchner E, Shrestha R. Rheumatic complications of human immunodeficiency virus infection in the era of highly active antiretroviral therapy: emergence of a new syndrome of immune reconstitution and changing patterns of disease. Semin Arthritis Rheum 2005;35:166–74.

[167] Bartke U, Venten I, Kreuter A, et al. Human immunodeficiency virus-associated psoriasis and psoriatic arthritis treated with infliximab. Br J Dermatol 2004;150:784–6 [erratum: Br J Dermatol 2004;150:1235].

[168] Aboulafia DM, Bundow D, Wilske K, et al. Etanercept for the treatment of human immunodeficiency virus-associated psoriatic arthritis. Mayo Clin Proc 2000;75:1093–8.

[169] Gaylis N. Infliximab in the treatment of an HIV positive patient with Reiter's syndrome. J Rheumatol 2003;30:407–11.

[170] Sha BE, Valdez H, Gelman RS, et al. Effect of etanercept (Enbrel) on interleukin 6, tumor necrosis factor alpha, and markers of immune activation in HIV-infected subjects receiving interleukin 2. AIDS Res Hum Retroviruses 2002;18:661–5.

[171] Colmegna I, Koehler JW, Garry RF, et al. Musculoskeletal and autoimmune manifestations of HIV, syphilis and tuberculosis. Curr Opin Rheumatol 2006;18:88–95.

ELSEVIER
SAUNDERS

Infect Dis Clin N Am
20 (2006) 963–968

INFECTIOUS
DISEASE CLINICS
OF NORTH AMERICA

Index

Note: Page numbers of article titles are in **boldface** type.

id.theclinics.com

Moving?

Make sure your subscription moves with you!

To notify us of your new address, find your **Clinics Account Number** (located on your mailing label above your name), and contact customer service at:

E-mail: elspcs@elsevier.com

800-654-2452 (subscribers in the U.S. & Canada)
407-345-4000 (subscribers outside of the U.S. & Canada)

Fax number: 407-363-9661

Elsevier Periodicals Customer Service
6277 Sea Harbor Drive
Orlando, FL 32887-4800

*To ensure uninterrupted delivery of your subscription, please notify us at least 4 weeks in advance of move.

United States Postal Service
Statement of Ownership, Management, and Circulation

1. Publication Title									2. Publication Number							3. Filing Date
Infectious Disease Clinics of North America									0 0 1 - 5 5 6							9/15/06

4. Issue Frequency	5. Number of Issues Published Annually	6. Annual Subscription Price
Mar, Jun, Sep, Dec	4	$170.00

7. Complete Mailing Address of Known Office of Publication (Not printer) (Street, city, county, state, and ZIP+4)

Elsevier Inc.
360 Park Avenue South
New York, NY 10010-1710

Contact Person
Sarah Carmichael

Telephone
(215) 239-3681

8. Complete Mailing Address of Headquarters or General Business Office of Publisher (Not printer)

Elsevier Inc., 360 Park Avenue South, New York, NY 10010-1710

9. Full Names and Complete Mailing Addresses of Publisher, Editor, and Managing Editor (Do not leave blank)

Publisher (Name and complete mailing address)

John Schrefer, Elsevier Inc., 1600 John F. Kennedy Blvd., Suite 1800, Philadelphia, PA 19103-2899

Editor (Name and complete mailing address)

Karen Sorensen, Elsevier Inc., 1600 John F. Kennedy Blvd., Suite 1800, Philadelphia, PA 19103-2899

Managing Editor (Name and complete mailing address)

Catherine Bewick, Elsevier Inc., 1600 John F. Kennedy Blvd., Suite 1800, Philadelphia, PA 19103-2899

10. Owner (Do not leave blank. If the publication is owned by a corporation, give the name and address of the corporation immediately followed by the names and addresses of all stockholders owning or holding 1 percent or more of the total amount of stock. If not owned by a corporation, give the names and addresses of the individual owners. If owned by a partnership or other unincorporated firm, give its name and address as well as those of each individual owner. If the publication is published by a nonprofit organization, give its name and address.)

Full Name	Complete Mailing Address
Wholly owned subsidiary of	4520 East-West Highway
Reed/Elsevier Inc., US holdings	Bethesda, MD 20814

11. Known Bondholders, Mortgages, and Other Security Holders Owning or Holding 1 Percent or More of Total Amount of Bonds, Mortgages, or Other Securities. If none, check box. ► None

Full Name	Complete Mailing Address
N/A	

12. Tax Status (For completion by nonprofit organizations authorized to mail at nonprofit rates) (Check one)
The purpose, function, and nonprofit status of this organization and the exempt status for federal income tax purposes:
☐ Has Not Changed During Preceding 12 Months
☐ Has Changed During Preceding 12 Months (Publisher must submit explanation of change with this statement)

(See Instructions on Reverse)

PS Form 3526, October 1999

13. Publication Title	14. Issue Date for Circulation Data Below
Infectious Disease Clinics of North America	June, 2006

15.	Extent and Nature of Circulation	Average No. Copies Each Issue During Preceding 12 Months	No. Copies of Single Issue Published Nearest to Filing Date
a.	Total Number of Copies (Net press run)	2,900	2,900
b. Paid and/or Requested Circulation	(1) Paid/Requested Outside-County Mail Subscriptions Stated on Form 3541. (Include advertiser's proof and exchange copies)	1,623	1,436
	(2) Paid In-County Subscriptions Stated on Form 3541 (Include advertiser's proof and exchange copies)		
	(3) Sales Through Dealers and Carriers, Street Vendors, Counter Sales, and Other Non-USPS Paid Distribution	450	441
	(4) Other Classes Mailed Through the USPS		
c.	Total Paid and/or Requested Circulation [Sum of 15b. (1), (2), (3), and (4)] ►	2,073	1,877
d. Free Distribution by Mail (Samples, complimentary, and other free)	(1) Outside-County as Stated on Form 3541	92	89
	(2) In-County as Stated on Form 3541		
	(3) Other Classes Mailed Through the USPS		
e.	Free Distribution Outside the Mail (Carriers or other means)		
f.	Total Free Distribution (Sum of 15d. and 15e.) ►	92	89
g.	Total Distribution (Sum of 15c. and 15f.) ►	2,165	1,966
h.	Copies not Distributed	735	934
i.	Total (Sum of 15g. and h.) ►	2,900	2,900
j.	Percent Paid and/or Requested Circulation (15c. divided by 15g. times 100)	95.75%	95.47%

16. Publication of Statement of Ownership
☐ Publication required. Will be printed in the December 2006 issue of this publication. ☐ Publication not required

17. Signature and Title of Editor, Publisher, Business Manager, or Owner

[signature]

John Famucci – Executive Director of Subscription Services

Date 9/15/06

I certify that all information furnished on this form is true and complete. I understand that anyone who furnishes false or misleading information on this form or who omits material or information requested on the form may be subject to criminal sanctions (including fines and imprisonment) and/or civil sanctions (including civil penalties).

Instructions to Publishers

1. Complete and file one copy of this form with your postmaster annually on or before October 1. Keep a copy of the completed form for your records.
2. In cases where the stockholder or security holder is a trustee, include in items 10 and 11 the name of the person or corporation for whom the trustee is acting. Also include the names and addresses of individuals who are stockholders who own or hold 1 percent or more of the total amount of bonds, mortgages, or other securities of the publishing corporation. In item 11, if none, check the box. Use blank sheets if more space is required.
3. Be sure to furnish all circulation information called for in item 15. Free circulation must be shown in items 15d, e, and f.
4. Item 15h., Copies not Distributed, must include (1) newsstand copies originally stated on Form 3541, and returned to the publisher, (2) estimated returns from news agents, and (3), copies for office use, leftovers, spoiled, and all other copies not distributed.
5. If the publication had Periodicals authorization as a general or requester publication, this Statement of Ownership, Management, and Circulation must be published; it must be printed in any issue in October or, if the publication is not published during October, the first issue printed after October.
6. In item 16, indicate the date of the issue in which this Statement of Ownership will be published.
7. Item 17 must be signed.

Failure to file or publish a statement of ownership may lead to suspension of Periodicals authorization.

PS Form 3526, October 1999 (Reverse)